The Food Counter's Pocket Companion

SIXTH EDITION

**Calories · Carbohydrates · Protein · Fats
Fiber · Sugar · Sodium · Iron · Calcium
Potassium · Vitamin D**

JANE STEPHENSON
REBECCA LINDBERG, MPH, RDN

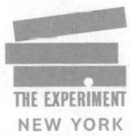

THE EXPERIMENT
NEW YORK

THE FOOD COUNTER'S POCKET COMPANION, SIXTH EDITION: *Calories, Carbohydrates, Protein, Fats, Fiber, Sugar, Sodium, Iron, Calcium, Potassium, and Vitamin D*
Copyright © 1999 by Jane Stephenson and Bridgett Wagener, RD
Copyright © 2001, 2003, 2004, 2008, 2010, 2012, 2014, 2016, 2018, 2019 by Jane Stephenson and Diane Bader
Copyright © 2022, 2024 by Jane Stephenson and Rebecca Lindberg, MPH, RDN

Originally published as *HealthCheques™: Carbohydrate, Fat & Calorie Guide* by Appletree Press, Inc., in 1999. First published in revised form by The Experiment, LLC, in 2022. This edition first published in 2024.

The authors and publisher have made every effort to provide accurate data based on values that are current as of 2023. Nutrient values and product availability are subject to change; in cases where the Nutrition Facts differ from the data provided, defer to the label. This book is sold with the understanding that the authors and publisher are not engaged in rendering medical, health, or any other kind of personal or professional services in the book. The author and publisher specifically disclaim all responsibility for any liability, loss, or risk—personal or otherwise—that is incurred as a consequence, directly or indirectly, of the use and application of any of the contents of this book.

The Experiment, LLC
220 East 23rd Street, Suite 600
New York, NY 10010-4658
theexperimentpublishing.com

THE EXPERIMENT and its colophon are registered trademarks of The Experiment, LLC. Many of the designations used by manufacturers and sellers to distinguish their products are claimed as trademarks. Where those designations appear in this book and The Experiment was aware of a trademark claim, the designations have been capitalized.

The Experiment's books are available at special discounts when purchased in bulk for premiums and sales promotions as well as for fundraising or educational use. For details, contact us at info@theexperimentpublishing.com.

Library of Congress Cataloging-in-Publication Data available upon request

ISBN 978-1-891011-36-8
Ebook ISBN 978-1-891011-37-5

Cover and text design by Jack Dunnington
Cover photo from Shutterstock/monticello

Manufactured in the United States of America

First printing January 2024
10 9 8 7 6 5 4 3 2 1

Contents

About This Book

The Food Counter's Pocket Companion, Sixth Edition, is a resource to help you make healthy food choices at home or on the go. The more you are aware of what is in the foods and beverages you choose, the better choices you can make for your overall well-being—no matter what type of eating pattern you follow.

This book lists the calories, fat, saturated fat, sodium, carbohydrate, fiber, sugar, protein, vitamin D, calcium, iron, and potassium content of over 4,500 common foods. Additionally, it highlights 13 important nutrients, and each summary includes practical tips to help you make healthier choices every day based on your individual needs. You can also learn how to customize your personal daily nutrient goals in three easy steps on page 2.

Keep this pocket companion in your purse, pocket, desk drawer, or glove compartment and pull it out whenever and wherever you need it. It's not a guide to restricting food or strictly counting calories—it's a tool for learning how to incorporate healthier food choices into whatever eating plan you follow, enjoy what you eat, nourish your body, and feel great.

Personalize Your Nutrition Goals

1. Estimate your calorie needs. Your calorie needs vary based on age, sex, body size, genetics, and activity level. This type of estimation is not a perfect science, but it will give you a good starting point for making informed decisions. You can use online calculators such as the Mifflin-St. Jeor (calculator.net/bmr-calculator .html) or National Institutes of Health Body Weight Planner (niddk.nih.gov/bwp) to calculate your personal needs.

Below are estimates of calorie needs based on the Dietary Guidelines for Americans, 2020–2025. Keep in mind that individual needs fluctuate. The best way to know how many calories your body needs is to monitor how you feel along with your food intake, activity, and weight.

Activity Level	Men (calories)	Women (calories)
Sedentary	2,000–2,600	1,600–2,000
Moderately Active	2,200–2,800	1,800–2,200
Active	2,400–3,200	2,000–2,400

2. Determine your nutrient needs. Your personal needs depend on the type of eating pattern you follow as well as your health history, goals, and activity level. Working with a registered dietitian is the most precise way to determine your needs. However, you can start by estimating using the table below.

Caloric goal	Fat (g) 20–35% daily calories	Saturated fat (g) <10% daily calories	Sodium (mg)	Carbohydrates (g) 45–65% daily calories	Fiber (g) 14 g per 1,000 calories	Sugar (g/tsp) <10% daily calories	Protein (g) 10–35% daily calories
1,600	36–62	18	2,300	180–260	22	40/10	40–140
1,800	40–70	20	2,300	203–293	25	45/11	45–158
2,000	44 78	22	2,300	225–325	28	50/13	50–175
2,400	53–93	27	2,300	270–390	34	60/15	60–210
2,800	62–109	31	2,300	315–455	39	70/18	70–245
3,200	71–124	36	2,300	360–520	45	80/20	80–280

3. Eat and drink to improve health and prevent disease.

Aim to increase fiber. Most people don't get enough fiber in their diets. For tips on boosting your intake, see page 167.

Cut down on sugar. Many experts recommend eating less sugar because a high sugar intake has been linked to obesity, high blood sugar, high blood pressure, inflammation, and fat buildup on artery walls. The American Heart Association suggests no more than 6 tsp for women and 9 tsp for men per day.

Choose good fats. You need fat to absorb vitamins, feel full after eating, and reduce disease risk. The key is eating good fats (like avocados, nuts, seeds, and olives, including oils from these foods) and staying clear of the bad fats (like trans fat). The American Heart Association recommends even less saturated fat than other guidelines: only 5 to 6 percent of calories. There's no need to monitor your cholesterol intake from food, as it has little to no effect on your blood cholesterol levels.

Reduce sodium. Most Americans eat too much sodium. Use herbs and spices in place of salt and limit processed and ultra-processed foods high in sodium. See page 173 for more tips.

Eat fruits and vegetables. You can reduce your risk of heart disease, stroke, and some types of cancers by eating at least 5 servings of fruits and vegetables every day.

Pick healthy drinks. Make water your beverage of choice—you can learn more about its importance on page 179. Limit alcohol intake to no more than 1 drink a day for women and 2 drinks a day for men.

Counting carbohydrates: Carbohydrate counting may be recommended for certain health conditions like diabetes. While some people stick to counting total grams of carbohydrate, there are others who count carbohydrate choices: One choice contains about 15 grams of carbohydrate.

Total carbohydrate in grams / 15 = Number of carb choices

MyPlate

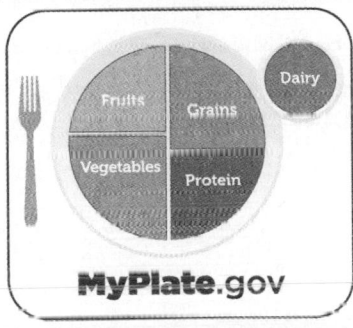

MyPlate is a visual way to design your breakfast, lunch, and dinner plates for better health. It recommends filling half your plate with fruits and vegetables, choosing whole grains over refined grains, and prioritizing high-quality, protein-rich foods. You can find resources for setting food goals, identifying tools to personalize your plate, and discovering new recipes at myplate.gov.

Abbreviations

Nutrient values have been rounded to the nearest calorie, gram, milligram, or microgram (with the exception of saturated fat values, which have been rounded to the nearest 0.5 gram). Apparent inconsistencies may result from rounding off numbers. Values may have been obtained from more than one source, recipe, or sample of the same food, and they may vary due to seasonal and manufacturer differences.

Nutrient values change as products and recipes are reformulated and reanalyzed. Menu items listed may not be available at all restaurants, and nutrient values for fast-food restaurants are meant for general information purposes only. Nutrient values are subject to change; values are current as of 2023. If the information you find on a label differs significantly from the data in this book, please use the label as your guide.

This book includes many trademarked company and product names. Where the authors and publisher were aware of a trademark, all such names have been capitalized.

Imperial	Metric
1 oz	28 g
1 fl oz	30 ml
1 in	2.5 cm

Abbreviation	Stands for . . .
fl oz	fluid ounce
g	gram
in	inch
mcg	microgram
mg	milligram
n/a	not available
oz	ounce
pc	piece
pkg	package
pkt	packet
tsp	teaspoon
T	tablespoon
IU	international unit
w/	with
w/o	without
/	or

RDA: The Recommended Dietary Allowance is the average daily level of intake sufficient to meet nutrient requirements for nearly all healthy people.

AI: Adequate Intakes are established when evidence is insufficient to develop an RDA; they are set at a level that ensures nutritional adequacy.

ALCOHOL

	Amount	Calories	Fat (g)	Saturated Fat (g)	Sodium (mg)	Carbohydrate (g)	Fiber (g)	Sugar (g)	Protein (g)	Vitamin D (mcg)	Calcium (mg)	Iron (mg)	Potassium (mg)
Alabama Slammer	5 fl oz	318	0	0.0	5	32	0	30	0	0	7	0	111
B-52	1.5 fl oz	154	2	1.0	14	17	0	15	0	0	0	0	5
Bahama Mama	5 fl oz	243	0	0.0	6	21	0	20	0	0	6	0	56
Beer	12 fl oz	146	0	0.0	11	11	0	0	1	0	14	0	118
light	12 fl oz	99	0	0.0	11	5	0	0	1	0	11	0	92
nonalcoholic	12 fl oz	133	0	0.0	47	29	0	29	1	0	25	0	29
Black Russian	4 fl oz	335	0	0.0	5	25	0	21	0	0	0	0	18
Bloody Mary	8 fl oz	165	1	0.0	497	8	1	5	2	0	24	1	439
Bourbon & club soda	6 fl oz	139	0	0.0	1	0	0	0	0	0	0	0	1
Brandy	1 fl oz	70	0	0.0	0	0	0	0	0	0	0	0	1
Brandy Alexander	3 fl oz	272	11	7.0	11	15	0	12	1	0	20	0	38
Champagne	4 fl oz	98	0	0.0	6	3	0	1	0	0	11	0	85
Cordials/liqueurs, 53-proof	1 fl oz	117	0	0.0	3	16	0	13	0	0	0	0	10
Cosmopolitan	6 fl oz	281	0	0.0	7	16	0	14	0	0	0	0	46
Daiquiri	6 fl oz	228	0	0.0	73	27	0	27	0	0	5	0	50
Fuzzy Navel	6 fl oz	380	0	0.0	6	48	0	45	1	0	10	0	166
Gimlet	2.5 fl oz	141	0	0.0	1	4	0	3	0	0	2	0	22
Gin & tonic	8 fl oz	187	0	0.0	20	15	0	15	0	0	2	0	1
Gin fizz	8 fl oz	158	0	0.0	38	5	0	5	0	0	10	0	22
Gin/rum/vodka/whiskey													
80-proof	1 fl oz	64	0	0.0	0	0	0	0	0	0	0	0	1
86-proof	1 fl oz	70	0	0.0	0	0	0	0	0	0	0	0	1
90-proof	1 fl oz	73	0	0.0	0	0	0	0	0	0	0	0	1
100-proof	1 fl oz	82	0	0.0	0	0	0	0	0	0	0	0	1
Grasshopper	4 fl oz	340	4	2.5	28	39	0	35	1	0	40	0	61
Harvey Wallbanger	6 fl oz	167	0	0.0	4	16	0	11	1	1	76	0	241
Highball	4 fl oz	71	0	0.0	19	0	0	0	0	0	5	0	2
Hot buttered rum	4 fl oz	191	5	3.5	5	6	0	6	0	0	10	0	13
Hot toddy	8 fl oz	158	0	0.0	10	18	0	17	0	0	6	0	22
Hurricane	8 fl oz	196	0	0.0	5	23	0	0	0	0	0	0	0
Irish coffee													
w/ whipped cream	8 fl oz	193	4	2.0	4	14	0	14	0	0	4	0	95
w/o whipped cream	8 fl oz	143	0	0.0	4	12	0	12	0	0	4	0	95
Irish cream	1 fl oz	97	4	2.5	24	7	0	6	1	0	5	0	10
Jack & Coke	6 fl oz	185	0	0.0	16	13	0	13	0	0	0	0	1
Kahlua	1 fl oz	101	0	0.0	2	14	0	11	0	0	0	0	9
Kamikaze	4 fl oz	241	0	0.0	6	10	0	8	0	0	4	0	24
Long Island Iced Tea	6 fl oz	193	0	0.0	29	16	0	15	0	0	2	0	13
Mai Tai	4 fl oz	187	0	0.0	6	21	0	17	0	0	8	0	81
Manhattan	2.5 fl oz	167	0	0.0	2	1	0	1	0	0	1	0	11

ALCOHOL

	Amount	Calories	Fat (g)	Saturated Fat (g)	Sodium (mg)	Carbohydrate (g)	Fiber (g)	Sugar (g)	Protein (g)	Vitamin D (mcg)	Calcium (mg)	Iron (mg)	Potassium (mg)
Margarita													
w/ salt	6 fl oz	220	0	0.0	369	29	0	29	0	0	4	0	40
w/o salt	6 fl oz	220	0	0.0	10	29	0	29	0	0	4	0	40
Martini	2.5 fl oz	151	0	0.0	2	0	0	0	0	0	1	0	10
Appletini	2.5 fl oz	142	0	0.0	1	5	0	4	0	0	2	0	20
chocolate	2.5 fl oz	142	0	0.0	1	5	0	4	0	0	2	0	20
Melon Ball	4 fl oz	205	0	0.0	16	20	0	15	1	0	8	0	177
Mimosa	8 fl oz	156	0	0.0	7	17	0	11	1	0	78	0	302
Mint julep	4 fl oz	223	0	0.0	5	7	0	7	0	0	0	0	1
Mojito	8 fl oz	205	0	0.0	4	28	1	26	0	0	34	1	50
Mudslide	4 fl oz	411	20	12.5	38	22	0	18	2	1	30	0	52
Old Fashioned	4 fl oz	194	0	0.0	5	7	0	7	0	0	12	0	42
Piña Colada	6 fl oz	272	4	3.5	11	35	0	32	1	0	14	0	162
Rob Roy	2.5 fl oz	165	0	0.0	3	3	0	2	0	0	2	0	22
Rum & cola	8 fl oz	214	0	0.0	7	19	0	18	0	0	2	0	10
Rusty Nail	4 fl oz	322	0	0.0	2	13	0	13	0	0	0	0	1
Screwdriver	8 fl oz	200	0	0.0	4	22	1	16	1	1	0	0	349
Sex on the Beach	6 fl oz	242	0	0.0	4	28	0	25	0	0	9	0	124
Singapore Sling	6 fl oz	170	0	0.0	27	14	0	12	0	0	9	0	66
Sloe Gin Fizz	8 fl oz	158	0	0.0	38	5	0	5	0	0	10	0	22
Sloe Screw	8 fl oz	223	0	0.0	5	21	0	15	1	1	27	0	322
Tequila Maria	8 fl oz	158	0	0.0	500	6	1	4	1	0	24	1	20
Tequila Sunrise	6 fl oz	202	0	0.0	7	24	0	17	1	0	68	0	220
Toasted Almond	4 fl oz	420	11	7.0	14	41	0	37	1	0	20	0	42
Tom Collins	8 fl oz	177	0	0.0	9	8	0	7	0	0	19	0	32
Vodka Red Bull	8 fl oz	203	0	0.0	67	17	0	17	1	0	10	0	6
Whiskey sour	4 fl oz	181	0	0.0	24	16	0	19	0	0	1	0	6
White Russian	4 fl oz	211	9	5.5	52	14	0	11	3	0	88	0	115
Wine													
cooking													
Marsala	2 T	25	0	0.0	170	2	0	2	0	0	2	0	28
red/white	2 T	20	0	0.0	190	1	0	0	0	0	3	0	26
sherry	2 T	45	0	0.0	190	2	0	2	0	0	2	0	26
table													
dessert, dry	4 fl oz	179	0	0.0	11	14	0	1	0	0	9	0	109
dessert, sweet	4 fl oz	189	0	0.0	11	16	0	9	0	0	9	0	109
red/rose	5 fl oz	122	0	0.0	5	3	0	1	0	0	9	1	149
sangria	8 fl oz	177	0	0.0	15	15	1	10	1	0	59	1	200
sherry, dry	5 fl oz	120	0	0.0	14	0	0	2	0	0	14	0	77
white, dry/medium	5 fl oz	121	0	0.0	7	4	0	1	0	0	13	0	104
Wine cooler	12 fl oz	245	0	0.0	18	36	0	35	0	0	14	0	97
Wine spritzer	8 fl oz	118	0	0.0	26	4	0	1	0	0	17	1	144

BEVERAGES

	Amount	Calories	Fat (g)	Saturated Fat (g)	Sodium (mg)	Carbohydrate (g)	Fiber (g)	Sugar (g)	Protein (g)	Vitamin D (mcg)	Calcium (mg)	Iron (mg)	Potassium (mg)
Café latte													
w/ skim milk	8 fl oz	68	0	0.0	76	10	0	9	6	2	190	0	373
w/ whole milk	8 fl oz	109	6	3.5	77	9	0	9	7	2	200	0	334
Café mocha w/ whipped cream													
w/ skim milk	8 fl oz	180	6	4.0	70	23	2	18	7	2	200	2	346
w/ whole milk	8 fl oz	207	11	6.0	73	23	2	19	7	2	200	2	317
Cappuccino													
w/ skim milk	8 fl oz	47	0	0.0	87	7	0	7	5	3	130	9	185
w/ water, flavored mix	8 fl oz	70	4	3.5	170	9	0	5	0	0	5	0	104
w/ whole milk	8 fl oz	72	4	2.0	54	6	0	6	4	2	130	0	185
Capri Sun													
orange	6 fl oz	50	0	0.0	15	14	0	13	0	0	0	0	0
Roarin' Waters	6 fl oz	30	0	0.0	15	8	0	8	0	0	0	0	0
Club soda/seltzer	8 fl oz	0	0	0.0	2.4	0	0	0	0	0	33	0	0
Coconut water	8 fl oz	46	1	0.5	252	9	3	6	2	0	58	1	600
Coffee													
brewed/instant	6 fl oz	1	0	0.0	1	0	0	0	0	0	1	0	9
flavored mixes	6 fl oz	60	2	0.5	40	10	0	0	0	0	5	0	111
Crystal Light	8 fl oz	5	0	0.0	75	3	0	0	0	0	0	0	175
Espresso	3 fl oz	3	0	0.0	4	0	0	0	0	0	5	0	34
Frappuccino	9.5 fl oz	180	3	2.0	95	33	0	0	6	0	260	0	0
Fruit2O flavored water	8 fl oz	0	0	0.0	38	0	0	0	0	0	0	0	0
Fruit punch	8 fl oz	90	0	0.0	15	25	0	24	0	0	0	1	0
Gatorade													
Bolt24	16.9 fl oz	45	0	0.0	230	11	0	9	0	0	0	0	60
G Series	12 fl oz	80	0	0.0	160	21	0	21	0	0	0	0	45
G2 Series	12 fl oz	30	0	0.0	160	8	0	7	0	0	0	0	45
Zero w/ protein	16.9 fl oz	50	0	0.0	230	1	0	0	10	0	0	0	70
Hawaiian Punch	8 fl oz	60	0	0.0	105	15	0	15	0	0	0	0	0
light	8 fl oz	10	0	0.0	105	2	0	2	0	0	0	0	0
Hi-C	8 fl oz	53	0	0.0	20	15	0	13	0	0	0	0	0
Hot cocoa													
homemade													
w/ 1% milk	8 fl oz	220	3	2.0	260	38	1	32	9	2	312	0	558
w/ whole milk	8 fl oz	260	8	5.0	248	38	1	32	9	3	308	0	558
mix													
sugar-free	8 fl oz	80	1	0.5	190	14	0	11	6	0	420	2	500
w/ water	8 fl oz	80	2	1.5	190	15	1	12	0	0	10	1	140
Kool-Aid	8 fl oz	60	0	0.0	0	16	0	16	0	0	0	0	0
sugar-free	8 fl oz	0	0	0.0	5	0	0	0	0	0	0	0	0

BEVERAGES

	Amount	Calories	Fat (g)	Saturated Fat (g)	Sodium (mg)	Carbohydrate (g)	Fiber (g)	Sugar (g)	Protein (g)	Vitamin D (mcg)	Calcium (mg)	Iron (mg)	Potassium (mg)
Lemonade	8 fl oz	110	0	0.0	15	29	0	28	0	0	5	0	25
sugar-free	8 fl oz	0	0	0.0	20	1	0	0	0	0	26	0	12
Quinine/tonic water	8 fl oz	90	0	0.0	0	23	0	23	0	0	2	0	0
Red Bull energy drink	8.4 fl oz	111	0	0.0	101	26	0	26	1	0	16	0	8
sugar-free	8.4 fl oz	13	0	0.0	208	2	0	0	1	0	33	0	8
Rockstar energy drink	8 fl oz	135	0	0.0	35	32	0	32	0	0	0	0	0
sugar-free	8 fl oz	13	0	0.0	120	1	0	0	0	0	0	0	0
Soda													
7 Up	12 fl oz	140	0	0.0	45	39	0	38	0	0	0	0	0
Coca-Cola/Coke	12 fl oz	140	0	0.0	45	39	0	39	0	0	0	0	0
cherry	12 fl oz	150	0	0.0	35	42	0	42	0	0	0	0	0
vanilla	12 fl oz	150	0	0.0	35	42	0	42	0	0	0	0	0
cream	12 fl oz	170	0	0.0	45	43	0	43	0	0	19	0	5
diet, most varieties	12 fl oz	0	0	0.0	35	0	0	0	0	0	0	0	0
Dr Pepper	12 fl oz	150	0	0.0	55	40	0	39	0	0	0	0	0
ginger ale	12 fl oz	140	0	0.0	50	36	0	36	0	0	11	1	4
grape	12 fl oz	150	0	0.0	51	38	0	38	0	0	0	0	0
Mello Yellow	12 fl oz	170	0	0.0	30	32	0	32	0	0	0	0	0
Mountain Dew	12 fl oz	170	0	0.0	65	46	0	46	0	0	0	0	0
Code Red	12 fl oz	168	0	0.0	108	46	0	46	0	0	0	0	0
Orange Crush	12 fl oz	160	0	0.0	70	43	0	43	0	0	0	0	0
Pepsi	12 fl oz	150	0	0.0	30	41	0	41	0	0	0	0	0
wild cherry	12 fl oz	160	0	0.0	30	42	0	42	0	0	0	0	0
root beer	12 fl oz	152	0	0.0	48	39	0	39	0	0	19	0	4
Sierra Mist	12 fl oz	140	0	0.0	35	37	0	37	0	0	6	0	4
Sprite	12 fl oz	140	0	0.0	70	38	0	38	0	0	0	0	0
Squirt	12 fl oz	140	0	0.0	55	39	0	38	0	0	0	0	0
Tang	8 fl oz	90	0	0.0	40	22	0	22	0	0	43	0	20
Tea													
brewed/instant	6 fl oz	0	0	0.0	0	0	0	0	0	0	0	0	0
iced													
diet, w/ lemon	8 fl oz	0	0	0.0	0	0	0	0	0	0	0	0	0
sweetened	8 fl oz	80	0	0.0	0	21	0	20	0	0	0	0	50
Vitaminwater	8 fl oz	40	0	0.0	0	11	0	11	0	0	110	0	220
Water, bottled	8 fl oz	0	0	0.0	0	0	0	0	0	0	0	0	0
Yoo-hoo, chocolate	8 fl oz	116	1	0.0	167	26	0	24	2	2	95	0	204

BREADS & BREAD PRODUCTS

Breads & Muffins

	Amount	Calories	Fat (g)	Saturated Fat (g)	Sodium (mg)	Carbohydrate (g)	Fiber (g)	Sugar (g)	Protein (g)	Vitamin D (mcg)	Calcium (mg)	Iron (mg)	Potassium (mg)
Bagels													
blueberry													
medium	1 (3 oz)	280	2	1.0	390	55	2	8	9	0	15	2	80
large	1 (5 oz)	382	3	0.0	616	78	5	17	14	0	47	4	173

BREADS & BREAD PRODUCTS

Breads & Muffins	Amount	Calories	Fat (g)	Saturated Fat (g)	Sodium (mg)	Carbohydrate (g)	Fiber (g)	Sugar (g)	Protein (g)	Vitamin D (mcg)	Calcium (mg)	Iron (mg)	Potassium (mg)
cinnamon raisin													
medium	1 (3 oz)	280	2	0.0	390	56	2	11	9	0	20	3	120
large	1 (5 oz)	381	3	0.0	596	79	5	17	14	0	48	4	194
egg													
medium	1 (3 oz)	236	2	0.5	430	45	2	6	9	0	11	3	58
large	1 (5 oz)	315	2	0.5	573	60	3	11	12	0	17	5	89
plain													
mini	1 (1.5 oz)	125	1	0.0	220	25	1	3	4	0	78	2	48
medium	1 (3 oz)	270	2	0.0	450	53	2	6	9	0	78	3	80
large	1 (5 oz)	394	3	0.5	716	75	3	8	15	0	78	6	96
Bialys	1 (2.5 oz)	180	1	0.0	240	38	3	1	7	0	0	1	0
Biscuits													
baking powder													
can	1 (2 oz)	180	6	2.5	450	26	1	5	4	0	0	2	260
homemade	1 (2 oz)	184	6	3.0	568	28	2	5	4	0	102	1	86
buttermilk													
can	1 (2 oz)	170	8	3.5	550	23	0	2	4	0	30	2	78
homemade	1 (2 oz)	201	9	2.5	328	25	1	1	4	0	102	2	66
Breads													
Boston brown, can	1 slice (1 oz)	55	0	0.0	179	12	1	1	1	0	20	1	90
challah/egg	1 slice (1 oz)	81	2	0.5	108	14	1	1	3	0	25	1	33
chapati	1 slice (1 oz)	84	2	0.5	116	13	1	1	3	0	26	1	75
cracked wheat	1 slice (1 oz)	74	1	0.5	153	14	2	0	2	0	12	1	50
French/Vienna	1 slice (1 oz)	77	1	0.0	170	15	1	1	3	0	15	1	33
Ezekiel/sprouted	1 slice (1 oz)	80	1	0.0	75	15	3	0	5	0	9	1	81
fruit	1 slice (1 oz)	103	5	0.5	87	13	0	7	2	0	41	1	47
garlic	1 slice (1 oz)	170	6	3.5	260	23	1	0	4	0	6	1	14
Irish soda	1 slice (1 oz)	84	3	1.5	139	14	1	5	2	0	29	1	73
Italian	1 slice (1 oz)	77	1	0.0	156	14	1	1	2	0	22	1	31
multigrain	1 slice (1 oz)	60	1	0.0	110	11	2	0	4	0	50	1	82
low-carb	1 slice (1 oz)	70	4	0.5	130	7	4	0	5	0	30	0	40
oatmeal	1 slice (1 oz)	74	1	0.0	96	11	1	2	3	0	23	1	40
pita													
white	1 (6 inch)	165	1	0.0	322	33	1	0	5	0	52	1	72
whole wheat	1 (6 inch)	168	1	0.0	337	36	4	2	6	0	10	2	109
pumpernickel	1 slice (1 oz)	71	1	0.0	169	13	2	0	2	0	19	1	59
raisin	1 slice (1 oz)	78	1	0.5	98	15	1	2	2	0	19	1	64
rye	1 slice (1 oz)	73	1	0.0	171	14	2	1	2	0	21	1	47
sourdough	1 slice (1 oz)	77	1	0.0	170	15	1	1	3	0	15	1	33
wheatberry	1 slice (1 oz)	76	1	0.0	144	14	2	2	3	0	38	1	50
white	1 slice (1 oz)	79	1	0.0	153	15	1	2	2	0	41	1	36
light	1 slice (0.8 oz)	40	0	0.0	111	9	2	1	3	0	58	0	18
whole wheat	1 slice (1 oz)	73	1	0.0	105	14	2	3	3	0	18	1	82
light	1 slice (0.8 oz)	40	0	0.0	90	9	3	1	3	0	26	0	37

BREADS & BREAD PRODUCTS

Breads & Muffins	Amount	Calories	Fat (g)	Saturated Fat (g)	Sodium (mg)	Carbohydrate (g)	Fiber (g)	Sugar (g)	Protein (g)	Vitamin D (mcg)	Calcium (mg)	Iron (mg)	Potassium (mg)
Breadsticks, soft	1 (2 oz)	150	5	1.0	270	23	1	2	4	0	10	2	59
Cornbread	1 (2 oz)	187	5	2.0	340	31	1	9	4	0	77	1	75
Croissants	1 (2 oz)	230	12	6.5	265	26	1	6	5	0	21	1	67
English muffins													
plain	1 medium	132	1	0.0	197	26	2	1	5	0	102	1	60
raisin	1 medium	136	1	0.0	170	27	2	8	5	0	73	3	99
whole wheat	1 medium	134	1	0.0	240	27	4	5	6	0	100	2	139
Melba toast	4	78	1	0.0	120	15	1	0	2	0	18	1	40
Muffins													
banana nut	1 (2 oz)	247	10	3.0	255	39	1	10	3	0	25	1	132
blueberry	1 (2 oz)	230	8	1.5	195	38	1	22	3	0	11	1	46
bran, w/ raisins	1 (2 oz)	153	4	0.5	223	27	3	5	4	0	36	2	287
chocolate chip	1 (2 oz)	275	10	3.0	200	43	1	25	4	0	15	2	87
corn	1 (2 oz)	173	5	1.0	265	29	2	10	3	0	42	2	39
cranberry nut	1 (2 oz)	212	9	1.5	191	30	1	18	3	0	25	1	69
lemon poppy seed	1 (2 oz)	229	12	2.5	178	27	1	16	3	0	23	1	18
pumpkin	1 (2 oz)	275	12	5.0	200	39	1	19	3	0	15	2	69
Popovers	1 (2 oz)	150	5	2.5	169	20	1	2	6	1	67	1	113
Rolls													
brown & serve	1 medium	78	2	0.5	134	13	1	2	3	0	45	1	35
crescent	1 medium	110	6	1.5	220	11	0	3	2	0	11	1	34
French	1 medium	105	2	0.5	231	19	1	0	3	0	41	1	51
hamburger/hot dog	1 medium	120	2	0.5	206	21	1	4	4	0	75	2	63
hard	1 medium	167	2	0.5	310	30	1	1	6	0	53	2	61
kaiser	1 medium	167	2	0.5	310	30	1	1	6	0	54	2	62
rye	1 medium	81	1	0.0	253	15	1	1	3	0	26	1	60
sesame seed	1 medium	140	3	1.5	240	23	0	0	5	0	36	1	59
sourdough	1 medium	100	1	0.0	240	19	1	2	4	0	16	1	36
submarine	1 (8 inch)	220	2	0.0	400	44	2	8	7	0	153	4	129
whole wheat	1 medium	75	1	0.0	136	14	2	1	2	0	76	2	49
yeast	1 medium	106	3	0.5	126	18	0	5	3	0	70	1	54
Scones	1 large	304	13	4.0	345	39	1	9	8	0	147	2	74

Bread Products

	Amount	Calories	Fat (g)	Saturated Fat (g)	Sodium (mg)	Carbohydrate (g)	Fiber (g)	Sugar (g)	Protein (g)	Vitamin D (mcg)	Calcium (mg)	Iron (mg)	Potassium (mg)
Corn fritters	1 (2 oz)	209	12	3.0	268	22	1	2	4	0	70	1	89
Crepes	1 (8 in)	144	7	2.0	187	14	0	3	6	1	60	1	101
Croutons	¼ cup	37	1	0.0	70	7	1	0	1	0	5	0	8
seasoned	¼ cup	47	2	0.5	109	6	1	0	1	0	10	0	18
French toast													
frozen	1 slice	130	3	0.5	200	22	1	5	5	0	60	4	80
homemade	1 slice	159	6	2.0	261	2	1	5	6	1	48	2	89

BREADS & BREAD PRODUCTS

Bread Products	Amount	Calories	Fat (g)	Saturated Fat (g)	Sodium (mg)	Carbohydrate (g)	Fiber (g)	Sugar (g)	Protein (g)	Vitamin D (mcg)	Calcium (mg)	Iron (mg)	Potassium (mg)
Lefse	1 (1.5 oz)	116	1	0.0	174	26	1	2	3	0	26	0	140
Pancakes													
blueberry, mix	2 (6 in)	342	14	3.0	634	45	2	10	9	0	317	3	213
buttermilk, mix	2 (6 in)	256	8	1.5	507	42	1	9	6	0	86	6	99
plain													
frozen	2 (6 in)	340	10	1.5	673	55	1	12	8	0	114	8	131
homemade	2 (6 in)	350	15	3.5	676	44	2	10	10	0	337	3	203
low-fat, homemade	2 (6 in)	296	2	0.0	472	63	1	9	6	0	63	2	107
whole wheat, mix	2 (6 in)	252	11	2.0	673	32	4	7	8	1	216	2	240
Pizza crust, Boboli	½ (8 in)	190	4	1.5	380	34	1	1	6	0	90	2	8
Pretzels, soft													
shopping mall, salted	1 large	340	5	3.0	990	65	2	10	8	0	20	1	90
SuperPretzel, frozen	1 medium	160	0	0.0	890	34	1	1	4	0	7	3	50
Stuffing, prepared													
bread, homemade	½ cup	177	9	1.5	472	22	1	2	3	0	30	1	72
cornbread, box	½ cup	179	9	2.0	526	22	3	0	3	0	26	1	62
Stove Top, box	½ cup	150	6	1.5	460	21	0	2	3	0	0	1	90
reduced sodium	½ cup	150	6	1.5	290	21	0	2	3	0	0	1	0
Taco shells, corn	3 (5 in)	189	9	3.0	129	25	3	1	3	0	39	1	92
Tortillas													
corn	2 (6 in)	100	2	0.0	10	20	3	2	2	0	60	1	80
flour	1 (8 in)	159	4	1.0	234	27	2	1	4	0	19	2	64
Waffles													
Belgian, mix	1 (8 in)	216	13	2.5	460	30	7	6	7	0	229	2	143
Eggo, frozen													
blueberry	1 (1.2 oz)	90	3	1.0	185	15	0	6	2	0	130	2	40
homestyle	1 (1.2 oz)	95	4	1.0	180	14	0	1	2	0	130	2	28
Nutrigrain	1 (1.2 oz)	70	1	0.5	190	14	2	3	2	0	130	2	45
plain													
homemade	1 (7 in)	218	11	2.0	383	25	1	2	6	0	191	2	119
low-fat, frozen	1 (1.2 oz)	80	1	0.5	137	16	0	2	2	0	132	2	31

CANDY

	Amount	Calories	Fat (g)	Saturated Fat (g)	Sodium (mg)	Carbohydrate (g)	Fiber (g)	Sugar (g)	Protein (g)	Vitamin D (mcg)	Calcium (mg)	Iron (mg)	Potassium (mg)
Almonds													
candy coated	10	200	6	0.5	13	35	2	21	3	0	33	1	90
chocolate covered	10	180	14	5.0	3	9	4	1	5	0	52	3	217
Bit-o-Honey	6 small	150	3	2.0	120	32	0	19	1	0	20	0	50
Bridge mix	¼ cup	200	12	8.0	16	24	2	20	2	0	40	1	133
Boston Baked Beans	½ cup	160	2	0.0	420	31	5	13	7	0	60	2	390
Cadbury Eggs, creme	1 (1.4 oz)	150	6	4.0	15	24	0	20	2	0	37	0	41

CANDY

	Amount	Calories	Fat (g)	Saturated Fat (g)	Sodium (mg)	Carbohydrate (g)	Fiber (g)	Sugar (g)	Protein (g)	Vitamin D (mcg)	Calcium (mg)	Iron (mg)	Potassium (mg)
Candy bars (average size)													
3 Musketeers	1 (1.4 oz)	240	7	5.0	90	42	1	36	1	0	20	0	80
5th Avenue	1 (1.4 oz)	260	12	4.5	115	38	2	29	4	0	31	1	170
100 Grand	1 (2.1 oz)	190	8	5.0	90	30	0	22	1	0	20	0	70
Almond Joy	1 (2 oz)	220	12	8.0	50	26	2	21	2	0	20	1	110
Baby Ruth	1 (1.5 oz)	280	14	8.0	140	39	1	33	4	0	40	1	149
Butterfinger	1 (2.1 oz)	250	10	5.0	100	39	1	24	3	0	0	0	143
Caramello	1 (1.7 oz)	180	8	5.0	35	24	0	21	2	0	70	0	14
Charleston Chew	1 (1.4 oz)	80	2	2.0	5	15	0	11	0	0	25	1	35
Chunky	1 (2.1 oz)	190	11	5.0	15	25	1	21	2	0	40	0	187
Heath Bar	1 (1.4 oz)	210	13	7.0	140	25	1	24	1	0	24	0	54
Hershey's													
Milk Chocolate	1 (1.4 oz)	220	13	8.0	35	26	1	26	3	1	60	1	100
Special Dark	1 (1.5 oz)	190	12	8.0	0	26	3	22	2	0	0	4	180
w/ almonds	1 (1.0 oz)	210	14	7.0	25	22	2	19	4	1	85	1	170
Kit Kat	1 (1.5 oz)	210	11	7.0	30	27	1	22	3	0	60	1	120
Milky Way	1 (1.5 oz)	240	9	7.0	75	37	1	31	2	0	40	0	72
Midnight	1 (1.8 oz)	220	8	5.0	65	38	1	29	1	0	20	0	98
Mounds	1 (2.1 oz)	230	13	10.0	55	29	3	21	2	0	10	2	120
Mr. Goodbar	1 (1.8 oz)	260	17	8.0	50	27	2	23	5	0	50	1	240
Nestle Crunch	1 (1.8 oz)	240	13	13.0	65	32	1	21	3	0	40	0	134
Pay Day	1 (1.6 oz)	240	13	2.5	120	27	2	21	7	0	51	1	200
Pearson's Nut Roll	1 (1.8 oz)	240	11	2.0	170	27	2	20	8	0	10	0	217
Skor	1 (1.9 oz)	210	12	7.0	135	25	0	24	1	0	26	1	94
Symphony	1 (1.4 oz)	200	12	7.0	40	22	1	21	3	0	91	0	163
Snickers	1 (1.8 oz)	250	12	4.5	120	33	1	27	4	0	50	0	150
Twix	1 (1.4 oz)	250	12	7.0	105	34	1	25	2	0	52	1	100
Whatchamacallit	1 (2.1 oz)	230	12	10.0	100	28	1	21	3	0	40	1	100
Candy corn	15	110	0	0.0	65	28	0	23	0	0	1	0	3
Caramels	4	156	3	1.0	100	31	0	26	2	0	56	0	87
Cherries, chocolate covered	2	150	4	2.0	0	30	0	26	1	0	0	1	0
Circus peanuts	6	220	0	0.0	0	54	0	50	2	0	0	0	2
Cotton candy	1 oz	110	0	0.0	0	28	0	28	0	0	0	0	0
Divinity, homemade	2 (0.4 oz)	83	0	0.0	8	20	0	10	0	0	2	0	10
Dots	12	150	0	0.0	15	36	0	23	0	0	1	0	2
Ferrero Rocher	3	230	16	5.0	25	18	1	15	3	0	31	1	132
Fondant	2 (0.5 oz ea)	106	0	0.0	3	26	0	25	0	0	1	0	1
Fudge, homemade													
chocolate													
w/ nuts	1 oz	131	5	2.0	11	19	1	18	1	0	16	0	52
w/o nuts	1 oz	117	3	2.0	13	22	1	13	1	0	14	1	38
vanilla													
w/ nuts	1 oz	123	4	1.0	12	21	0	20	1	0	13	0	29
w/o nuts	1 oz	109	2	1.0	13	23	0	23	0	0	11	0	14

CANDY

	Amount	Calories	Fat (g)	Saturated Fat (g)	Sodium (mg)	Carbohydrate (g)	Fiber (g)	Sugar (g)	Protein (g)	Vitamin D (mcg)	Calcium (mg)	Iron (mg)	Potassium (mg)
Ghirardelli Chocolate Squares													
dark	4 squares	213	16	9.0	0	23	4	16	3	0	27	1	227
milk	4 squares	220	13	8.0	30	26	0	23	3	0	80	0	180
w/ caramel	3 squares	225	12	7.5	68	27	0	24	3	0	75	0	135
Goobers	¼ cup	220	13	5.0	10	22	2	18	5	0	40	0	187
Good & Plenty	33	131	0	0.0	18	33	0	25	0	0	5	0	5
Gum, regular/sugar-free	1 stick	5	0	0.0	0	2	0	0	0	0	0	0	0
Gumdrops	10	143	0	0.0	16	36	0	21	0	0	1	0	2
Gummy bears	15	131	0	0.0	15	33	0	20	0	0	1	0	2
Hard candies	3 small	71	0	0.0	7	18	0	11	0	0	1	0	1
sugar-free	3 small	34	0	0.0	0	8	0	0	0	0	0	0	0
Hershey's													
Hugs	7	160	9	6.0	30	19	0	16	2	0	60	0	105
Kisses	7	160	9	6.0	25	19	1	18	2	1	40	1	120
w/ almonds	7	160	10	5.0	20	16	3	15	3	0	40	1	130
Hot Tamales	16	110	0	0.0	0	27	0	18	0	0	0	0	0
Jelly beans	35 small	140	0	0.0	15	37	0	28	0	0	1	0	14
Jolly Ranchers	3	70	0	0.0	0	17	0	11	0	0	1	0	0
Junior Mints	12	130	3	1.5	0	26	0	25	0	0	6	1	62
Licorice, black/red	3 (8 in)	120	1	0.0	70	27	0	16	1	0	0	0	15
Lifesavers	4	60	0	0.0	0	15	0	12	0	0	0	0	0
Lollipops													
Blow Pop	1	70	0	0.0	0	17	0	13	0	0	123	0	0
Dum • Dum	2	50	0	0.0	0	13	0	10	0	0	0	0	0
Saf-T-Pop	1	43	0	0.0	0	11	0	9	0	0	0	0	0
Tootsie Pop	1	60	0	0.0	0	15	0	11	0	0	0	0	1
M&M's	1 pkg	230	9	6.0	35	35	1	31	2	0	40	1	94
crispy	1 pkg	200	7	4.5	60	31	1	25	2	0	40	0	0
peanut	1 pkg	250	13	5.0	25	30	2	23	5	0	40	6	0
Malted milk balls	13	140	5	5.0	70	23	0	17	1	0	46	1	100
Marshmallows	4 large	100	0	0.0	25	24	0	17	1	0	1	0	1
Mike and Ike	16	110	0	0.0	10	27	0	18	0	0	0	0	0
Milk Duds	10	130	5	2.5	75	22	0	16	1	0	0	0	94
Mints													
Altoids	3	10	0	0.0	0	2	0	2	0	0	0	0	0
Breath Savers	1	5	0	0.0	0	2	0	0	0	0	0	0	0
butter	7	50	0	0.0	0	12	0	11	0	0	0	0	0
Nips, caramel	2	60	2	1.0	10	12	0	7	0	0	10	0	0
Nonpareils	5	180	9	5.0	0	23	2	17	1	0	1	2	0
Orange slices	2	90	0	0.0	0	23	0	19	0	0	1	0	0
Peanut brittle	1.5 oz	210	7	2.0	113	30	2	23	3	0	12	0	71
Peanuts, chocolate covered	10 pcs	208	13	6.0	16	20	2	15	5	0	42	1	201
Peeps	4	110	0	0.0	0	28	0	25	0	0	0	0	1

CANDY

CANDY	Amount	Calories	Fat (g)	Saturated Fat (g)	Sodium (mg)	Carbohydrate (g)	Fiber (g)	Sugar (g)	Protein (g)	Vitamin D (mcg)	Calcium (mg)	Iron (mg)	Potassium (mg)
Pez	1 roll (12)	35	0	0.0	0	9	0	9	0	0	0	0	0
Praline, homemade	1 (1.4 oz)	189	10	1.0	19	23	1	22	1	0	17	1	85
Raisinets	10	40	2	0.5	4	7	1	0	1	0	0	0	51
Raisins, yogurt covered	¼ cup	120	4	4.0	15	21	1	18	1	0	20	0	160
Reese's													
Peanut Butter Cups	2 (0.8 oz)	210	12	4.5	150	24	2	22	5	0	39	1	150
Pieces	38	150	7	6.0	35	19	1	16	3	0	10	1	90
Rolos	5	140	6	4.5	50	20	0	19	1	0	40	0	70
Skittles	27	110	1	1.0	5	26	0	21	0	0	0	0	3
Sour Patch Kids	12	110	0	0.0	25	27	0	24	0	0	10	0	2
Starburst	6	120	3	2.5	0	24	0	16	0	0	0	0	0
Sugar Babies	21	120	1	0.5	25	28	0	22	0	0	0	0	0
Sugar Daddy	1 (1.7 oz)	200	3	1.5	70	44	0	29	1	0	20	0	31
Swedish Fish													
small	12 (1 in)	110	0	0.0	25	27	0	23	0	0	0	0	0
medium	19 (2 in)	140	0	0.0	30	36	0	29	0	0	0	0	0
SweeTARTS	13	60	0	0.0	0	14	0	13	0	0	0	0	0
Taffy													
Airheads	2 (4 in)	130	1	0.0	5	30	0	21	0	0	0	0	0
saltwater	1 (0.5 oz)	60	1	0.5	8	14	0	10	0	0	1	0	1
Tic Tacs	2	4	0	0.0	0	0	0	0	0	0	0	0	0
Toblerone	4 pcs	190	10	6.0	20	22	1	21	2	0	60	1	100
Tootsie Rolls	6 small	140	3	0.5	15	28	0	20	1	0	20	1	46
Truffles	3	183	12	6.5	25	16	1	14	2	0	57	1	107
Turtles	2	170	10	4.0	40	19	1	16	2	0	40	0	125
Whoppers	18	190	7	7.0	95	31	0	24	1	0	63	1	140
York Peppermint Pattie	1 (1.4 oz)	150	3	1.5	10	32	1	26	1	0	0	1	48

CEREAL BARS & CEREALS

Cereal Bars

	Amount	Calories	Fat (g)	Saturated Fat (g)	Sodium (mg)	Carbohydrate (g)	Fiber (g)	Sugar (g)	Protein (g)	Vitamin D (mcg)	Calcium (mg)	Iron (mg)	Potassium (mg)
Fiber One Oats & Chocolate	1 bar	140	4	1.5	95	29	9	9	2	0	140	1	0
Kashi Chewy Granola													
chocolate almond sea salt	1 bar	130	5	1.0	125	23	4	7	3	0	20	1	120
chocolate peanut butter	1 bar	140	6	1.5	140	21	5	6	3	0	10	1	130
trail mix	1 bar	130	5	0.0	105	24	3	7	3	0	20	1	110
Milk 'n Cereal													
Cinnamon Toast Crunch	1 bar	180	4	2.0	150	33	1	14	3	0	290	2	110
Honey Nut Cheerios	1 bar	160	4	2.0	90	13	1	13	3	1	280	1	120
Nature Valley													
Crunchy Granola													
cinnamon	1 bar	90	4	0.0	75	15	1	6	2	0	0	1	0
maple brown sugar	1 bar	100	4	0.0	75	15	1	6	2	0	0	1	0
oats 'n honey	1 bar	100	4	0.0	70	15	1	6	2	0	0	1	0
peanut butter	1 bar	100	4	0.0	80	14	1	5	2	0	0	1	0

CEREAL BARS & CEREALS

Cereal Bars	Amount	Calories	Fat (g)	Saturated Fat (g)	Sodium (mg)	Carbohydrate (g)	Fiber (g)	Sugar (g)	Protein (g)	Vitamin D (mcg)	Calcium (mg)	Iron (mg)	Potassium (mg)
Sweet & Salty Nut Granola													
almond	1 bar	160	7	2.0	140	22	2	8	3	0	30	1	100
dark chocolate peanut & almond	1 bar	170	8	3.0	125	22	2	9	3	0	0	1	0
peanut	1 bar	170	8	2.5	140	20	1	7	4	0	0	0	0
Nutri-Grain Soft Baked													
apple cinnamon	1 bar	130	4	0.5	125	25	1	13	2	0	130	2	80
blueberry	1 bar	130	4	0.5	130	25	1	13	2	0	130	2	80
strawberry	1 bar	130	4	0.5	140	25	1	13	2	0	130	2	80
Power Bar Protein Plus													
chocolate peanut butter	1 bar	210	6	3.0	200	25	4	12	20	0	96	1	100
vanilla	1 bar	210	5	3.0	130	23	4	14	20	0	96	1	120
Quaker Chewy Granola													
chocolate chip	1 bar	100	4	1.5	70	17	1	7	1	0	80	1	60
cookies & cream, 25% less sugar	1 bar	90	3	0.5	85	18	3	5	1	0	110	1	50
oatmeal raisin	1 bar	90	2	0.0	80	19	1	7	1	0	90	1	60
peanut butter/chocolate chip	1 bar	100	3	1.0	95	17	1	7	2	0	100	1	60
Rice Krispies Treats	1 bar	90	2	0.5	105	17	0	8	0	0	0	1	0
Special K													
cranberry almond chewy nut	1 bar	140	6	1.5	55	20	2	12	3	0	20	1	120
chocolate almond chewy nut	1 bar	170	10	3.0	45	16	2	9	4	0	20	1	130
stawberry pastry crisps	1 bar	100	2	1.0	80	20	0	7	0	0	10	1	20
Hot Cereal (prepared)													
Cream of Rice	1 cup	150	0	0.0	0	35	0	0	2	5	340	13	30
Cream of Wheat	1¼ cups	120	0	0.0	100	25	1	0	3	4	260	9	30
Grits, corn													
instant	1 pkt	100	0	0.0	310	22	1	0	2	0	130	8	40
old fashioned	⅓ cup	140	1	0.0	0	32	2	0	3	0	0	2	60
quick	⅓ cup	130	1	0.0	0	29	2	0	3	0	0	2	50
Maltex	1 cup	180	1	0.0	0	38	5	2	5	0	0	9	200
Malt-O-Meal	1 cup	130	0	0.0	0	27	0	0	4	0	100	11	30
Maypo	1 cup	180	3	0.5	105	34	4	4	5	0	180	14	150
Oat bran	1 cup	88	2	0.5	2	25	6	0	7	0	22	2	202
Oatmeal													
apples & cinnamon, instant	1 pkt	160	2	0.5	160	33	4	11	4	0	108	4	150
cinnamon & spice, instant	1 pkt	160	3	0.5	200	32	3	10	4	0	20	1	130
maple & brown sugar, instant	1 pkt	160	2	0.5	260	33	3	12	4	0	20	1	110
regular													
instant	1 pkt	100	2	0.5	75	18	3	0	4	0	120	8	100
old fashioned/quick	1 cup	150	3	0.5	0	27	4	1	5	0	20	2	150
steel cut, cooked	1 cup	166	4	1.0	9	28	4	1	6	0	21	2	164
Wheatena	1 cup	143	1	0.0	5	30	5	1	5	0	22	1	200

CEREAL BARS & CEREALS

Ready-to-Eat Cereal (w/o milk)	Amount	Calories	Fat (g)	Saturated Fat (g)	Sodium (mg)	Carbohydrate (g)	Fiber (g)	Sugar (g)	Protein (g)	Vitamin D (mcg)	Calcium (mg)	Iron (mg)	Potassium (mg)
All-Bran	½ cup	110	2	0.0	300	36	17	12	5	2	30	5	430
buds	½ cup	110	2	0.0	300	36	17	12	5	2	30	5	430
Amaranth flakes	1 cup	130	2	0.0	5	25	3	4	4	0	20	1	130
Apple Jacks	1 cup	120	1	0.0	146	29	3	15	2	2	0	5	50
Basic 4	1 cup	200	2	1.0	280	43	5	12	4	1	300	5	170
Bran flakes	1 cup	110	1	0.0	278	32	7	7	4	1	15	9	200
Cap'n Crunch	1 cup	150	2	0.5	290	33	0	17	2	0	0	8	50
Crunch Berries	1 cup	150	2	0.5	270	32	0	16	2	0	0	8	50
peanut butter crunch	1 cup	170	4	1.0	300	32	0	13	3	0	0	7	70
Cheerios	1½ cups	140	3	0.5	190	29	4	2	5	2	130	13	250
apple cinnamon	1 cup	150	3	0.0	150	30	3	12	3	2	130	4	99
banana nut	¾ cup	110	2	0.0	120	22	2	8	2	1	120	5	80
frosted	1 cup	140	2	0.0	200	29	3	12	3	2	130	4	94
honey nut	1 cup	140	2	0.0	210	30	3	12	3	2	130	4	152
multigrain	1⅓ cups	150	2	0.0	150	32	3	8	3	2	130	18	170
Chex													
cinnamon	1 cup	170	4	0.0	250	33	2	8	2	2	130	11	49
corn	1¼ cups	150	1	0.0	280	33	2	4	3	2	130	11	61
honey nut	1 cup	170	1	0.0	270	38	2	12	2	2	130	4	88
rice	1¼ cups	160	1	0.0	330	36	2	3	3	2	130	13	51
wheat	1 cup	210	1	0.0	340	51	8	6	6	2	130	18	190
Cinnamon Toast Crunch	1 cup	170	4	0.0	230	33	2	12	2	2	130	4	80
Cocoa Pebbles	1 cup	140	2	0.0	220	31	0	12	2	2	9	3	60
Cocoa Puffs	¾ cup	100	2	0.0	100	23	1	9	1	1	120	5	85
Cocoa Rice Krispies	1 cup	160	1	0.0	140	37	0	13	3	2	190	5	70
Cookie Crisp	1 cup	140	2	0.0	150	31	2	2	2	1	120	4	81
Corn flakes	1½ cups	150	0	0.0	300	36	1	4	3	3	1	12	60
Corn Pops	1⅓ cups	150	0	0.0	160	36	0	15	2	2	2	5	30
Cracklin' Oat Bran	¾ cup	200	0	0.5	65	41	7	16	4	3	20	5	210
Crispix	1⅓ cups	150	0	0.0	260	34	0	5	3	3	3	11	20
Crunchy Oatmeal Squares	1 cup	210	3	0.5	190	44	5	9	6	0	30	17	200
Fiber One	⅔ cup	90	1	0.0	140	34	18	0	3	0	130	4	148
honey clusters	1 cup	170	2	0.0	200	45	10	10	4	0	130	16	193
Froot Loops	1⅓ cups	150	2	0.5	210	34	2	12	2	2	3	5	60
Frosted Flakes	1 cup	130	0	0.0	190	33	1	12	2	2	1	7	30
Fruity Pebbles	1 cup	140	2	0.0	190	31	0	12	1	2	8	1	20
Golden Crisp	1 cup	150	1	0.0	85	34	0	21	2	0	4	1	70
Golden Grahams	¾ cup	110	1	0.0	230	25	1	9	2	1	120	5	70
Granola, Bear Naked													
fruit & nut	½ cup	270	12	3.0	0	39	5	13	6	0	30	2	190
peanut butter	⅔ cup	290	13	2.0	55	42	5	13	6	0	20	2	210
protein original cinnamon	½ cup	260	12	1.0	100	31	5	12	11	0	40	2	240

Ready-to-Eat Cereal (w/o milk)	Amount	Calories	Fat (g)	Saturated Fat (g)	Sodium (mg)	Carbohydrate (g)	Fiber (g)	Sugar (g)	Protein (g)	Vitamin D (mcg)	Calcium (mg)	Iron (mg)	Potassium (mg)
Granola, Simply	⅔ cup	260	7	1.0	30	48	7	13	7	0	60	2	190
w/ raisins	⅔ cup	270	7	0.5	30	51	7	17	7	0	60	2	230
Grape-Nuts	½ cup	200	1	0.0	280	47	7	5	6	0	20	17	260
flakes	1 cup	150	2	0.0	200	34	5	7	4	2	10	13	160
Great Grains													
banana nut crunch	1 cup	230	5	0.5	240	45	5	10	6	2	20	17	295
blueberry nut crunch	1 cup	220	3	0.0	200	48	4	16	4	2	20	3	150
cranberry almond crunch	1 cup	210	3	0.0	200	44	5	12	5	2	20	5	180
crunchy pecan	¾ cup	210	5	0.5	160	39	5	8	5	2	20	16	190
raisins, dates & pecans	¾ cup	200	4	0.0	140	40	5	13	4	2	20	11	210
Honey Bunches of Oats													
honey roasted	1 cup	160	2	0.0	190	34	2	9	3	2	10	16	60
w/ almonds	1 cup	170	3	0.0	180	34	2	9	3	2	10	16	80
Honeycomb	1¾ cups	110	1	0.0	70	25	0	12	1	0	110	0	20
Kashi	1¼ cups	180	2	0.0	115	40	13	8	12	0	40	2	390
GO													
cinnamon crisp	1 cup	210	5	0.5	200	37	11	11	13	0	60	3	350
Organic													
blueberry clusters	1 cup	210	3	0.0	130	44	3	11	5	0	10	1	120
honey toasted oat	1 cup	150	2	0.0	65	35	6	7	4	0	10	12	100
Strawberry Fields	1 cup	200	0	0.0	180	46	3	11	5	0	0	1	110
Whole Wheat Biscuits													
cinnamon harvest	31 biscuits	200	1	0.0	0	48	7	9	7	0	10	2	190
simply raisin	30 biscuits	190	1	0.0	0	47	7	7	7	0	20	2	280
Kix	1½ cups	160	1	0.0	220	34	3	4	3	2	130	11	54
honey	1½ cups	160	2	0.0	190	34	2	3	2	2	130	11	100
Life	1 cup	160	2	0.0	210	33	3	8	4	0	150	13	110
Lucky Charms	1 cup	140	1	0.0	160	31	1	12	1	2	130	4	80
Mini-Wheats													
blueberry	25 biscuits	210	1	0.0	10	50	6	12	5	0	10	18	210
frosted bite-size	25 biscuits	210	2	0.0	10	51	6	12	5	0	0	18	160
Mueslix	1 cup	250	4	0.0	150	50	5	17	6	0	30	2	200
Nature's Path Flax Plus													
maple pecan crunch	1 cup	230	7	1.0	210	39	6	10	6	0	30	3	250
multibran	1 cup	150	2	0.0	180	31	7	5	5	0	22	2	190
Oat bran flakes	1 cup	179	1	0.5	179	37	4	10	5	0	34	1	160
Oatmeal Squares w/ brown sugar	1 cup	210	3	0.5	190	44	5	9	6	0	30	17	200
Puffed rice	1 cup	56	0	0.0	0	13	0	0	1	0	1	4	16
Puffed wheat	1 cup	44	0	0.0	1	10	1	0	2	0	3	4	42
Raisin Bran	1 cup	190	1	0.0	200	47	7	17	5	0	20	2	280
Crunch	1 cup	190	1	0.0	200	46	4	19	4	0	20	1	280
Reese's Puffs	¾ cup	120	3	0.5	160	22	1	9	2	1	120	5	70
Rice Krispies	1½ cups	150	0	0.0	200	36	0	4	3	3	0	11	30

CEREAL BARS & CEREALS

Ready-to-Eat Cereal (w/o milk)	Amount	Calories	Fat (g)	Saturated Fat (g)	Sodium (mg)	Carbohydrate (g)	Fiber (g)	Sugar (g)	Protein (g)	Vitamin D (mcg)	Calcium (mg)	Iron (mg)	Potassium (mg)
Shredded Wheat													
Big Biscuit	2 biscuits	170	1	0.0	0	41	7	0	6	0	20	2	230
Spoon Size	1⅓ cups	210	2	0.0	0	49	8	0	7	0	20	2	250
Wheat 'N Bran	1⅓ cups	210	2	0.0	0	49	8	0	7	0	20	2	240
Smart Start Antioxidants	1¼ cups	240	1	0.0	260	56	3	18	5	2	10	8	130
Special K	1¼ cups	150	1	0.0	270	29	0	5	7	2	10	11	10
fruit & yogurt	1 cup	160	1	0.0	190	36	3	13	3	2	10	11	90
red berries	1 cup	140	1	0.0	250	34	3	11	3	2	10	11	80
Total whole grain	1 cup	140	1	0.0	190	33	4	6	3	2	40	18	140
Trix	1¼ cups	160	2	0.0	180	33	1	12	2	2	130	4	0
Weetabix	3 biscuits	180	1	0.0	190	43	6	2	5	0	20	7	230
Wheat bran flakes	1 cup	110	1	0.0	190	29	7	7	4	2	10	9	210
Wheat germ	3 T	60	1	0.0	0	8	2	1	4	0	10	1	141
Wheaties	1 cup	130	1	0.0	240	30	4	5	3	2	0	13	130

CHEESE

	Amount	Calories	Fat (g)	Saturated Fat (g)	Sodium (mg)	Carbohydrate (g)	Fiber (g)	Sugar (g)	Protein (g)	Vitamin D (mcg)	Calcium (mg)	Iron (mg)	Potassium (mg)
American	1 oz	106	9	5.0	474	1	0	1	6	1	300	0	37
fat-free	1 oz	36	0	0.0	373	3	0	1	6	1	220	0	110
low-fat	1 oz	68	4	2.5	340	3	0	2	5	2	150	0	94
singles	1 slice	95	6	4.0	297	3	0	1	5	1	270	0	59
fat-free	1 slice	37	0	0.0	373	3	0	2	6	0	224	0	83
reduced fat	1 slice	67	4	2.0	343	3	0	3	6	2	208	0	69
Blue	1 oz	100	8	5.0	325	1	0	0	6	0	150	0	73
Brick	1 oz	105	8	5.0	159	1	0	0	7	0	191	0	38
Brie	1 oz	95	8	5.0	178	0	0	0	6	0	52	0	43
Camembert	1 oz	85	7	4.0	239	0	0	0	6	0	110	0	53
Caraway	1 oz	107	8	5.0	196	1	0	0	7	0	191	0	26
Cheddar	1 oz	115	9	5.0	185	1	0	0	7	0	201	0	22
fat-free	1 oz	45	0	0.0	283	2	0	0	9	0	253	0	19
low-fat	1 oz	50	2	1.0	247	1	0	0	7	0	118	0	19
shredded	¼ cup	114	9	5.0	184	1	0	0	6	0	201	0	21
spread	2 T	80	7	5.0	150	1	0	1	2	0	40	0	69
Cheez Whiz	2 T	80	5	1.0	430	6	0	3	3	0	78	0	94
Colby	1 oz	112	9	6.0	171	1	0	0	7	0	194	0	36
& Monterey Jack	1 oz	111	9	5.0	172	1	0	0	7	0	152	0	30
Cottage													
1% fat	½ cup	81	1	0.5	459	3	0	3	14	0	67	0	97
2% fat	½ cup	92	3	1.5	348	5	0	5	12	0	125	0	141
fat-free	½ cup	80	0	0.0	390	8	0	6	13	1	100	0	159
Cream cheese	2 T	102	10	6.0	91	2	0	1	2	0	28	0	38
fat-free	2 T	38	0	0.0	253	3	0	2	6	0	126	0	100
flavored													
onion & chive	2 T	80	7	5.0	150	2	0	1	2	0	40	0	68
strawberry	2 T	80	6	4.0	105	5	0	4	1	0	40	0	39
light	2 T	60	5	2.5	108	2	0	2	2	0	44	0	74

CHEESE

	Amount	Calories	Fat (g)	Saturated Fat (g)	Sodium (mg)	Carbohydrate (g)	Fiber (g)	Sugar (g)	Protein (g)	Vitamin D (mcg)	Calcium (mg)	Iron (mg)	Potassium (mg)
Easy Cheese, American	2 T	80	6	1.0	430	3	0	2	4	0	260	0	90
Edam	1 oz	101	8	5.0	230	0	0	0	7	0	207	0	53
Feta	1 oz	75	6	4.0	260	1	0	1	4	0	140	0	18
Fondue	¼ cup	148	11	6.5	163	1	0	0	10	0	343	0	46
Fontina	1 oz	110	9	5.5	227	0	0	0	7	0	156	0	18
Goat, soft	1 oz	75	6	4.0	130	0	0	0	5	0	40	1	7
Gorgonzola	1 oz	100	8	5.5	325	1	0	0	6	0	150	0	73
Gouda	1 oz	101	8	5.0	232	1	0	1	7	0	198	0	34
Gruyère	1 oz	117	9	5.5	202	0	0	0	8	0	287	0	23
Havarti	1 oz	105	8	5.0	159	1	0	0	7	0	191	0	39
Jarlsberg	1 oz	111	9	5.0	53	0	0	0	8	0	252	0	20
Limburger	1 oz	93	8	5.0	227	0	0	0	6	0	141	0	36
Mascarpone	1 oz	120	12	7.0	10	0	0	0	2	0	40	0	70
Monterey Jack	1 oz	101	9	5.0	192	0	0	0	6	0	203	0	23
Mozzarella													
part-skim	1 oz	84	6	3.0	189	2	0	0	7	0	198	0	53
whole milk	1 oz	90	7	4.5	201	1	0	0	6	0	163	0	21
Muenster	1 oz	104	9	5.5	178	0	0	0	7	0	203	0	38
Neufchatel	1 oz	72	6	3.5	95	1	0	1	3	0	33	0	43
Parmesan, grated	1 T	30	2	1.5	113	0	0	0	3	0	90	0	9
reduced fat	1 T	19	1	1.0	107	0	0	0	1	0	78	0	9
Pepper Jack	1 oz	111	9	5.0	192	0	0	0	7	0	203	0	23
Port wine, cold pack	2 T	80	6	3.0	160	3	0	3	4	0	100	0	73
Provolone	1 oz	100	8	5.0	248	1	0	0	7	0	214	0	39
Ricotta													
fat-free	½ cup	100	0	0.0	130	10	0	4	10	0	200	0	316
low-fat	½ cup	120	6	4.0	140	6	0	4	14	0	200	0	280
part-skim	½ cup	140	9	6.0	170	6	0	6	12	0	200	0	155
whole milk	½ cup	180	12	8.0	150	6	0	6	14	0	300	0	219
Romano, grated	1 T	30	2	1.5	113	0	0	0	3	0	90	0	11
Roquefort	1 oz	105	9	5.5	513	1	0	0	6	0	188	0	26
Soy	1 oz	43	2	0.5	6	2	0	0	4	0	53	2	56
String	1 oz	83	6	3.0	189	2	0	1	7	0	198	0	53
Swiss													
natural	1 oz	111	9	5.0	53	1	0	0	8	0	252	0	20
processed	1 oz	92	7	4.5	440	1	0	0	6	0	205	0	81
Velveeta	1 oz	70	4	1.0	390	3	0	2	4	0	230	0	0
Yogurt cheese	1 oz	26	2	1.0	22	2	0	2	1	0	50	0	61

COMBINATION FOODS, FROZEN ENTRÉES & MEALS

	Amount	Calories	Fat (g)	Saturated Fat (g)	Sodium (mg)	Carbohydrate (g)	Fiber (g)	Sugar (g)	Protein (g)	Vitamin D (mcg)	Calcium (mg)	Iron (mg)	Potassium (mg)
Bagel Bites, frozen													
cheese & pepperoni	4 pcs	190	6	2.5	420	27	1	2	7	0	100	2	160
mozzarella	4 pcs	170	4	2.0	370	28	1	2	7	0	110	2	130
three cheese	4 pcs	180	5	3.0	360	28	1	3	6	0	100	2	140
Baked beans w/ pork, can	½ cup	150	1	0.0	550	29	7	7	7	0	67	2	391
Beans & rice	1 cup	279	7	1.0	393	43	6	0	11	0	92	4	556
Beef goulash w/ noodles	1 cup	361	14	3.5	130	27	2	2	30	0	45	4	525
Beef stroganoff w/ noodles	1 cup	344	19	7.5	468	23	2	3	20	0	74	2	374
Beefaroni, can	1 cup	200	7	2.5	730	27	1	5	6	0	0	1	150
Burritos, frozen													
bean & cheese	1 (6 oz)	413	11	2.5	941	66	18	6	13	0	97	5	393
beef & bean	1 (6 oz)	352	11	4.0	866	51	6	1	11	0	47	4	307
Casseroles													
chicken w/ cheese sauce	1 cup	368	16	6.5	739	9	0	4	44	1	120	2	284
green bean	1 cup	115	5	1.0	736	16	4	6	4	0	92	1	366
seafood Newburg	1 cup	613	50	29.5	551	10	0	6	30	2	266	1	481
tuna noodle	1 cup	376	16	8.0	571	35	2	5	23	2	146	3	316
Chicken cacciatore w/ pasta	1 cup	320	18	4.5	172	39	1	12	29	0	42	2	586
Chicken cordon bleu	6 oz	281	13	4.0	886	27	3	1	15	0	136	2	356
Chicken divan	6 oz	249	16	7.0	479	10	1	2	16	0	165	1	350
Chicken nuggets, frozen	4 pcs	210	15	3.5	360	9	1	1	11	0	33	1	146
Chicken parmigiana, frozen	1 (6 oz)	364	17	5.5	867	17	2	4	34	0	247	2	477
Chicken tetrazzini	1 cup	290	12	5.0	954	17	1	1	29	0	44	1	317
Chili w/ beans, can													
beef	1 cup	263	7	3.0	1220	34	7	4	16	0	93	9	934
turkey	1 cup	193	3	1.0	1200	26	5	6	17	0	81	3	706
Chimichangas, frozen													
beef	1 (4.5 oz)	360	20	5.0	470	37	3	4	9	0	179	3	337
chicken	1 (4.5 oz)	340	16	4.0	540	39	2	3	11	0	173	3	298
Chipped beef, creamed	1 (6 oz)	187	10	6.0	801	12	1	8	13	2	188	1	295
Chop suey, can													
beef & noodle	1 cup	286	9	2.0	803	27	3	5	23	0	48	4	453
chicken & noodle	1 cup	290	9	1.5	825	27	3	5	23	0	42	2	436
pork & noodle	1 cup	317	12	3.5	799	27	3	5	22	0	48	3	480
Chow mein, can													
beef & noodle	1 cup	286	9	2.0	803	27	3	5	23	0	48	4	453
chicken & noodle	1 cup	290	9	1.5	825	27	3	5	23	0	42	2	436
Corn dogs, frozen	1 (2.7 oz)	180	9	2.5	470	18	1	6	7	0	30	1	130
Egg rolls													
pork	1 (6 oz)	220	11	2.5	390	24	2	3	5	0	21	1	128
shrimp	1 (6 oz)	180	7	1.5	490	25	2	4	5	0	30	1	134
Eggplant parmigiana	1 cup	311	22	8.0	701	17	4	6	13	0	312	1	428
Enchiladas													
beef	1 (6 oz)	211	7	2.0	724	28	4	1	9	0	58	2	236
chicken	1 (6 oz)	213	9	2.5	314	24	3	1	9	0	107	2	140

COMBINATION FOODS, FROZEN ENTRÉES & MEALS

	Amount	Calories	Fat (g)	Saturated Fat (g)	Sodium (mg)	Carbohydrate (g)	Fiber (g)	Sugar (g)	Protein (g)	Vitamin D (mcg)	Calcium (mg)	Iron (mg)	Potassium (mg)
Fajitas													
beef	1 (6 oz)	305	14	4.0	241	27	2	5	17	0	105	3	413
chicken	1 (6 oz)	277	9	1.5	262	34	4	5	15	0	96	2	340
Frozen breakfasts													
cinnamon French toast w/ sausage	1 (6.5 oz)	414	21	6.5	797	34	1	11	22	2	199	3	372
egg, steak & cheese bagel	1 (8.6 oz)	691	35	13.5	1570	56	0	7	39	1	228	5	355
pancakes w/ sausage	1 (6 oz)	459	23	6.0	976	47	1	16	15	1	82	3	291
sausage, egg & cheese biscuit	1 (4.5 oz)	415	28	11.0	756	28	3	4	12	1	174	2	344
scrambled eggs (2) & bacon (2)	1 (5.3 oz)	267	20	6.5	493	3	0	2	17	2	83	2	254
scrambled eggs & sausage w/ hash browns	1 (6.3 oz)	364	27	7.5	779	17	1	2	13	2	60	2	490
Frozen dinners													
baked chicken	1 (8.9 oz)	260	11	5.0	860	18	1	4	21	0	50	1	660
chicken à la king	1 (11.5 oz)	400	15	4.0	950	48	1	4	19	0	120	2	580
chicken fettuccine Alfredo	1 (10.5 oz)	540	31	11.0	940	43	3	5	23	0	220	1	430
chicken Marsala	1 (9 oz)	300	7	3.0	850	40	2	6	20	0	20	1	400
chicken Parmesan	1 (12 oz)	470	19	5.0	1050	52	4	8	24	3	190	3	610
chicken pot pie	1 (10 oz)	630	37	12.0	920	55	2	7	18	0	140	4	570
fettuccine Alfredo	1 (11.5 oz)	640	37	14.0	970	58	3	6	18	0	310	1	250
fish filet	1 (9 oz)	490	21	5.0	750	49	0	3	26	0	130	2	530
fried chicken	1 (8.9 oz)	380	18	6.0	1040	32	1	2	22	0	50	2	340
green pepper steak	1 (10.5 oz)	290	9	3.0	810	34	1	4	18	0	60	2	840
Healthy Choice													
chicken margherita w/ balsamic	1 (9.5 oz)	270	6	1.0	360	36	5	7	17	0	0	2	470
crustless chicken pot pie	1 (9.6 oz)	300	6	2.0	600	40	3	6	21	0	40	2	700
grilled chicken pesto w/ vegetables	1 (9.9 oz)	290	7	2.0	590	36	3	2	20	0	90	2	570
Mexican-style street corn	1 (9.2 oz)	240	5	2.0	520	30	8	6	18	0	80	2	760
lasagna													
cheese	1 (10.7 oz)	350	12	6.0	770	43	3	10	18	0	390	2	680
meat	1 (10 oz)	420	20	8.0	780	40	3	6	20	0	190	2	720
Lean Cuisine													
chicken fried rice	1 (9 oz)	310	8	2.0	720	43	3	2	17	0	50	2	610
lasagna w/ meat sauce	1 (10.5 oz)	310	7	3.5	610	45	4	8	17	0	210	2	800
glazed turkey tenderloins	1 (9 oz)	300	6	2.0	530	47	3	24	14	0	110	1	510
shrimp scampi	1 (10 oz)	350	9	3.0	660	50	2	4	16	0	90	1	600
meatloaf	1 (9.9 oz)	330	16	7.0	900	25	3	6	22	0	90	2	1020
roast turkey	1 (9.6 oz)	280	10	4.0	770	29	2	3	18	0	60	1	550
Salisbury steak	1 (9.6 oz)	340	16	8.0	1000	26	2	4	23	0	180	2	520
stuffed peppers w/ beef	1 (10 oz)	200	8	3.0	770	22	3	7	10	0	50	2	490
Swedish meatballs w/ pasta	1 (11.5 oz)	500	23	10.0	1100	48	3	5	26	1	120	2	530
three cheese ravioli	1 (10 oz)	370	13	6.0	840	43	3	7	21	0	290	3	430
turkey Tetrazzini	1 (12 oz)	470	24	10.0	980	42	2	5	21	0	120	1	610

COMBINATION FOODS, FROZEN ENTRÉES & MEALS

	Amount	Calories	Fat (g)	Saturated Fat (g)	Sodium (mg)	Carbohydrate (g)	Fiber (g)	Sugar (g)	Protein (g)	Vitamin D (mcg)	Calcium (mg)	Iron (mg)	Potassium (mg)
Hamburger Helper, box, prepared													
beef pasta	1 cup	280	11	4.5	575	25	1	1	3	0	78	3	376
cheeseburger macaroni	1 cup	310	12	5.0	713	30	0	3	3	1	130	3	376
cheesy enchilada	1 cup	320	12	4.5	552	33	1	3	3	0	104	3	376
lasagna	1 cup	310	12	4.0	644	30	1	6	3	0	52	3	376
stroganoff	1 cup	300	12	5.0	575	30	1	3	4	2	130	2	376
Hot Pockets, frozen													
chicken bacon ranch	1 (4.3 oz)	270	9	4.5	620	37	1	3	11	0	210	2	260
four cheese pizza	1 (4.3 oz)	270	10	4.0	700	37	2	4	9	0	260	2	180
hickory ham & cheddar	1 (4.5 oz)	270	9	4.0	690	39	1	3	9	0	160	2	170
Italian style meatballs & mozzarella	1 (4.5 oz)	290	12	4.0	630	37	2	3	11	1	180	3	270
Philly steak & cheese	1 (4.5 oz)	290	10	5.0	750	40	1	0	11	0	170	2	190
Lasagna													
w/ meat	6 oz	272	11	5.5	272	28	2	6	16	0	139	1	352
w/ vegetables	6 oz	239	7	4.5	284	31	2	4	12	0	458	1	350
Lo mein, pork	6 oz	241	12	2.0	121	10	2	4	17	0	34	2	286
Macaroni & cheese													
frozen	1 (12 oz)	500	24	10.0	1200	51	2	5	21	0	390	1	440
three cheese, box	1 cup	360	12	4.0	750	50	1	8	10	0	180	3	310
Manicotti w/ red sauce	2 large	580	28	12.0	1520	66	6	4	20	1	398	3	564
Meatballs	1 medium	58	3	1.0	83	2	0	0	5	0	10	1	62
Meatloaf	3 oz	169	9	3.5	101	5	0	2	15	0	56	2	236
Moussaka	1 cup	238	13	4.5	460	13	4	6	17	0	118	2	457
Pasta Roni, box, prepared													
butter & garlic	1 cup	250	9	2.0	667	36	2	2	7	0	104	2	180
butter & herb Italiano	1 cup	300	14	3.0	759	39	2	2	7	0	130	2	160
shells & white cheddar	1 cup	290	15	4.0	644	36	2	3	7	0	130	1	260
Pepper steak	1 cup	320	20	4.0	563	6	1	4	28	0	37	3	438
Pizza, frozen													
cheese	1 slice (5.2 oz)	341	15	5.5	663	36	2	5	15	0	335	3	296
French bread	1 (5.2 oz)	360	16	6.0	700	40	2	5	15	0	290	2	280
pepperoni	1 slice (5.2 oz)	378	20	4.5	912	35	2	5	13	0	320	3	300
French bread	1 (5.6 oz)	400	20	7.0	950	40	2	4	15	0	200	3	310
Pot pies, frozen													
beef	½ pie (7 oz)	400	21	9.0	660	40	4	4	13	0	40	3	410
chicken	½ pie (7 oz)	440	26	11.0	650	40	2	2	11	0	30	4	190
Ravioli w/ red sauce													
cheese	6 oz	232	10	4.5	390	26	2	6	10	0	117	1	348
meat	6 oz	268	12	4.0	122	25	2	3	15	0	48	3	364
Salmon loaf	3 oz	168	9	2.5	410	7	0	12	14	7	167	1	243
Salmon patties	1 (4.2 oz)	259	15	3.5	502	14	1	1	16	8	229	1	293

COMBINATION FOODS, FROZEN ENTRÉES & MEALS

	Amount	Calories	Fat (g)	Saturated Fat (g)	Sodium (mg)	Carbohydrate (g)	Fiber (g)	Sugar (g)	Protein (g)	Vitamin D (mcg)	Calcium (mg)	Iron (mg)	Potassium (mg)
Sandwiches (w/ bread/bun)													
BBQ beef	1 (6 oz)	376	9	3.0	697	44	1	15	28	0	107	4	330
BLT w/ mayonnaise	1 (5 oz)	314	10	3.0	542	41	2	2	15	0	321	3	284
bologna & cheese w/ mayonnaise	1 (4 oz)	336	18	7.0	898	30	1	6	13	2	464	2	228
cheeseburger	1 (6 oz)	459	22	9.0	1068	43	3	9	23	0	209	4	313
chicken													
breaded & fried	1 (6 oz)	425	19	4.0	1280	36	2	6	28	0	99	3	417
roasted/grilled	1 (6 oz)	250	5	1.0	539	25	2	7	23	0	53	2	322
chicken salad w/ mayonnaise	1 (6 oz)	392	17	3.0	599	34	2	4	25	0	112	3	316
corned beef	1 (6 oz)	350	12	5.0	1365	34	2	4	24	0	104	4	184
egg salad w/ mayonnaise	1 (6 oz)	503	35	7.0	675	29	2	4	15	2	126	3	178
grilled cheese	1 (4 oz)	386	20	7.0	912	39	2	6	13	2	597	3	195
ham & cheese w/ mustard & mayonnaise	1 (6 oz)	364	18	7.0	1374	29	2	6	20	2	507	3	359
ham salad w/ mayonnaise	1 (6 oz)	376	17	3.5	1240	34	2	5	20	1	111	3	349
hamburger	1 (6 oz)	412	17	6.0	653	45	2	10	22	0	129	5	369
hot dog	1 (3.5 oz)	299	16	5.0	791	27	1	5	10	0	132	2	191
peanut butter & jelly	1 (3 oz)	326	14	3.0	376	42	3	13	10	0	92	2	209
Reuben w/ dressing	1 (6 oz)	485	29	9.5	1214	33	4	7	21	0	281	3	231
roast beef w/ cheese	1 (6 oz)	555	34	14.5	849	29	2	4	31	1	264	4	390
salami & cheese w/ mustard	1 (6 oz)	555	34	15.0	849	29	2	4	31	1	263	4	390
sloppy Joe, beef	1 (6 oz)	396	11	3.5	1202	56	2	28	17	0	116	3	390
tuna salad w/ mayonnaise	1 (6 oz)	340	18	2.5	410	30	5	6	19	0	85	3	191
turkey club w/ bacon	1 (8 oz)	463	24	8.0	1497	33	2	2	25	0	227	3	300
Scalloped potatoes & ham	1 cup	241	7	2.0	956	33	3	5	12	1	107	2	823
Shepherd's pie	1 cup	265	8	2.0	578	34	3	3	15	0	36	2	714
Spaghetti w/ meatballs	1 cup	332	11	2.5	682	43	4	6	14	0	42	3	472
SpaghettiOs, can	1 cup	170	1	0.5	600	33	3	12	6	0	30	2	270
w/ franks	1 cup	220	7	2.0	600	29	3	10	9	0	30	2	370
w/ meatballs	1 cup	230	7	2.5	570	30	2	8	11	0	80	2	320
Stew													
beef													
can	1 cup	200	10	4.0	990	17	1	3	10	0	0	1	281
homemade	1 cup	191	10	5.0	989	17	1	3	9	0	0	0	280
chicken & vegetables	1 cup	170	6	2.0	850	17	2	2	12	0	24	2	168
turkey & vegetables	1 cup	170	6	2.0	850	17	2	2	12	0	24	2	168
Stuffed cabbage rolls	1 (8 oz)	196	7	2.5	818	25	4	10	9	0	44	1	414
Stuffed green peppers w/ rice	1 (6 oz)	274	19	5.0	320	20	2	3	6	0	146	1	218
Stuffed shells w/ red sauce	2 (3 oz)	832	55	32.0	1727	49	2	10	37	0	307	1	83
Suddenly Pasta Salad	¾ cup	250	9	1.0	500	39	1	3	6	0	0	2	360
creamy Italian	¾ cup	360	24	2.5	460	38	2	3	6	0	26	2	170
creamy Parmesan	¾ cup	350	27	2.6	368	31	2	2	5	0	26	2	110
Sweet & sour pork	1 cup	438	19	3.5	893	41	2	21	26	0	72	2	597

COMBINATION FOODS, FROZEN ENTRÉES & MEALS

	Amount	Calories	Fat (g)	Saturated Fat (g)	Sodium (mg)	Carbohydrate (g)	Fiber (g)	Sugar (g)	Protein (g)	Vitamin D (mcg)	Calcium (mg)	Iron (mg)	Potassium (mg)
Tacos, soft shell													
beef & bean	1 (4 oz)	299	13	4.5	851	33	5	4	13	0	164	3	368
chicken & bean	1 (4 oz)	226	9	3.0	607	26	4	2	11	0	127	2	271
Tamales, bean & cheese	1 (3 oz)	215	13	3.5	393	18	3	1	8	0	190	1	168
Tortellini w/ red sauce													
cheese	1 cup	373	9	4.0	720	57	4	7	15	0	178	2	403
meat	1 cup	281	10	3.0	1292	33	2	3	14	1	78	3	258
Totino's Pizza Rolls, frozen													
pepperoni	6	220	8	2.0	380	30	1	2	6	0	20	2	140
triple cheese	6	210	8	2.0	320	31	1	2	5	0	52	2	188
Tuna Helper, box													
cheesy pasta	1 cup	280	12	8.0	667	28	0	1	3	1	130	1	282
creamy pasta	1 cup	260	11	6.0	713	28	0	0	3	1	130	1	282
fettuccine Alfredo	1 cup	290	11	6.0	552	33	1	2	4	1	130	1	376
Veal Marsala	6 oz	232	15	7.0	245	11	1	1	28	0	17	2	479
Veal parmigiana	6 oz	345	24	7.5	730	14	1	3	26	2	168	2	413
Veal scallopini	6 oz	408	30	8.0	634	3	1	1	31	1	66	2	444
Velveeta Skillets													
chicken & broccoli	1 cup	390	11	3.0	610	40	2	5	33	0	150	3	490
chicken Alfredo	1 cup	340	11	3.0	880	29	1	4	31	0	160	2	340
creamy beef stroganoff	1 cup	390	16	6.0	810	30	1	7	28	1	210	4	570
ultimate cheeseburger mac	1 cup	380	17	6.0	930	27	0	5	28	0	160	4	510
Welsh rarebit, frozen	1 (3 oz)	138	10	4.5	242	5	0	4	6	1	201	0	117
Yorkshire pudding	2 oz	150	5	2.5	169	20	1	2	6	1	67	1	113
Ziti w/ meat sauce	1 cup	361	18	7.0	787	30	2	3	20	0	138	3	385

CONDIMENTS, SAUCES & BAKING INGREDIENTS

Condiments & Sauces

	Amount	Calories	Fat (g)	Saturated Fat (g)	Sodium (mg)	Carbohydrate (g)	Fiber (g)	Sugar (g)	Protein (g)	Vitamin D (mcg)	Calcium (mg)	Iron (mg)	Potassium (mg)
Alfredo sauce	¼ cup	160	14	7.0	780	6	0	2	2	1	60	0	40
BBQ sauce	1 T	20	0	0.0	185	5	0	4	0	0	2	0	7
Bearnaise sauce	2 T	161	17	10.0	124	0	0	0	2	0	15	0	16
Béchamel sauce	2 T	45	4	2.0	130	2	0	1	1	0	20	0	51
Cheese sauce	2 T	55	4	2.0	261	2	0	0	2	0	58	0	9
Chili sauce	2 T	40	0	0.0	460	10	0	6	0	0	2	0	63
Chipotle hot sauce	1 tsp	0	0	0.0	120	0	0	0	0	0	0	0	21
Chipotle salsa	2 T	10	0	0.0	140	14	1	1	0	0	9	0	123
Chutney	2 T	51	0	0.0	81	13	1	11	0	0	13	0	124
Clam sauce													
red	½ cup	70	3	0.0	760	6	1	3	5	0	20	1	70
white	½ cup	160	15	2.0	540	3	0	1	4	0	25	1	115
Cocktail sauce	2 T	37	0	0.0	294	8	1	4	0	0	8	0	93
Cranberry-orange relish	2 T	40	0	0.0	11	10	1	9	0	0	4	0	13
Cranberry sauce	2 T	55	0	0.0	5	13	0	11	0	0	1	0	10
Duck sauce	2 T	81	0	0.0	150	20	0	10	0	0	4	0	29

CONDIMENTS, SAUCES & BAKING INGREDIENTS

Condiments & Sauces	Amount	Calories	Fat (g)	Saturated Fat (g)	Sodium (mg)	Carbohydrate (g)	Fiber (g)	Sugar (g)	Protein (g)	Vitamin D (mcg)	Calcium (mg)	Iron (mg)	Potassium (mg)
Enchilada sauce													
green	2 T	13	1	0.0	140	2	0	1	0	0	3	0	124
red	2 T	10	0	0.0	145	2	0	1	0	0	3	0	49
Fish sauce	1 T	6	0	0.0	1413	1	0	1	1	0	8	0	52
Hoisin sauce	1 T	35	1	0.0	258	7	0	4	1	0	5	0	19
Hollandaise sauce	2 T	161	17	10.5	124	0	0	0	2	0	15	0	16
Horseradish	1 T	7	0	0.0	63	2	1	1	0	0	8	0	37
sauce	1 T	75	6	0.0	105	3	0	0	0	0	2	0	7
Ketchup/catsup	1 T	20	0	0.0	160	5	0	4	0	0	3	0	48
Liquid smoke	1 tsp	0	0	0.0	10	0	0	0	0	0	0	0	0
Lobster sauce	1 T	24	2	0.5	131	1	0	0	1	0	3	0	23
Manwich sauce	¼ cup	35	0	0.0	310	8	1	6	0	0	0	0	150
Mole poblano	2 T	47	3	0.5	113	4	1	2	1	0	11	0	75
Mustard													
brown/yellow	1 tsp	0	0	0.0	55	0	0	0	0	0	3	0	8
Dijon	1 tsp	5	0	0.0	120	0	0	0	0	0	3	0	8
honey	1 tsp	10	0	0.0	45	1	0	1	0	0	6	0	15
Olives													
black	5	24	2	0.5	169	1	1	0	0	0	21	1	2
green w/ pimiento	5	25	2	0.5	265	1	1	0	0	0	9	0	7
Oyster sauce	1 T	9	0	0.0	492	2	0	0	0	0	6	0	10
Pasta sauce, red													
arrabbiata, Rao's	½ cup	100	7	1.0	420	6	1	4	2	0	20	0	370
chunky garden combination, Ragú	½ cup	90	3	0.0	470	14	2	10	2	0	26	1	430
four cheese, Classico	½ cup	60	1	0.0	500	10	2	6	2	0	40	1	350
fra diavolo	½ cup	80	4	2.0	460	9	3	6	1	0	20	2	280
marinara													
homemade	½ cup	90	6	1.0	520	5	1	3	1	0	20	1	350
Newman's Own	½ cup	80	2	0.0	490	12	3	7	3	0	26	1	705
Old World Style meat flavored, Ragú	½ cup	90	4	1.0	480	12	2	7	2	0	22	1	428
primavera, Botticelli	½ cup	90	5	2.0	320	9	3	6	2	0	25	0	250
Sockarooni, Newman's Own	½ cup	70	2	0.0	500	12	3	6	3	0	26	1	705
tomato & basil, Barilla	½ cup	50	1	0.0	460	10	3	5	2	0	78	1	435
traditional													
Barilla	½ cup	50	1	0.0	450	10	3	5	2	0	52	1	428
Old World Style, Ragú	½ cup	60	1	0.0	480	11	3	8	2	0	30	1	600
Prego	½ cup	70	1	0.0	470	12	3	9	2	0	30	1	330
vodka, Classico	½ cup	80	4	1.5	460	9	2	5	2	0	60	1	280
Peanut sauce	2 T	72	5	1.0	374	6	1	5	2	0	6	0	66
Pesto sauce	2 T	171	18	3.0	304	2	0	0	3	0	61	1	60

CONDIMENTS, SAUCES & BAKING INGREDIENTS

Condiments & Sauces

	Amount	Calories	Fat (g)	Saturated Fat (g)	Sodium (mg)	Carbohydrate (g)	Fiber (g)	Sugar (g)	Protein (g)	Vitamin D (mcg)	Calcium (mg)	Iron (mg)	Potassium (mg)
Pickles													
bread & butter	3 chips	10	0	0.0	170	2	0	2	0	0	14	0	23
dill	1 medium	8	0	0.0	526	2	1	1	0	0	37	0	76
sweet	1 medium	23	0	0.0	114	5	0	5	0	0	15	0	25
Pico de gallo	2 T	10	0	0.0	150	3	0	2	0	0	7	0	94
Pizza sauce	¼ cup	50	0	0.0	360	10	1	8	2	0	0	1	223
Plum sauce	2 T	70	0	0.0	205	16	0	15	0	0	5	1	98
Relish, sweet pickle	1 T	20	0	0.0	95	5	0	3	0	0	0	0	4
Salsa	2 T	10	0	0.0	220	2	1	1	0	0	9	0	82
Salt	1 tsp	0	0	0.0	2325	0	0	0	0	0	1	0	0
substitute	¼ tsp	0	0	0.0	0	0	0	0	0	0	0	0	690
Sauerkraut, can	2 T	5	0	0.0	180	1	1	0	0	0	9	0	50
Soy sauce	1 T	10	0	0.0	1250	2	0	1	1	0	0	0	65
light	1 T	20	0	0.0	550	40	0	2	1	0	0	0	000
substitute, liquid aminos	1 tsp	5	0	0.0	310	0	0	0	1	0	0	0	0
Steak sauce													
A.1.	1 tsp	15	0	0.0	290	3	0	2	0	0	0	0	0
Heinz 57	1 T	20	0	0.0	160	4	0	3	0	0	0	0	0
Stir-fry sauce	1 T	20	0	0.0	520	4	0	3	1	0	6	0	54
Sweet & sour sauce	2 T	60	0	0.0	130	13	0	12	0	0	0	0	31
Szechuan sauce	1 T	30	1	0.0	610	6	0	3	1	0	0	0	30
Tabasco sauce	1 tsp	0	0	0.0	35	0	0	0	0	0	0	0	7
Taco sauce	1 T	8	0	0.0	130	2	0	1	0	0	2	0	18
Tamari sauce	1 T	11	0	0.0	1005	1	0	0	2	0	4	0	38
Tartar sauce	1 T	60	6	1.0	110	2	0	1	0	0	26	0	68
Teriyaki sauce	1 T	16	0	0.0	690	3	0	3	1	0	5	0	41
Tomato sauce, can	½ cup	29	0	0.0	581	7	2	4	2	0	17	1	364
Vinegar													
balsamic	1 T	14	0	0.0	4	3	0	2	0	0	4	0	18
cider/white	1 T	3	0	0.0	1	0	0	0	0	0	1	0	11
raspberry/red wine	1 T	3	0	0.0	1	0	0	0	0	0	1	0	6
Worcestershire sauce	1 tsp	0	0	0.0	60	0	0	0	0	0	6	0	43

Baking Ingredients

	Amount	Calories	Fat (g)	Saturated Fat (g)	Sodium (mg)	Carbohydrate (g)	Fiber (g)	Sugar (g)	Protein (g)	Vitamin D (mcg)	Calcium (mg)	Iron (mg)	Potassium (mg)
Agave nectar													
amber	1 T	60	0	0.0	0	16	0	16	0	0	0	0	0
light	1 T	60	0	0.0	0	16	0	16	0	0	0	0	0
Baking powder	¼ tsp	0	0	0.0	120	0	0	0	0	0	40	0	0
Baking soda	¼ tsp	0	0	0.0	315	0	0	0	0	0	0	0	0
Bisquick, dry	⅓ cup	140	2	0.5	380	30	0	2	3	0	80	2	0
gluten-free	¼ cup	150	0	0.0	390	33	0	3	3	0	70	0	0
Bread crumbs	¼ cup	100	1	0.0	150	18	2	2	4	0	50	1	56
seasoned	¼ cup	100	1	0.0	400	18	2	2	4	0	60	1	0

CONDIMENTS, SAUCES & BAKING INGREDIENTS

Baking Ingredients	Amount	Calories	Fat (g)	Saturated Fat (g)	Sodium (mg)	Carbohydrate (g)	Fiber (g)	Sugar (g)	Protein (g)	Vitamin D (mcg)	Calcium (mg)	Iron (mg)	Potassium (mg)
Butterscotch chips	1 T	80	4	3.5	10	9	0	9	0	0	20	0	30
Carob chips, unsweetened	1 T	35	2	1.5	25	4	1	3	1	0	40	0	44
Chocolate, baking													
semisweet	1 oz	70	5	3.0	0	8	1	6	0	0	5	1	61
unsweetened	1 oz	70	7	4.5	0	4	3	0	2	0	0	3	150
Chocolate chips													
milk chocolate	1 T	70	5	3.0	10	9	0	8	1	0	20	1	60
semisweet	1 T	70	4	2.5	10	10	0	9	0	0	0	1	40
Cocoa powder	1 T	10	1	0.0	0	3	2	0	1	0	10	1	220
Corn flake crumbs	¼ cup	80	0	0.0	160	19	0	2	2	1	0	6	40
Cornstarch	1 T	30	0	0.0	0	7	0	0	0	0	0	0	0
Corn syrup, dark/light	1 T	60	0	0.0	15	15	0	5	0	0	3	0	0
Cornmeal	2 T	55	1	0.0	5	12	1	0	1	0	0	1	44
Flour													
all-purpose/white	¼ cup	110	0	0.0	0	23	0	0	3	0	0	1	34
bread	¼ cup	110	0	0.0	0	23	0	0	4	0	0	1	34
buckwheat	¼ cup	140	1	0.0	0	29	9	0	4	0	21	1	184
cake	¼ cup	120	0	0.0	0	25	1	0	4	0	0	1	36
carob	¼ cup	57	0	0.0	9	23	10	13	1	0	90	1	213
coconut	¼ cup	120	2	1.0	10	9	5	3	3	0	3	1	309
corn	¼ cup	106	1	0.0	1	22	2	0	2	0	2	1	92
potato	¼ cup	143	0	0.0	22	33	2	1	3	0	26	1	400
rice, white	¼ cup	145	1	0.0	0	32	1	0	2	0	4	0	30
rye, medium	¼ cup	89	0	0.0	1	19	3	0	3	0	6	1	95
soy	¼ cup	130	5	1.0	0	10	4	2	12	0	59	2	579
fat-free	¼ cup	86	0	0.0	5	9	5	4	14	0	63	2	626
white, self-rising	¼ cup	110	0	0.0	390	23	1	0	3	0	80	1	88
whole wheat	¼ cup	102	1	0.0	1	22	3	0	4	0	10	1	109
Graham cracker crumbs	3 T	80	2	0.0	125	14	1	3	1	0	0	1	23
Honey	1 T	64	0	0.0	1	17	0	17	0	0	1	0	11
Matzo meal, unsalted	¼ cup	110	0	0.0	0	23	1	1	3	0	0	1	62
Molasses	1 T	58	0	0.0	7	15	0	15	0	0	41	1	293
Phyllo dough	3 sheets	170	3	1.0	275	30	1	0	4	0	6	2	42
Pie crusts													
graham	⅛ pie	100	5	3.0	115	14	0	6	1	0	5	0	10
chocolate	⅛ pie	100	5	3.0	105	14	0	6	1	0	5	1	20
reduced fat	⅛ pie	100	4	2.5	100	15	0	6	1	0	5	1	10
pastry, homemade	⅛ pie	113	7	2.0	116	10	1	0	1	2	0	1	14
Pie fillings, canned													
apple	⅓ cup	100	0	0.0	5	27	1	23	0	0	0	0	27
blueberry	⅓ cup	80	0	0.0	0	21	0	16	0	0	0	0	99
cherry	⅓ cup	90	0	0.0	20	22	1	18	0	0	0	0	78
lemon	⅓ cup	120	2	0.0	2	27	0	20	0	0	0	0	65
pumpkin	½ cup	140	1	0.0	5	10	3	5	1	0	39	1	187

CONDIMENTS, SAUCES & BAKING INGREDIENTS

Baking Ingredients	Amount	Calories	Fat (g)	Saturated Fat (g)	Sodium (mg)	Carbohydrate (g)	Fiber (g)	Sugar (g)	Protein (g)	Vitamin D (mcg)	Calcium (mg)	Iron (mg)	Potassium (mg)
Shake 'n Bake, box	⅛ pkt	30	0	0.0	180	6	0	0	0	0	0	0	0
Sugar													
brown/raw/white	¼ cup	195	0	0.0	1	50	0	50	0	0	1	0	1
powdered	¼ cup	120	0	0.0	0	30	0	29	0	0	0	0	0
Sweeteners, artificial													
Equal	1 pkt	0	0	0.0	0	0	0	0	0	0	0	0	0
Purecane sweetener	1 tsp	0	0	0.0	0	4	0	0	0	0	0	0	0
Splenda	1 pkt	0	0	0.0	0	0	0	0	0	0	0	0	0
Stevia	1 tsp	0	0	0.0	0	1	0	0	0	0	0	0	0
Sugar Twin, brown/white	1 tsp	0	0	0.0	0	0	0	0	0	0	0	0	0
Sweet 'N Low	1 pkt	0	0	0.0	0	0	0	0	0	0	0	0	0
Swerve													
brown/granular	1 tsp	0	0	0.0	0	4	0	0	0	0	0	0	0
confectioners'	1 tsp	0	0	0.0	0	3	0	0	0	0	0	0	0
Truvia	1 pkt	0	0	0.0	0	2	0	0	0	0	0	0	0
Yeast	1 pkt	0	0	0.0	0	1	0	0	0	0	0	0	14

CRACKERS, DIPS & SNACKS

Crackers	Amount	Calories	Fat (g)	Saturated Fat (g)	Sodium (mg)	Carbohydrate (g)	Fiber (g)	Sugar (g)	Protein (g)	Vitamin D (mcg)	Calcium (mg)	Iron (mg)	Potassium (mg)
Ak-mak	5	110	2	0.0	220	19	3	1	5	0	9	1	102
Animal	16	120	2	0.0	105	25	0	7	2	0	10	1	28
Better Cheddars	18	150	8	1.0	240	17	0	0	3	0	30	1	40
Cheese & peanut butter	3	190	9	1.5	310	24	1	4	4	0	20	1	70
Cheez-It	27	150	8	1.5	230	17	0	0	3	0	30	1	30
reduced fat	27	140	6	1.5	250	19	0	0	3	0	30	1	30
white cheddar	27	150	8	1.5	230	17	0	0	3	0	30	1	30
Chicken in a Biskit	12	160	8	1.0	230	19	0	2	2	0	0	1	20
Club	4	70	3	0.0	125	9	0	1	0	0	0	0	10
mini	34	140	6	0.5	300	20	0	3	2	0	10	1	30
multi-grain	4	60	3	0.0	140	10	0	2	0	0	0	0	10
reduced fat	5	70	2	0.0	150	12	0	2	1	0	0	1	10
Goldfish	55	140	6	0.5	230	20	0	0	3	0	20	1	30
grahams s'mores	52	140	5	1.0	125	23	1	10	2	0	10	1	80
parmesan	60	140	5	1.0	260	20	0	0	3	0	32	1	40
pizza	55	140	5	0.5	230	20	0	0	3	0	20	1	80
pretzel	43	130	3	0.0	280	24	0	1	3	0	10	1	20
Graham	2 sheets	130	3	0.0	160	24	1	8	2	0	13	1	48
reduced fat	2 sheets	140	2	0.0	170	28	2	8	2	0	17	1	62
Matzos, lightly salted	1 sheet	110	1	0.0	100	23	1	0	3	0	5	0	38
Oyster	22	60	2	0.0	160	11	0	0	1	0	2	1	16
Popchips, sea salt	1 bag	100	4	0.0	150	16	0	0	1	0	10	0	330
Ritz	5	80	5	1.0	130	10	0	1	1	0	20	1	10
peanut butter sandwiches	1 pack	200	11	2.0	310	22	0	4	4	0	40	1	80
roasted vegetable	5	80	4	1.0	150	10	0	1	1	0	20	1	30
whole wheat	5	70	3	0.5	120	10	0	2	1	0	20	1	30

CRACKERS, DIPS & SNACKS

Crackers	Amount	Calories	Fat (g)	Saturated Fat (g)	Sodium (mg)	Carbohydrate (g)	Fiber (g)	Sugar (g)	Protein (g)	Vitamin D (mcg)	Calcium (mg)	Iron (mg)	Potassium (mg)
Saltines	5	70	2	0.0	135	12	0	0	1	0	3	1	19
whole grain	5	70	2	0.0	125	12	1	0	1	0	30	1	50
Sociables	5	70	3	0.0	140	9	0	0	0	0	20	1	20
Table Water	4	50	1	0.0	80	10	0	0	1	0	31	1	29
Teddy Grahams													
chocolate	24	130	4	0.0	70	22	2	7	2	0	130	1	80
cinnamon	24	130	4	0.0	85	22	2	7	2	0	130	1	50
honey	24	130	4	0.0	90	22	1	7	2	0	130	1	50
Toasteds													
buttercrisp	5	80	4	0.5	180	10	0	1	0	0	0	1	10
harvest wheat	5	80	4	0.0	150	10	0	1	1	0	0	1	20
Town House	5	80	5	1.0	150	9	0	1	0	0	0	0	10
dipping thins, sea salt	7	80	4	0.0	160	11	0	1	0	0	20	0	20
flatbread crisps, Italian herb	8	70	2	0.0	120	11	0	0	1	0	0	1	20
FlipSides	5	70	4	0.5	190	10	0	1	1	0	0	1	10
pita, sea salt	6	70	3	0.0	140	11	0	0	1	0	0	1	20
Triscuit	6	120	4	0.0	160	20	3	0	3	0	10	1	120
reduced fat	6	110	3	0.0	150	21	4	0	3	0	10	2	120
Wasa													
Crisp'n Light 7 Grain	3	60	1	0.0	90	13	2	1	2	0	5	0	58
light rye	2	40	0	0.0	70	11	4	0	2	0	9	1	87
sourdough	1	30	0	0.0	50	7	2	0	1	0	4	0	50
whole grain	1	30	0	0.0	50	8	3	0	1	0	7	0	59
Wheat Thins	16	140	5	0.0	200	22	3	5	2	0	30	1	90
hint of salt low sodium	16	140	5	0.5	55	22	3	4	2	0	9	1	90
reduced fat	16	120	4	0.0	200	22	3	4	2	0	30	1	90
sundried tomato & basil	15	140	5	0.5	160	21	2	4	2	0	31	1	99
Dips													
Fritos bean	2 T	35	1	0.0	190	5	2	0	2	0	0	0	94
Good & Gather													
Buffalo-style chicken	2 T	60	5	2.0	250	1	0	1	3	0	26	0	0
classic onion	2 T	70	7	4.5	170	2	0	1	1	0	26	0	0
spinach artichoke	2 T	60	5	2.5	160	2	0	1	1	0	26	0	0
Hidden Valley ranch	2 T	100	11	1.5	270	2	0	1	0	0	9	0	15
Lay's French onion	2 T	60	5	0.5	190	2	0	0	0	0	0	0	0
Marzetti													
classic caramel	2 T	140	5	2.0	75	24	0	19	0	0	0	0	50
cream cheese fruit	2 T	60	3	2.0	95	9	0	8	0	0	0	0	0
Sabra classic hummus	2 T	70	5	1.0	130	4	1	0	2	0	0	1	94
Tostitos salsa con queso	2 T	40	3	1.0	280	5	1	1	1	0	26	0	0
Nutrition Bars													
ALOHA													
chocolate chip cookie dough	1 bar	240	11	2.5	105	25	10	5	14	0	36	6	111
coconut chocolate almond	1 bar	260	13	7.0	70	22	6	4	14	0	32	2	186
peanut butter chocolate chip	1 bar	240	12	3.0	90	24	10	5	14	0	16	1	173

CRACKERS, DIPS & SNACKS

Nutrition Bars

	Amount	Calories	Fat (g)	Saturated Fat (g)	Sodium (mg)	Carbohydrate (g)	Fiber (g)	Sugar (g)	Protein (g)	Vitamin D (mcg)	Calcium (mg)	Iron (mg)	Potassium (mg)
Atlas													
almond chocolate chip	1 bar	210	10	3.5	200	18	10	1	20	1	104	1	115
peanut butter chocolate chip	1 bar	210	9	3.5	200	19	10	1	20	1	139	1	135
vanilla almond	1 bar	210	10	3.0	200	18	10	1	20	1	171	1	125
Barebells													
caramel cashew	1 bar	200	8	3.0	80	18	3	1	20	0	160	1	150
cookies & cream	1 bar	200	7	3.0	75	20	3	1	20	0	140	1	130
salty peanut	1 bar	200	8	3.0	105	18	3	1	20	0	160	1	140
BUILT													
cookies 'n cream	1 bar	130	3	2.0	75	19	6	4	17	0	108	1	213
peanut butter brownie	1 bar	180	6	2.0	100	20	6	4	19	0	101	2	247
raspberry	1 bar	130	3	1.5	70	19	5	4	17	0	97	1	215
Bulletproof collagen protein													
chocolate chip cookie dough	1 bar	190	12	6.0	85	12	8	2	11	0	22	2	110
fudge brownie	1 bar	180	11	5.0	85	13	8	2	11	0	22	2	123
vanilla shortbread	1 bar	190	12	5.0	90	12	8	2	11	0	21	1	140
CLIF													
Bars													
chocolate brownie	1 bar	250	6	1.5	180	43	5	17	10	0	46	2	268
chocolate chip	1 bar	250	6	2.0	130	43	5	17	10	0	45	2	258
crunchy peanut butter	1 bar	260	8	1.0	230	40	5	17	11	0	39	2	253
white chocolate macadamia nut	1 bar	260	7	1.5	230	42	5	17	9	0	44	2	228
Builders protein													
chocolate mint	1 bar	280	9	6.0	200	31	3	17	20	0	42	4	234
crunchy peanut butter	1 bar	300	11	6.0	330	29	2	16	20	0	40	3	198
vanilla almond	1 bar	290	11	6.0	200	29	2	16	20	0	46	3	212
FITCRUNCH													
chocolate peanut butter	1 bar	190	8	4.0	200	14	1	3	16	0	40	1	140
milk & cookies	1 bar	210	11	8.0	135	15	1	3	16	0	70	1	100
peanut butter & jelly	1 bar	190	8	4.0	200	14	1	3	16	0	39	1	135
GoMacro MacroBars													
coconut + almond butter + chocolate chips	1 bar	280	10	3.5	15	36	3	12	11	0	26	1	188
oatmeal chocolate chip	1 bar	270	9	2.0	60	35	3	13	12	0	26	2	188
peanut butter chocolate chip	1 bar	290	11	2.0	10	39	2	14	11	0	26	1	188
KIND													
energy bars													
chocolate chunk	1 bar	230	7	2.0	160	34	5	13	10	0	52	2	188
peanut butter	1 bar	250	10	1.5	190	32	5	13	10	0	52	2	188
nut bars													
caramel almond & sea salt	1 bar	170	15	3.0	125	16	7	5	6	0	72	1	188
cranberry almond	1 bar	160	12	1.0	20	19	5	8	5	0	72	1	188
dark chocolate cherry cashew	1 bar	170	10	3.0	20	22	6	10	4	0	24	1	188
dark chocolate nuts & sea salt	1 bar	180	15	3.0	140	16	7	5	6	0	48	2	188
peanut butter dark chocolate	1 bar	200	14	4.0	20	17	3	9	7	0	24	1	188

CRACKERS, DIPS & SNACKS

Nutrition Bars

	Amount	Calories	Fat (g)	Saturated Fat (g)	Sodium (mg)	Carbohydrate (g)	Fiber (g)	Sugar (g)	Protein (g)	Vitamin D (mcg)	Calcium (mg)	Iron (mg)	Potassium (mg)
protein bars													
crunchy peanut butter	1 bar	250	18	4.0	135	17	6	8	12	0	26	1	188
dark chocolate nut	1 bar	240	17	4.0	125	18	5	8	12	0	52	2	282
Kirkland													
chocolate brownie	1 bar	190	7	2.5	140	22	10	2	21	0	107	1	96
chocolate chip cookie dough	1 bar	190	7	2.5	190	22	10	2	21	0	108	1	117
No Cow													
birthday cake	1 bar	190	5	2.0	150	27	16	1	20	0	27	3	17
chocolate chip cookie dough	1 bar	200	5	2.0	210	26	15	1	20	0	30	4	40
maple	1 bar	200	5	2.0	200	25	14	1	22	0	46	3	25
ONE													
almond bliss	1 bar	240	9	7.0	115	22	3	1	20	0	147	1	122
birthday cake	1 bar	220	8	6.0	140	23	3	1	20	0	110	0	83
maple glazed doughnut	1 bar	230	8	6.0	150	23	3	1	20	0	102	0	80
peanut butter pie	1 bar	220	9	5.0	140	23	8	1	20	0	88	1	124
Pure Protein													
birthday cake	1 bar	200	5	3.5	150	18	0	3	20	0	160	1	80
chewy chocolate chip	1 bar	200	5	3.5	110	18	2	3	20	0	150	1	90
lemon cake	1 bar	200	7	4.0	130	16	0	2	20	0	190	0	110
PaleoPro Primal													
cherry cashew	1 bar	260	14	3.5	200	26	12	6	15	0	20	2	200
coconut cacao	1 bar	270	17	5.0	190	23	15	4	15	0	70	2	110
Perfect Bar													
dark chocolate chip peanut butter	1 bar	330	20	4.0	105	24	4	18	15	0	110	1	400
peanut butter	1 bar	340	19	3.0	50	27	3	19	17	0	140	1	450
pumpkin pie	1 bar	310	19	3.0	35	24	3	16	14	0	110	1	460
salted caramel	1 bar	310	19	3.5	130	25	2	17	12	0	130	2	370
Power Crunch													
French vanilla crème	1 bar	220	13	7.0	125	11	0	5	14	0	60	1	120
lemon meringue	1 bar	220	14	7.0	125	11	0	7	13	0	60	0	100
PRO													
birthday cake	1 bar	340	23	11.0	170	12	0	7	20	0	100	0	100
peanut butter fudge	1 bar	300	21	10.0	220	15	2	4	20	0	80	1	220
Quest													
birthday cake	1 bar	180	7	4.0	250	25	12	0	20	0	160	0	90
blueberry muffin	1 bar	180	7	2.0	220	23	13	2	20	0	160	0	90
caramel chocolate chunk	1 bar	180	6	2.0	300	25	15	1	20	0	150	1	110
RXBAR													
banana chocolate walnut	1 bar	210	9	2.0	130	25	3	17	12	0	40	2	430
blueberry	1 bar	210	7	1.0	140	24	4	15	12	0	60	1	460
chocolate sea salt	1 bar	210	9	2.0	260	23	5	13	12	0	60	2	480
mixed berry	1 bar	210	7	1.0	140	24	5	15	12	0	60	1	480
peanut butter	1 bar	200	7	1.0	310	25	5	15	12	0	40	1	480

CRACKERS, DIPS & SNACKS

Nutrition Bars	Amount	Calories	Fat (g)	Saturated Fat (g)	Sodium (mg)	Carbohydrate (g)	Fiber (g)	Sugar (g)	Protein (g)	Vitamin D (mcg)	Calcium (mg)	Iron (mg)	Potassium (mg)
think!													
high protein brownie crunch	1 bar	230	8	3.0	190	23	1	0	20	0	120	2	170
keto protein chocolate peanut butter pie	1 bar	180	14	4.5	95	14	3	2	10	0	70	1	180
vegan high protein peanut butter chocolate chip	1 bar	190	6	3.0	160	23	2	5	13	0	50	2	150
Snacks													
Bugles	1⅓ cups	150	8	6.0	320	18	0	2	1	0	0	0	0
Cheetos													
crunchy	21	160	10	1.5	250	15	0	0	2	0	10	0	50
puffs	13	160	10	1.5	270	16	0	1	2	0	20	0	60
Cheez Doodles													
baked puffs	23	150	8	2.0	320	17	0	2	2	0	195	0	0
extra crunchy	23	150	9	2.5	230	17	0	1	1	0	195	0	0
Cheez-It snack mix	½ cup	130	5	1.0	300	20	0	3	3	0	10	1	30
Chex Mix	½ cup	120	4	0.5	260	22	1	2	2	0	0	1	0
Combos, cheddar	9 pcs	140	7	3.0	310	18	0	4	2	0	0	1	100
pretzel	9 pcs	130	5	3.0	300	19	0	4	2	0	30	1	130
Cracker Jack	1 cup	120	2	0.0	70	23	1	15	2	0	0	0	0
Doritos nacho chips													
cool ranch	12	150	8	1.0	190	18	1	0	2	0	30	0	50
nacho cheese	12	150	8	1.0	210	18	1	1	2	0	40	0	50
spicy sweet chili	12	140	7	1.0	270	18	1	1	2	0	26	0	50
Fritos corn chips	32	160	10	1.5	170	16	1	0	2	0	30	0	30
Funyuns	13	140	6	1.0	280	19	0	0	2	0	10	1	40
Good Sense sesame oat bran sticks	⅓ cup	170	12	1.5	340	13	1	0	3	0	64	2	56
Jax	20	150	10	2.5	290	14	0	2	2	0	30	0	20
Mission chicharrones pork rinds	0.5 oz	80	5	2.0	270	0	0	0	9	0	0	0	0
Popcorn													
Angie's BOOMCHICKAPOP													
cheddar cheese	2⅔ cups	160	10	1.5	310	14	2	3	3	0	60	0	100
real butter	3½ cups	160	11	4.0	190	15	0	3	2	0	0	0	0
sweet & salty kettle corn	2 cups	140	8	0.5	110	18	2	8	1	0	0	1	0
Jiffy Pop	4 cups	140	7	3.5	220	20	3	0	3	0	0	0	0
oil popped, salted	3 cups	165	9	1.5	292	19	3	0	3	0	30	1	74
Old Dutch	3 cups	180	12	1.0	150	14	4	0	2	0	0	0	48
Orville Redenbacher's													
kettle corn	4½ cups	160	8	4.0	160	20	3	0	3	0	0	1	0
SmartPop!, butter	3 cups	120	2	0.5	340	26	4	0	4	0	0	1	0
Pop Secret, butter	3 cups	130	8	4.0	270	12	2	0	2	0	0	0	50
Skinny Pop	3¾ cups	150	10	1.0	75	15	3	0	2	0	0	0	40

Snacks	Amount	Calories	Fat (g)	Saturated Fat (g)	Sodium (mg)	Carbohydrate (g)	Fiber (g)	Sugar (g)	Protein (g)	Vitamin D (mcg)	Calcium (mcg)	Iron (mg)	Potassium (mg)
Skinny Pop popcorn mini cakes													
cinnamon & sugar	20	120	3	0.0	60	20	4	3	3	0	10	1	40
sea salt	22	120	4	0.0	170	18	4	0	3	0	0	1	50
sharp cheddar	20	120	4	0.0	135	18	4	0	3	0	0	1	50
Smartfood													
caramel & cheddar	1½ cups	140	8	3.0	150	27	1	6	1	0	10	0	0
sweet & salty kettle corn	1½ cups	140	6	0.5	110	20	2	12	1	0	0	0	0
white cheddar	2½ cups	160	10	2.0	240	13	2	2	4	0	60	1	60
Potato chips													
Lay's	15	160	10	1.5	170	15	0	0	2	0	10	1	350
BBQ	15	150	9	1.5	150	16	1	2	2	0	10	1	330
Old Dutch, sour cream & onion	15	160	10	1.0	160	15	1	1	2	0	26	0	350
Pringles	15	150	9	2.5	150	16	0	0	1	0	0	0	110
BBQ	14	150	9	2.5	135	16	0	1	1	0	0	0	110
cheddar cheese	14	150	9	2.5	180	16	0	0	1	0	10	0	110
sour cream & onion	14	150	9	2.5	160	16	0	0	1	0	0	0	110
Ruffles, baked	12	120	3	0.0	135	22	1	2	2	0	10	0	230
Pretzels													
Dot's Homestyle original seasoned	1 oz	130	6	0.0	360	18	0	0	2	0	10	0	52
Snack Factory crisps	11	110	0	0.0	270	24	0	2	2	0	0	1	0
Snyder's													
butter snaps	24	120	1	0.0	270	25	0	0	3	0	0	1	0
mini	20	110	0	0.0	250	25	0	0	3	0	0	1	0
rods	3	120	1	0.0	290	24	0	0	3	0	0	1	0
sourdough, hard	1 oz	110	0	0.0	90	23	0	0	3	0	0	1	0
Quaker rice cakes													
caramel corn	1	50	0	0.0	25	11	0	3	0	0	0	0	20
chocolate	1	60	1	0.0	35	12	0	4	1	0	0	0	40
lightly salted	1	35	0	0.0	15	7	0	0	0	0	0	0	30
Stacy's Everything Bagel Chips	12	130	4	0.0	330	19	0	2	4	0	10	1	10
Sunchips	16	140	6	0.5	110	19	2	2	2	0	10	1	70
Tostitos tortilla chips	7	140	7	1.0	115	19	1	0	2	0	30	0	40
bite size	22	150	7	1.0	115	18	1	0	2	0	20	0	40
crispy rounds	13	150	7	1.0	115	18	1	0	2	0	20	0	40
hint of lime	6	150	7	1.0	125	18	1	0	2	0	30	0	40
Scoops!	11	140	7	1.0	115	19	1	0	2	0	30	0	40
simply organic blue corn	6	140	6	0.5	80	19	1	0	2	0	30	0	40
Veggie Straws, sea salt	38	130	7	0.5	220	17	0	0	0	0	80	1	210

DESSERTS, SWEETS & TOPPINGS

Bars

Bars	Amount	Calories	Fat (g)	Saturated Fat (g)	Sodium (mg)	Carbohydrate (g)	Fiber (g)	Sugar (g)	Protein (g)	Vitamin D (mcg)	Calcium (mg)	Iron (mg)	Potassium (mg)
Brownies													
fudge, iced	1 (2 in)	180	6	2.5	120	32	1	22	2	0	7	1	113
w/ nuts	1 (2 in)	210	12	5.0	70	27	2	19	4	0	0	3	200
w/o nuts	1 (2 in)	175	8	3.0	63	28	3	18	2	0	0	3	215
Lemon	1 (2 in)	180	7	4.0	60	27	0	20	2	0	30	0	30
Nutty Buddy	2 cookies	310	18	8.0	110	32	1	20	4	0	10	1	110
Rice Krispies Treats													
homemade	1 (2 in)	70	2	1.0	53	14	0	7	1	0	2	4	20
packaged	1	90	2	0.5	105	17	0	8	0	0	0	1	0
strawberry	1	90	2	0.5	105	17	0	8	0	0	0	1	0
Seven layer	1 (2 in)	257	15	8.0	103	21	1	17	2	0	10	1	84

Cakes, Pastries & Sweet Breads

Cakes, Pastries & Sweet Breads	Amount	Calories	Fat (g)	Saturated Fat (g)	Sodium (mg)	Carbohydrate (g)	Fiber (g)	Sugar (g)	Protein (g)	Vitamin D (mcg)	Calcium (mg)	Iron (mg)	Potassium (mg)
Angel food cake	1/14 cake	159	0	0.0	72	34	0	26	6	0	5	1	152
Apple dumplings	1 (6 oz)	504	24	5.5	354	72	6	40	4	0	17	2	189
Apple fritters	1 (3 oz)	248	9	3.0	243	40	2	23	3	0	62	1	110
Baklava	1 (2 in)	213	15	5.5	48	21	1	15	2	0	14	1	54
Banana bread	1/12 loaf	172	1	0.5	170	37	2	18	4	0	23	1	175
Black forest cake	1/10 cake	447	14	3.0	441	78	3	41	6	0	73	2	247
Caramel rolls	1/12 recipe	251	12	6.0	178	34	1	14	4	0	30	1	72
Carrot cake, iced	1/12 cake	569	36	7.0	470	59	3	40	6	0	60	2	470
Cheesecake													
amaretto	1/12 cake	417	26	15.5	314	37	0	29	7	0	86	1	314
chocolate	1/12 cake	527	37	21.5	343	43	2	32	10	0	74	3	140
regular, New York–style	1/12 cake	556	37	22.0	408	47	1	33	11	0	114	2	194
Chocolate cake, iced	1/12 cake	528	19	7.0	491	84	2	64	6	0	76	2	77
Cinnamon rolls	1/12 recipe	376	19	12.0	437	46	1	21	6	0	52	2	105
Cobbler, fruit	1/4 recipe	384	13	8.0	371	65	1	47	4	0	136	1	119
Coffee cake													
apple crumble	1/8 recipe	631	34	13.0	435	76	3	34	10	0	122	3	254
regular w/ crumb topping	1/24 recipe	255	14	2.0	220	31	1	22	3	0	60	1	79
Cream puffs	1/8 recipe	257	16	7.5	91	26	1	14	4	0	18	1	44
Crepes	1/8 recipe	163	8	3.5	235	17	0	5	6	0	66	1	115
Cupcakes, iced													
chocolate	1	220	10	2.5	180	32	2	19	3	0	14	1	76
chocolate filled	1	284	16	3.0	193	35	1	24	3	0	33	1	59
vanilla lemon filled	1	379	19	9.0	237	50	0	43	3	0	37	1	48
Danish													
cheese	1/10 recipe	498	29	14.0	582	51	0	32	8	0	40	2	60
kringle	1/18 recipe	411	30	15.0	157	35	1	23	4	0	46	1	104
Devil Dogs	1 cake	180	7	3.0	135	28	1	17	2	0	10	1	80
Ding Dongs	2 cakes	310	16	11.0	310	43	1	31	2	0	0	2	120
Donuts													
cake	1 medium	200	11	6.0	220	23	0	11	2	0	0	1	30
holes, glazed	4 medium	220	10	5.0	170	31	0	17	2	0	70	1	40
raised, glazed	1 medium	190	11	4.5	90	21	1	10	2	0	78	1	46

DESSERTS, SWEETS & TOPPINGS

Cakes, Pastries & Sweet Breads	Amount	Calories	Fat (g)	Saturated Fat (g)	Sodium (mg)	Carbohydrate (g)	Fiber (g)	Sugar (g)	Protein (g)	Vitamin D (mcg)	Calcium (mg)	Iron (mg)	Potassium (mg)
Eclairs, chocolate	1 (5 in)	210	12	11.0	120	25	0	20	2	0	52	1	33
Funnel cake	1 (6 in)	278	14	2.5	117	29	1	14	7	1	124	2	148
Funny Bones	2 cakes	340	17	11.0	260	41	2	28	5	0	60	2	220
Gingerbread cake	1/12 cake	359	14	2.0	353	56	4	31	6	0	90	1	374
Ho Hos	3 cakes	380	20	13.0	300	52	1	40	2	0	0	2	120
Honey buns, iced	1 (1.8 oz)	220	12	6.0	170	26	0	14	3	0	90	1	50
Lemon cake, iced	1/12 cake	335	13	8.0	161	53	0	41	3	0	47	1	39
Marble cake	1/12 cake	276	11	2.0	398	41	1	25	4	0	10	0	24
Pecan caramel roll	1/12 recipe	327	13	5.0	293	47	2	18	6	0	72	2	120
Pineapple upside down cake	1/12 cake	506	25	8.0	384	69	2	53	4	0	116	2	207
Pop Tarts													
frosted raspberry	1 pkg	370	9	3.0	320	70	1	30	3	0	0	2	40
unfrosted blueberry	1 pkg	380	10	3.0	360	69	1	24	4	0	0	1	40
Pound cake	1/12 cake	580	26	16.0	172	79	1	55	8	0	65	2	115
Pumpkin bread	1/12 loaf	257	9	2.0	274	42	2	23	4	0	86	2	171
Ring Dings	1 cake	180	9	6.0	140	24	1	16	1	0	10	1	90
Snoballs	1 cake	160	5	3.0	180	29	1	20	1	0	10	1	55
Spice cake, iced	1/16 cake	275	13	8.0	222	36	1	19	4	0	115	1	90
Sponge cake	1/14 cake	148	3	1.0	37	28	0	22	4	0	16	1	53
Strudel w/ fruit	1/6 recipe	501	17	4.0	130	88	4	62	6	0	70	2	406
Toaster Strudel, strawberry	2 pastries	340	12	4.5	320	54	1	19	5	0	0	2	0
Turnovers w/ fruit	1 (3 oz)	380	25	7.0	210	34	1	10	4	0	26	1	70
Twinkies	2 cakes	280	9	4.0	370	47	0	32	2	0	0	1	0
Yankee Doodles	1 cake	140	5	2.5	150	22	1	13	1	0	10	1	90
Yellow cake, iced	1/12 cake	253	10	3.0	285	37	1	22	4	0	99	1	69
Yodels	2 cakes	280	14	9.0	150	36	1	27	2	0	20	2	160
Zingers	2 cakes	290	10	4.5	230	49	0	39	1	0	23	1	41
Cookies													
Animal	7	77	2	0.5	70	13	0	2	1	0	0	0	21
iced	7	150	8	7.0	50	20	0	12	1	0	10	1	20
Arrowroot biscuit	1	20	1	0.0	5	3	0	1	0	0	0	1	5
Biscotti													
almond, mini	2	120	5	2.0	50	16	0	9	2	0	20	1	40
chocolate dipped, mini	2	150	7	3.0	55	21	0	12	3	0	30	1	60
dark chocolate almond	1	170	7	3.0	35	26	1	14	3	0	26	1	40
toffee almond dipped	1	110	5	2.0	80	17	0	10	2	0	20	1	40
Chocolate chip													
Chips Ahoy!	3	160	8	3.0	105	22	0	11	1	0	10	1	50
chewy	2	140	6	3.0	85	21	0	11	1	0	0	1	30
chunky	2	160	8	3.0	75	21	0	11	1	0	10	1	50
thins	4	150	7	2.5	50	21	0	12	1	0	0	1	40
homemade	1	170	9	4.0	150	21	0	11	2	0	6	2	51
Chocolate wafers	5	140	5	0.5	180	23	0	9	2	0	0	2	70

DESSERTS, SWEETS & TOPPINGS

Cookies

	Amount	Calories	Fat (g)	Saturated Fat (g)	Sodium (mg)	Carbohydrate (g)	Fiber (g)	Sugar (g)	Protein (g)	Vitamin D (mcg)	Calcium (mg)	Iron (mg)	Potassium (mg)
E.L. Fudge	2	180	9	3.5	100	24	1	13	2	0	0	2	50
Fig Newtons	2	200	4	1.0	180	41	2	24	2	0	40	1	140
strawberry	2	100	2	0.0	95	21	1	12	0	0	10	0	50
Fudge Stripes	2	140	7	4.0	70	19	0	9	1	0	0	1	60
Ginger snaps	4	120	4	1.5	120	22	0	10	1	0	10	1	30
Girl Scout cookies													
Caramel deLites	2	140	6	5.0	50	19	0	12	0	0	0	1	0
Lemonades	2	150	7	4.5	70	20	0	9	1	0	0	1	0
Peanut Butter Patties	2	130	7	4.0	90	15	0	8	2	0	0	1	0
Peanut Butter Sandwiches	3	170	8	2.5	105	22	1	9	3	0	0	1	0
S'mores	2	150	7	3.5	110	21	1	10	2	0	0	1	50
Thin Mints	4	160	7	5.0	105	22	0	10	1	0	0	2	0
Trefoils	4	120	5	2.0	110	19	0	6	1	0	0	1	0
Ladyfingers	4	110	1	0.0	30	23	0	13	3	0	0	0	0
Lorna Doone shortbread	1 pkg	210	10	3.0	220	29	0	8	2	0	0	1	30
LU Le Pim's milk chocolate biscuits	2	120	6	3.5	65	17	0	10	2	0	20	1	60
Macaroons	2	100	4	1.0	10	13	1	12	2	0	16	0	51
Mallomars	2	120	5	2.5	35	17	0	11	1	0	10	1	50
Milano, dark chocolate	3	180	9	4.0	60	22	1	11	2	0	10	1	70
Iced molasses	3	120	2	0.0	180	25	0	13	1	0	0	1	90
Nutter Butter	2	130	5	1.5	100	20	0	8	2	0	10	1	40
Oatmeal raisin	1	150	5	2.0	80	24	1	13	2	0	11	1	43
Oreo	3	160	7	2.0	135	25	0	14	1	0	10	1	50
Doublestuf	2	140	7	2.0	90	21	0	13	0	0	10	1	40
golden	3	170	7	2.0	120	25	0	12	1	0	0	1	20
thins	1 pkg	140	6	2.0	95	21	0	12	1	0	0	1	40
Peanut butter	2	120	4	1.0	150	20	0	12	2	0	0	0	25
Sandies													
classic shortbread	2	160	9	4.0	95	20	0	7	2	0	0	1	10
pecan shortbread	2	170	10	3.0	110	19	0	7	1	0	0	1	20
Social Tea biscuits	7	140	4	1.0	120	24	0	7	2	0	0	1	20
Sugar	2	160	7	2.5	95	24	0	13	1	0	11	1	26
Sugar wafers	3	150	7	1.5	30	22	0	16	0	0	2	0	8
Vanilla wafers	8	140	6	1.5	115	21	0	11	1	0	0	1	30
Vienna Fingers, creme filled	2	150	6	2.5	95	23	0	11	1	0	0	1	20
Frozen Yogurt													
Chocolate	½ cup	111	3	2.0	55	19	2	17	3	0	87	0	204
Flavored	½ cup	111	3	2.0	55	19	0	17	3	0	87	0	136
fat-free	½ cup	110	0	0.0	60	23	0	15	3	0	150	0	230
Premium	½ cup	136	32	1.0	50	27	0	6	4	0	95	1	136
Soft serve													
chocolate	½ cup	115	4	2.5	71	18	2	16	3	0	106	1	188
vanilla	½ cup	115	4	2.5	63	17	0	17	3	0	103	0	152

DESSERTS, SWEETS & TOPPINGS

Ice Cream

	Amount	Calories	Fat (g)	Saturated Fat (g)	Sodium (mg)	Carbohydrate (g)	Fiber (g)	Sugar (g)	Protein (g)	Vitamin D (mcg)	Calcium (mg)	Iron (mg)	Potassium (mg)
Butter pecan	½ cup	122	7	3.0	112	15	1	14	3	0	88	0	130
Cherry Garcia	½ cup	255	15	10.0	41	27	0	23	4	1	113	2	180
Cookie dough	½ cup	181	9	5.0	73	23	0	16	3	0	69	0	120
Chocolate fudge brownie	½ cup	172	7	4.0	60	25	1	18	3	0	78	1	224
Chocolate/strawberry/vanilla	½ cup	140	7	4.5	50	19	1	17	3	0	72	1	164
fat-free, 98%	½ cup	94	2	1.0	51	21	4	14	3	0	86	1	162
light	½ cup	140	5	3.5	53	19	1	19	4	0	119	1	128
no added sugar	½ cup	130	4	3.0	56	20	1	4	3	0	91	0	147
premium	½ cup	186	13	7.5	42	15	1	13	4	0	105	1	176
Gelato	½ cup	170	10	7.0	50	18	0	17	3	0	99	0	138
Italian ice	½ cup	130	0	0.0	25	32	0	22	0	0	3	0	4
Mint chocolate chip	½ cup	133	5	3.0	46	19	0	17	3	0	109	0	55
Rocky road	½ cup	160	6	3.0	58	24	1	15	3	0	83	1	183
Sherbet	½ cup	107	2	1.0	34	23	1	18	1	0	40	0	71
Sorbet	½ cup	100	0	0.0	0	25	1	24	0	0	3	0	28

Ice Cream Cones

	Amount	Calories	Fat (g)	Saturated Fat (g)	Sodium (mg)	Carbohydrate (g)	Fiber (g)	Sugar (g)	Protein (g)	Vitamin D (mcg)	Calcium (mg)	Iron (mg)	Potassium (mg)
Cake/wafer	1	20	0	0.0	5	4	0	0	0	0	0	0	10
Sugar	1	60	1	0.0	20	13	0	4	1	0	10	1	20
Waffle	1	60	1	0.0	20	12	0	4	0	0	0	1	10

Ice Cream Novelties

	Amount	Calories	Fat (g)	Saturated Fat (g)	Sodium (mg)	Carbohydrate (g)	Fiber (g)	Sugar (g)	Protein (g)	Vitamin D (mcg)	Calcium (mg)	Iron (mg)	Potassium (mg)
Chocolate eclair bar	1 (3 oz)	150	7	3.5	65	21	1	12	2	0	30	0	0
Creamsicle	1 (2.5 oz)	100	2	1.0	30	20	0	12	1	0	50	0	0
Crunch bars	2 (1 oz)	170	11	7.0	50	19	0	13	1	0	40	1	50
Dove													
bar	1 (2.5 oz)	250	16	11.0	40	24	1	22	3	0	100	0	150
minis	1 (0.6 oz)	60	4	2.5	5	6	1	5	0	0	0	0	0
Drumstick crunch	1 (3 oz)	280	15	8.0	90	34	2	21	4	0	40	1	110
Fruit juice bar	1 (2 oz)	45	0	0.0	3	10	0	8	0	0	2	0	22
Fudgesicle	2 (2.8 oz)	80	2	1.0	90	18	4	5	3	0	200	1	0
Ice cream sandwich	1 (2.3 oz)	180	6	3.5	150	29	1	14	3	0	60	1	152
Klondike bar	1 (3 oz)	250	14	11.0	65	29	0	23	3	0	90	0	180
cookies & creme	1 (2.6 oz)	240	13	10.0	110	29	0	19	2	0	70	1	140
Heath	1 (2.6 oz)	220	13	10.0	70	25	0	14	2	0	70	0	140
no sugar added	1 (2.6 oz)	170	9	8.0	65	22	0	5	3	0	100	0	190
M&M's cookie sandwich	1 (3 oz)	230	9	5.0	140	35	0	23	3	0	70	1	130
Nondairy, vanilla													
almond milk	⅔ cup (3.6 oz)	210	10	7.0	85	28	0	21	2	0	10	0	20
cashew milk	⅔ cup (3.6 oz)	190	9	5.0	130	26	0	19	2	0	10	1	90
coconut milk	⅔ cup (3.6 oz)	200	12	11.0	5	23	1	18	0	0	0	0	50
oat milk	⅔ cup (3.6 oz)	220	13	8.0	40	24	1	19	1	0	0	0	0
soy milk	⅔ cup (3.6 oz)	160	4	0.5	10	31	4	16	2	1	10	0	80
Popsicle	1 (1.7 oz)	40	0	0.0	0	10	0	7	0	0	0	0	5
sugar-free	1 (1.7 oz)	15	0	0.0	0	4	0	0	0	0	0	0	3
Push-Up, sherbet	1 (2.5 oz)	70	1	0.0	15	16	0	12	0	0	0	0	15

DESSERTS, SWEETS & TOPPINGS

Ice Cream	Amount	Calories	Fat (g)	Saturated Fat (g)	Sodium (mg)	Carbohydrate (g)	Fiber (g)	Sugar (g)	Protein (g)	Vitamin D (mcg)	Calcium (mg)	Iron (mg)	Potassium (mg)
Snickers bar	1 (1.7 oz)	180	11	6.0	50	18	0	15	3	0	60	0	120
Snow cone	1 (6 oz)	30	0	0.0	5	8	0	5	0	0	0	0	0
Tofutti Cutie, vanilla	1 (1.4 oz)	90	3	1.5	95	17	0	8	1	0	4	0	20
Yasso Greek yogurt bar, chocolate fudge	1 (2.3 oz)	80	0	0.0	55	15	1	12	5	0	110	1	200
Other Sweets													
Caramel apple	1	424	7	2.0	198	95	6	77	4	0	125	0	429
Chocolate mousse	½ cup	247	15	8.0	437	28	0	21	3	0	73	1	271
Custard	½ cup	147	7	3.0	86	16	0	16	7	0	151	1	209
Flan w/ caramel													
homemade	½ cup	222	6	3.0	81	35	0	35	7	0	127	1	181
mix	½ cup	117	2	1.0	129	22	0	22	3	1	129	0	186
Gelatin, prepared	½ cup	81	0	0.0	101	19	0	10	2	0	4	0	1
sugar-free	½ cup	23	0	0.0	56	5	0	0	1	0	4	0	1
Marshmallows	4 large	100	0	0.0	25	24	0	17	0	0	1	0	1
Pudding													
bread, homemade	½ cup	189	4	2.0	95	36	1	28	4	0	104	1	190
chocolate													
instant, sugar-free, w/ skim milk	½ cup	70	0	0.0	173	15	0	6	4	5	150	1	125
instant, w/ 2% milk	½ cup	160	3	1.5	490	31	0	25	5	2	150	1	220
regular, ready-to-eat	1 (4 oz)	153	5	1.5	164	25	0	19	2	0	55	1	199
rice, regular, ready-to-eat	½ cup	122	2	1.5	110	21	0	13	4	0	107	0	141
tapioca, ready-to-eat	½ cup	143	4	1.0	160	24	0	16	2	0	78	0	101
vanilla													
instant, sugar-free, w/ skim milk	½ cup	65	0	0.0	58	18	0	6	4	5	150	0	125
instant, w/ 2% milk	½ cup	229	4	2.0	361	42	0	25	7	0	245	0	311
regular, ready-to-eat	1 (4 oz)	126	4	1.0	138	22	0	17	1	0	48	0	63
Pies*													
Apple/cherry	1 slice	413	19	4.5	327	58	1	27	4	0	11	2	123
Banana cream	1 slice	387	20	5.0	340	47	1	17	6	1	108	2	238
Boston cream	⅙ pie (8 in)	231	8	2.0	234	40	1	33	2	0	21	0	36
Chocolate cream	1 slice	360	13	7.0	302	58	2	45	6	0	127	1	159
Coconut cream	1 slice	259	17	8.0	309	27	1	26	4	0	68	0	133
Grasshopper	1 slice	270	17	7.0	211	28	0	15	2	0	32	1	76
Hostess fruit	4	410	15	8.0	460	64	1	25	3	0	7	1	35
Key lime	1 slice	345	13	4.5	237	52	1	43	7	0	158	1	249
Lemon meringue	1 slice	382	12	5.0	387	67	0	51	4	0	20	1	73
Pecan	1 slice	582	38	10.5	383	57	3	37	6	0	57	2	214
Pumpkin	1 slice	323	13	3.0	318	46	2	25	5	0	85	1	222
Rhubarb	1 slice	315	13	5.5	177	47	2	27	3	0	63	2	199
Shoofly	1 slice	376	11	4.0	323	66	1	36	4	0	104	4	659
Strawberry cream	1 slice	353	21	12.0	203	37	2	26	3	0	47	1	175
Sweet potato	1 slice	530	22	10.5	348	80	2	57	6	0	89	1	227

* Based on a 10-in pie (8 slices) unless indicated.

DESSERTS, SWEETS & TOPPINGS

Syrups & Toppings	Amount	Calories	Fat (g)	Saturated Fat (g)	Sodium (mg)	Carbohydrate (g)	Fiber (g)	Sugar (g)	Protein (g)	Vitamin D (mcg)	Calcium (mg)	Iron (mg)	Potassium (mg)
Apple butter	1 T	29	0	0.0	3	7	0	6	0	0	2	0	16
Butterscotch/caramel	2 T	103	0	0.0	143	27	0	27	1	0	22	0	34
Chocolate syrup	2 T	112	0	0.0	29	26	1	20	1	0	6	1	90
light	2 T	54	0	0.0	35	12	0	10	1	0	4	0	66
Coffee syrup	2 T	80	0	0.0	0	20	0	20	0	0	0	0	0
Frosting/icing													
chocolate	2 T	159	7	2.0	73	25	0	23	0	0	3	1	78
sugar-free	2 T	100	6	3.0	85	16	1	0	0	0	0	1	97
vanilla	2 T	140	5	2.5	70	23	0	19	0	0	0	0	15
sugar-free	2 T	100	6	3.0	60	17	0	0	0	0	0	0	0
Fruit spread	1 T	45	0	0.0	0	11	0	10	0	0	2	0	13
Grenadine syrup	1 T	54	0	0.0	5	13	0	9	0	0	1	0	6
Honey	1 T	64	0	0.0	1	17	0	17	0	0	1	0	11
Hot fudge	2 T	133	3	1.5	132	24	1	13	2	0	19	1	108
sugar-free	2 T	90	1	0.0	40	24	1	0	1	0	0	1	0
Jam/jelly/marmalade	1 T	56	0	0.0	6	14	0	10	0	0	4	0	15
Maple syrup	1 T	52	0	0.0	2	13	0	12	0	0	20	0	42
Marshmallow crème	2 T	81	0	0.0	20	20	0	12	0	0	1	0	1
Pancake syrup	1 T	47	0	0.0	16	12	0	4	0	0	1	0	3
low-calorie	1 T	25	0	0.0	27	7	0	5	0	0	2	0	1
Whipped cream, homemade	2 T	116	11	7.0	11	4	0	3	1	0	19	0	23
Whipped toppings													
Cool Whip	2 T	20	2	1.0	0	3	0	2	0	0	0	0	0
pressurized	2 T	15	1	1.0	1	1	0	1	0	0	6	0	9
Reddi Wip	2 T	15	1	0.5	0	1	0	0	0	0	0	0	0
fat-free	2 T	5	0	0.0	0	1	0	0	0	0	0	0	0

EGGS, EGG DISHES & EGG SUBSTITUTES

Eggs	Amount	Calories	Fat (g)	Saturated Fat (g)	Sodium (mg)	Carbohydrate (g)	Fiber (g)	Sugar (g)	Protein (g)	Vitamin D (mcg)	Calcium (mg)	Iron (mg)	Potassium (mg)
Chicken													
boiled/poached	1 large	73	5	1.5	147	0	0	0	6	1	27	0	67
deviled w/ filling	½ egg	60	5	1.0	166	1	0	0	3	0	17	1	36
Eggland's Best	1 large	60	4	1.0	65	0	0	0	6	6	30	1	70
fried w/ ½ tsp fat	1 large	90	7	2.0	95	0	0	0	6	1	29	1	70
powdered													
whites	2 T	20	0	0.0	120	0	0	0	8	0	0	0	120
whole	2 T	89	7	2.0	71	0	0	0	7	1	36	1	81
scrambled w/ 1 tsp fat	2 large	182	13	4.0	178	2	0	2	12	2	81	1	161
whites	1	21	0	0.0	66	0	0	0	4	0	3	0	65
yolk	1	55	5	1.5	8	1	0	0	3	1	22	1	19
Duck	1	130	10	3.0	102	1	0	1	9	0	44	3	155
Goose	1	266	19	5.0	199	2	0	1	20	2	86	5	302
Quail	1	14	1	0.5	13	0	0	0	1	0	6	0	12
Turkey	1	135	9	3.0	119	1	0	0	11	0	78	3	112

EGGS, EGG DISHES & EGG SUBSTITUTES

Egg Dishes

	Amount	Calories	Fat (g)	Saturated Fat (g)	Sodium (mg)	Carbohydrate (g)	Fiber (g)	Sugar (g)	Protein (g)	Vitamin D (mcg)	Calcium (mg)	Iron (mg)	Potassium (mg)
Frittatas, plain (10 in)													
caramelized onion sausage	¼ pie	367	29	12.0	690	6	1	3	19	2	71	2	341
egg white	¼ pie	170	11	4.0	879	7	2	4	11	0	124	1	350
Omelets													
cheese	1 (2 egg)	299	24	9.0	325	1	0	0	19	2	247	2	160
egg white	1 (4 egg white)	171	12	7.0	376	1	0	1	15	0	13	0	220
ham & cheese	1 (2 egg)	354	28	12.0	708	2	0	1	23	4	226	2	248
vegetable & cheese	1 (2 egg)	320	25	9.0	542	3	0	1	20	4	226	2	278
Quiche (9 in)													
ham & cheese	⅙ pie	327	23	10.0	538	16	1	2	14	0	219	2	167
Lorraine	⅙ pie	761	68	30.5	1022	19	1	1	19	0	224	2	285
spinach	⅙ pie	613	48	27.0	1155	24	3	6	23	0	563	3	393
Soufflés													
cheese	1 cup	439	33	19.0	721	23	0	2	14	0	191	2	130
spinach	1 cup	440	29	17.0	661	14	4	2	34	0	774	4	591
Egg Substitutes													
Egg Beaters	3 T	25	0	0.0	90	0	0	0	5	0	0	1	0
Liquid egg whites	3 T	25	0	0.0	75	0	0	0	5	0	0	0	75

FATS, OILS, CREAM & GRAVY

	Amount	Calories	Fat (g)	Saturated Fat (g)	Sodium (mg)	Carbohydrate (g)	Fiber (g)	Sugar (g)	Protein (g)	Vitamin D (mcg)	Calcium (mg)	Iron (mg)	Potassium (mg)
Bacon fat	1 T	116	13	5.0	19	0	0	0	0	0	0	0	0
Beef fat/tallow	1 T	116	13	6.5	0	0	0	0	0	0	0	0	0
Benecol spread	1 T	70	8	1.0	105	0	0	0	0	0	0	0	0
light	1 T	50	5	1.0	95	0	0	0	0	0	0	0	0
Butter													
stick	1 tsp	34	4	2.5	30	0	0	0	0	0	1	0	1
	1 T	102	12	7.0	91	0	0	0	0	0	3	0	3
stick, unsalted	1 tsp	34	4	2.5	1	0	0	0	0	0	1	0	1
whipped	1 tsp	23	3	1.5	21	0	0	0	0	0	1	0	1
Butter flavored sprinkles	1 tsp	5	0	0.0	180	1	0	0	0	0	0	0	0
Chicken fat	1 T	115	13	4.0	0	0	0	0	0	1	0	0	0
Coconut milk creamer	1 T	30	1	1.0	15	4	0	4	0	0	0	0	0
Coffee-Mate	1 T	20	1	0.0	5	2	0	0	0	0	0	0	0
liquid, flavored	1 T	35	2	0.0	5	5	0	5	0	0	0	0	0
fat-free	1 T	25	0	0.0	5	5	0	5	0	0	0	0	30
zero sugar	1 T	15	1	0.0	5	1	0	0	0	0	0	0	0
powder	1 tsp	10	1	0.5	5	1	0	0	0	0	0	0	0
fat-free	1 tsp	10	0	0.0	0	2	0	0	0	0	0	0	0
flavored	1 tsp	10	0	0.0	5	2	0	1	0	0	0	0	0
sugar-free, flavored	1 tsp	15	1	1.0	5	0	0	0	0	0	0	0	0
Coffee Rich	1 T	10	1	1.0	0	1	0	0	0	0	0	0	20
Cooking spray	⅓ second	2	0	0.0	0	0	0	0	0	0	0	0	0
	2 seconds	14	1	0.0	1	0	0	0	0	0	0	0	0

FATS, OILS, CREAM & GRAVY

	Amount	Calories	Fat (g)	Saturated Fat (g)	Sodium (mg)	Carbohydrate (g)	Fiber (g)	Sugar (g)	Protein (g)	Vitamin D (mcg)	Calcium (mg)	Iron (mg)	Potassium (mg)
Cream													
heavy	1 T	52	6	3.5	6	0	0	0	0	0	10	0	11
light	1 T	44	5	3.0	5	0	0	0	0	0	10	0	15
Gravy, beef													
au jus, jar	¼ cup	5	0	0.0	230	0	0	0	1	0	0	0	0
brown, mix	¼ cup	20	0	0.0	251	4	0	0	1	0	16	0	16
fat-free, can	¼ cup	20	0	0.0	300	3	0	0	1	0	0	0	0
homemade	¼ cup	51	1	0.0	740	10	1	1	2	0	21	0	40
regular, can	¼ cup	31	1	0.5	326	3	0	0	2	0	4	0	47
Gravy, chicken													
dry	1 T	31	1	0.0	332	5	0	0	1	0	12	0	32
fat-free, can	¼ cup	15	0	0.0	310	3	0	0	1	0	0	0	0
giblet, homemade	¼ cup	49	3	0.5	341	3	0	0	3	0	12	2	117
regular, can	¼ cup	47	3	1.0	252	3	0	1	1	0	12	0	65
Gravy, other													
mushroom, can	¼ cup	30	2	0.0	339	3	0	0	1	0	4	0	63
onion, mix	¼ cup	19	0	0.0	251	4	0	0	1	0	17	0	16
pork, can	¼ cup	45	3	1.5	310	3	0	1	1	0	0	0	0
sausage, can	¼ cup	70	6	1.5	270	3	0	1	2	0	0	0	120
turkey, can	¼ cup	30	1	0.5	344	3	0	0	2	0	2	0	65
turkey, mix	¼ cup	24	1	0.0	274	4	0	0	1	0	8	0	221
Half & half	1 T	20	2	1.0	6	1	0	1	0	0	16	0	20
fat-free	1 T	9	0	0.0	15	1	0	1	0	0	14	0	31
Lard/pork fat	1 T	116	13	5.0	0	0	0	0	0	0	0	0	0
Margarine													
fat-free	1 tsp	2	0	0.0	42	0	0	0	0	0	2	0	3
	1 T	7	0	0.0	125	0	0	0	0	0	6	0	8
light	1 tsp	16	2	0.5	27	0	0	0	0	0	0	0	2
	1 T	47	5	1.0	81	0	0	0	0	0	0	0	5
regular, soft/tub	1 tsp	33	4	1.0	31	0	0	0	0	0	0	0	1
	1 T	101	11	2.0	93	0	0	0	0	0	0	0	2
regular, soft/tub, unsalted	1 T	101	11	2.0	4	0	0	0	0	0	0	0	2
regular, stick	1 tsp	33	4	1.0	38	0	0	0	0	0	0	0	1
	1 T	100	11	2.0	105	0	0	0	0	0	0	0	3
regular, stick, unsalted	1 T	102	12	2.0	0	0	0	0	0	0	0	0	3
Mayonnaise	1 T	94	10	1.5	88	0	0	0	0	0	1	0	3
light	1 T	36	3	0.5	124	1	0	0	0	0	1	0	5
low-fat	1 T	15	1	0.0	130	2	0	0	0	0	0	0	0
vegan	1 T	47	8	1.0	100	0	0	0	0	0	0	0	0
Miracle Whip	1 T	40	4	0.5	95	2	0	1	0	0	0	0	0
light	1 T	20	2	0.0	130	2	0	0	0	0	0	0	0
Mocha Mix	1 T	20	2	0.0	5	1	0	0	0	0	0	0	20
fat-free	1 T	10	0	0.0	5	1	0	0	0	0	0	0	0

FATS, OILS, CREAM & GRAVY

	Amount	Calories	Fat (g)	Saturated Fat (g)	Sodium (mg)	Carbohydrate (g)	Fiber (g)	Sugar (g)	Protein (g)	Vitamin D (mcg)	Calcium (mg)	Iron (mg)	Potassium (mg)
Oils													
avocado	1 T	124	14	1.5	0	0	0	0	0	0	0	0	0
canola	1 T	124	14	1.0	0	0	0	0	0	0	0	0	0
chili, flavored	1 T	130	14	3.0	0	0	0	0	0	0	0	0	0
coconut	1 T	117	14	12.0	0	0	0	0	0	0	0	0	0
cod liver/fish	1 T	123	14	3.0	0	0	0	0	0	34	0	0	0
corn	1 T	122	14	2.0	0	0	0	0	0	0	0	0	0
cottonseed	1 T	120	14	3.5	0	0	0	0	0	0	0	0	0
flaxseed/linseed	1 T	120	14	1.0	0	0	0	0	0	0	0	0	0
grapeseed	1 T	120	14	1.5	0	0	0	0	0	0	0	0	0
olive	1 T	119	14	2.0	0	0	0	0	0	0	0	0	0
palm	1 T	120	14	6.5	0	0	0	0	0	0	0	0	0
palm kernel	1 T	116	14	11.0	0	0	0	0	0	0	0	0	0
peanut	1 T	119	14	2.5	0	0	0	0	0	0	0	0	0
safflower	1 T	120	14	1.0	0	0	0	0	0	0	0	0	0
sesame	1 T	120	14	2.0	0	0	0	0	0	0	0	0	0
soybean	1 T	120	14	2.0	0	0	0	0	0	0	0	0	0
sunflower	1 T	120	14	1.5	0	0	0	0	0	0	0	0	0
walnut	1 T	120	14	1.0	0	0	0	0	0	0	0	0	0
wheat germ	1 T	120	14	2.5	0	0	0	0	0	0	0	0	0
Popcorn topping	1 T	120	14	2.0	0	0	0	0	0	0	0	0	0
Silk creamer													
almond, vanilla	1 T	25	1	0.0	15	4	0	4	0	0	0	0	0
oat, vanilla	1 T	25	1	0.0	15	4	0	4	0	0	0	0	0
soy													
original	1 T	20	2	0.5	0	2	0	1	0	0	0	0	0
vanilla	1 T	30	2	0.5	0	4	0	3	0	0	0	0	0
Sour cream	1 T	23	2	1.0	6	0	0	0	0	0	13	0	17
fat-free	1 T	11	0	0.0	21	2	0	0	1	0	19	0	19
imitation, soy	1 T	31	3	3.0	15	1	0	1	0	0	1	0	24
light	1 T	20	2	1.0	13	1	0	0	1	0	21	0	32
Vegetable shortening	1 T	110	12	3.0	0	0	0	0	0	0	0	0	0
Yogurt spread	1 T	46	5	1.0	88	0	0	0	0	0	7	0	9

FISH & SEAFOOD

	Amount	Calories	Fat (g)	Saturated Fat (g)	Sodium (mg)	Carbohydrate (g)	Fiber (g)	Sugar (g)	Protein (g)	Vitamin D (mcg)	Calcium (mg)	Iron (mg)	Potassium (mg)
Abalone													
baked/broiled	3 oz	119	1	0.0	341	7	0	0	19	0	27	3	213
flour fried	3 oz	161	6	1.5	503	9	0	0	17	0	32	3	241
Anchovies, oil pack, can	3	25	1	0.5	440	0	0	0	4	0	28	1	65
Anchovy paste	1 T	25	2	0.5	1130	0	0	0	3	4	20	2	33
Bass, freshwater	3 oz	124	4	1.0	77	0	0	0	21	3	88	2	388
Bluefish	3 oz	135	5	1.0	66	0	0	0	22	11	23	1	406
Burbot	3 oz	98	1	0.0	105	0	0	0	21	1	54	1	440
Butterfish	3 oz	159	9	2.5	97	0	0	0	19	11	24	1	409

FISH & SEAFOOD	Amount	Calories	Fat (g)	Saturated Fat (g)	Sodium (mg)	Carbohydrate (g)	Fiber (g)	Sugar (g)	Protein (g)	Vitamin D (mcg)	Calcium (mg)	Iron (mg)	Potassium (mg)
Calamari/squid													
baked/broiled	3 oz	78	1	0.0	37	3	0	0	16	0	28	1	209
flour fried	3 oz	149	6	1.5	260	7	0	0	15	0	33	1	237
Carp													
baked/broiled	3 oz	138	6	1.0	54	0	0	0	19	26	44	1	363
flour fried	3 oz	239	13	3.0	175	11	0	0	18	26	46	1	370
Catfish													
farmed													
baked/broiled	3 oz	122	6	1.5	101	0	0	0	16	8	8	0	311
flour fried	3 oz	195	11	3.0	238	7	1	1	15	8	37	1	289
wild	3 oz	89	2	0.5	43	0	0	0	16	11	9	0	356
Caviar, black/red	1 T	42	3	0.5	240	1	0	0	4	1	44	2	29
Chilean sea bass, grilled	3 oz	105	2	0.5	74	0	0	0	20	6	11	0	279
Cisco, smoked	3 oz	151	10	1.5	409	0	0	0	14	11	22	0	249
Clams													
breaded & fried	10 small	190	11	2.5	342	10	0	0	13	0	59	13	306
raw	6 large	103	1	0.0	721	4	0	0	18	0	47	2	55
stuffed, frozen	3 oz	142	5	0.0	467	13	0	3	7	0	33	1	0
Cod, Atlantic/Pacific													
baked/broiled	3 oz	89	1	0.0	66	0	0	0	19	1	12	0	208
breaded & fried	3 oz	150	7	1.5	320	12	1	2	10	1	0	1	260
dried & salted	3 oz	247	2	0.5	5976	0	0	0	53	3	136	2	1239
Crab													
Alaska king	3 oz	83	1	0.0	912	0	0	0	16	0	50	1	223
blue													
can	1 cup	112	1	0.5	760	0	0	0	24	0	123	1	350
fresh	3 oz	74	1	0.0	249	0	0	0	15	0	75	1	280
Dungeness	3 oz	94	1	0.0	322	1	0	0	19	0	50	0	347
imitation	3 oz	24	0	0.0	132	4	0	2	2	0	3	0	23
snow	3 oz	100	2	0.0	590	0	0	0	20	0	20	0	170
soft shell, flour fried	1 crab	358	24	3.5	76	25	1	2	9	0	64	2	149
Crab cakes	1 (2 oz)	160	10	2.0	491	5	0	0	11	0	202	1	162
Crawdads/crayfish	3 oz	70	1	0.0	80	0	0	0	14	0	51	1	252
Croaker, breaded & fried	3 oz	188	11	3.0	296	6	0	0	16	1	27	1	289
Cusk	3 oz	95	1	0.0	34	0	0	0	21	1	11	1	428
Cuttlefish	3 oz	134	1	0.0	633	1	0	0	28	0	153	9	541
Dolphinfish/mahi mahi	3 oz	93	1	0.0	96	0	0	0	20	12	16	1	453
Drum, freshwater	3 oz	130	5	1.0	82	0	0	0	19	1	66	1	300
Eel	3 oz	201	13	2.5	55	0	0	0	20	25	22	1	297
Escargot/snails	3 oz	77	1	0.0	59	2	0	0	14	0	9	3	325
Fish cakes, breaded, pan fried	1 (3 oz)	75	3	3.0	263	15	1	0	6	1	30	1	71
Fish fillets, frozen	1 (3.5 oz)	156	7	2.0	311	9	0	1	9	0	58	0	212
Fish sticks, frozen	3 oz	223	9	1.0	516	24	2	2	9	0	41	1	200

FISH & SEAFOOD

FISH & SEAFOOD	Amount	Calories	Fat (g)	Saturated Fat (g)	Sodium (mg)	Carbohydrate (g)	Fiber (g)	Sugar (g)	Protein (g)	Vitamin D (mcg)	Calcium (mg)	Iron (mg)	Potassium (mg)
Flounder													
baked/broiled	3 oz	73	2	0.5	309	0	0	0	21	3	21	0	168
breaded & fried	3 oz	200	12	2.5	347	14	0	3	10	3	17	1	150
Gefilte fish	3 oz	71	2	0.5	445	6	0	0	8	8	20	2	77
Grouper	3 oz	100	1	0.5	45	0	0	0	21	6	18	1	404
Haddock													
baked/broiled	3 oz	77	1	0.0	222	0	0	0	17	1	12	0	298
breaded & fried	3 oz	108	4	1.0	126	10	0	1	8	1	24	1	200
smoked	3 oz	99	1	0.0	649	0	0	0	21	1	42	1	353
Halibut													
Atlantic/Pacific	3 oz	94	2	0.5	70	0	0	0	19	5	8	0	449
Greenland	3 oz	203	15	2.5	88	0	0	0	16	3	3	1	292
Herring													
Atlantic													
baked/broiled	3 oz	173	10	2.0	98	0	0	0	20	5	63	1	356
pickled	3 oz	223	15	2.0	740	8	0	7	12	2	66	1	59
Pacific	3 oz	213	15	3.5	81	0	0	0	18	5	90	1	461
Ling/lingcod	3 oz	93	1	0.0	65	0	0	0	19	1	15	0	476
Lobster													
tail	3 oz	90	1	0.0	399	2	0	0	21	0	75	0	170
Northern, broiled/steamed	3 oz	76	1	0.0	413	0	0	0	16	0	82	0	196
spiny, steamed	3 oz	122	2	0.5	193	3	0	0	23	0	54	1	177
Lox/smoked salmon	3 oz	150	9	1.5	810	0	0	0	15	15	0	0	149
Mackerel													
Atlantic	3 oz	223	15	3.5	71	0	0	0	20	17	13	1	341
Jack/Pacific	3 oz	171	9	2.5	94	0	0	0	22	17	25	1	443
king	3 oz	114	2	0.5	173	0	0	0	22	17	34	2	474
Spanish	3 oz	134	5	1.5	56	0	0	0	20	17	11	1	471
Milkfish	3 oz	162	7	2.0	78	0	0	0	22	5	55	0	318
Monkfish	3 oz	83	2	0.5	20	0	0	0	16	1	9	0	436
Mullet, striped	3 oz	128	4	1.0	60	0	0	0	21	2	26	1	389
Mussels	3 oz	146	4	0.5	314	6	0	0	20	0	28	6	228
Octopus	3 oz	139	2	0.5	391	4	0	0	25	0	90	8	536
Orange roughy	3 oz	89	1	0.0	59	0	0	0	19	1	9	1	154
Oysters													
Eastern													
breaded & fried	6 (3 oz)	175	11	3.0	367	10	0	0	8	0	55	6	215
raw	6 (3 oz)	43	1	0.5	71	5	0	0	5	0	50	4	131
Pacific, raw	3 (3 oz)	69	2	0.5	90	4	0	0	8	0	7	4	143
smoked, oil pack, can	3 oz	320	29	14.0	192	3	0	0	11	0	32	7	230
Perch													
baked/broiled	3 oz	100	1	0.0	67	0	0	0	21	4	87	1	292
breaded & fried	3 oz	226	15	2.0	465	11	0	0	21	3	83	1	250
Pollock, Atlantic	3 oz	100	1	0.0	94	0	0	0	21	1	66	1	388

FISH & SEAFOOD

	Amount	Calories	Fat (g)	Saturated Fat (g)	Sodium (mg)	Carbohydrate (g)	Fiber (g)	Sugar (g)	Protein (g)	Vitamin D (mcg)	Calcium (mg)	Iron (mg)	Potassium (mg)
Pompano, Florida	3 oz	179	10	4.0	65	0	0	0	20	12	37	1	541
Rockfish, Pacific	3 oz	93	1	0.5	76	0	0	0	19	4	15	0	397
Roe	3 oz	174	7	1.5	100	2	0	0	24	12	24	1	241
Sablefish	3 oz	213	17	3.5	61	0	0	0	15	12	38	1	390
Salmon													
Atlantic	3 oz	155	7	1.0	48	0	0	0	22	14	13	1	534
Chinook	3 oz	197	11	2.5	51	0	0	0	22	14	24	1	429
coho	3 oz	156	6	1.5	45	0	0	0	23	14	39	1	387
pink, can	3 oz	109	4	0.5	342	0	0	0	17	12	183	1	293
sockeye, can	3 oz	142	6	1.0	347	0	0	0	20	18	197	1	267
Sardines, oil pack, can	2	50	3	0.5	74	0	0	0	6	1	92	1	95
Scallops													
bay/sea, steamed	3 oz	94	1	0.0	567	5	0	0	18	0	9	1	267
imitation	3 oz	84	0	0.0	676	9	0	0	11	0	7	0	88
sea, breaded & fried	6 large	201	10	2.5	432	9	0	0	17	0	39	1	310
Scup	3 oz	115	3	1.0	46	0	0	0	21	1	43	1	313
Shad	3 oz	214	15	4.0	55	0	0	0	19	4	51	1	418
Shad roe	3 oz	173	7	1.5	100	2	0	0	24	13	24	1	241
Shark	3 oz	194	12	2.5	104	5	0	0	16	1	43	1	132
Shrimp													
baked/broiled/raw	10 large	66	1	0.5	521	1	0	0	13	0	50	2	94
breaded & fried	10 large	376	23	4.0	1373	27	1	1	16	0	51	2	132
Smelt, rainbow													
baked/broiled	3 oz	105	3	0.5	66	0	0	0	19	1	1	1	316
flour fried	3 oz	217	11	2.5	188	11	0	0	18	1	1	1	340
Snapper	3 oz	109	2	0.5	49	0	0	0	22	1	34	0	444
Sole													
baked/broiled	3 oz	67	1	0.5	236	11	1	3	5	3	28	0	45
breaded & fried	3 oz	189	9	0.5	411	21	2	0	8	3	13	1	154
Sturgeon													
baked/broiled	3 oz	115	4	1.0	59	0	0	0	18	11	15	1	309
smoked	3 oz	147	4	1.0	629	0	0	0	27	14	15	1	322
Sucker, white	3 oz	101	3	0.5	43	0	0	0	18	18	77	1	414
Sunfish	3 oz	97	1	0.0	88	0	0	0	21	2	88	1	382
Swordfish	3 oz	146	7	1.5	83	0	0	0	20	14	5	0	424
Tilefish	3 oz	125	4	0.5	50	0	0	0	21	11	22	0	435
Trout, rainbow													
baked/broiled	3 oz	128	5	1.5	48	0	0	0	20	20	73	0	381
parmesan crusted	3 oz	263	13	2.5	253	2	0	1	33	20	90	2	578
Tuna, can													
light													
oil pack	3 oz	168	7	1.5	354	0	0	0	25	6	11	1	176
water pack	3 oz	73	1	0.0	210	0	0	0	17	1	15	1	152
low sodium, water pack	3 oz	109	3	0.5	43	0	0	0	20	3	12	1	202

FISH & SEAFOOD

	Amount	Calories	Fat (g)	Saturated Fat (g)	Sodium (mg)	Carbohydrate (g)	Fiber (g)	Sugar (g)	Protein (g)	Vitamin D (mcg)	Calcium (mg)	Iron (mg)	Potassium (mg)
white													
oil pack	3 oz	158	7	1.0	337	0	0	0	23	1	3	1	283
water pack	¼ cup	108	3	0.5	321	0	0	0	20	2	12	1	202
Tuna, fresh													
bluefin	3 oz	156	5	1.5	43	0	0	0	25	5	9	1	275
yellowfin	3 oz	111	1	0.0	46	0	0	0	25	3	3	1	448
Turbot	3 oz	104	3	0.5	163	0	0	0	18	3	20	0	259
Walleye	3 oz	94	1	0.0	356	0	0	0	20	1	61	1	366
Whitefish	3 oz	146	6	1.0	55	0	0	0	21	17	28	0	345
Whiting	3 oz	99	1	0.5	112	0	0	0	20	2	53	0	369
Yellowtail	3 oz	159	6	1.0	43	0	0	0	25	11	25	1	457

FRUIT & VEGETABLE JUICES

Fruit Juices & Nectars

	Amount	Calories	Fat (g)	Saturated Fat (g)	Sodium (mg)	Carbohydrate (g)	Fiber (g)	Sugar (g)	Protein (g)	Vitamin D (mcg)	Calcium (mg)	Iron (mg)	Potassium (mg)
Apple cider/juice	1 cup	120	0	0.0	30	20	0	30	0	0	0	0	240
Ceres 100% juice blend													
peach	8 oz	120	0	0.0	5	21	0	20	1	0	10	0	360
pear	8 oz	110	0	0.0	5	19	0	18	0	0	10	0	290
Dole pineapple, unsweetened	1 can	100	0	0.0	0	24	0	22	0	0	0	1	240
Grapefruit													
100%	1 cup	100	0	0.0	10	25	0	21	0	0	20	0	300
white	1 cup	90	0	0.0	15	24	0	17	0	0	0	0	315
Jumex apricot nectar	1 can	170	0	0.0	55	42	2	40	0	0	26	0	0
Iberia guava nectar	1 bottle	150	0	0.0	10	43	0	41	0	0	0	0	0
Lemon	1 tsp	0	0	0.0	0	0	0	0	0	0	0	0	0
Lime	1 tsp	0	0	0.0	0	0	0	0	0	0	0	0	0
Mango	1 cup	140	0	0.0	10	33	0	32	0	0	0	0	166
Mott's apple-cherry	8 oz	120	0	0.0	30	29	0	28	0	0	0	1	300
Naked													
Blue Machine	1 bottle	320	0	0.0	20	76	3	55	2	0	50	1	700
Green Machine	1 bottle	270	0	0.0	25	63	0	53	4	0	40	1	760
Mighty Mango	1 bottle	290	0	0.0	20	68	0	57	2	0	40	1	650
Strawberry Banana	1 bottle	270	0	0.0	5	52	5	38	2	0	40	1	920
Ocean Spray													
cranberry cocktail													
red, diet	1 cup	5	0	0.0	40	2	0	1	0	0	0	0	0
red, regular	1 cup	110	0	0.0	5	28	0	25	0	0	0	0	45
white, regular	1 cup	100	0	0.0	40	26	0	25	0	0	0	0	0
Cran•Apple	1 cup	100	0	0.0	45	27	0	26	0	0	0	0	0
Cran•Pomegranate	1 cup	100	0	0.0	30	28	0	26	0	0	0	1	0
Cran•Raspberry	1 cup	100	0	0.0	35	28	0	26	0	0	0	0	0
diet	1 cup	5	0	0.0	35	2	0	1	0	0	0	0	0
White Cran•Peach	1 cup	100	0	0.0	40	28	0	26	0	0	0	0	0
Orange	1 cup	110	0	0.0	0	26	0	22	2	0	20	0	450

FRUIT & VEGETABLE JUICES

Fruit Juices & Nectars	Amount	Calories	Fat (g)	Saturated Fat (g)	Sodium (mg)	Carbohydrate (g)	Fiber (g)	Sugar (g)	Protein (g)	Vitamin D (mcg)	Calcium (mg)	Iron (mg)	Potassium (mg)
Pom Wonderful, 100%													
pomegranate	1 cup	160	0	0.0	5	39	0	34	0	0	20	0	550
pomegranate cherry	1 cup	160	0	0.0	10	38	0	32	1	0	30	0	570
Sunsweet Amaz!n prune	1 cup	180	0	0.0	30	44	4	24	1	0	30	0	530
Welch's grape													
100%	1 cup	140	0	0.0	10	37	0	35	1	0	30	0	140
white	1 cup	140	0	0.0	15	37	0	36	1	0	30	0	140
light	1 cup	45	0	0.0	80	12	0	11	0	0	0	0	110
white, sparkling	1 cup	110	0	0.0	15	28	0	28	0	0	0	0	0
Vegetable Juices													
Bolthouse carrot	1 cup	70	0	0.0	150	15	1	13	2	0	42	0	547
Clamato tomato cocktail	1 cup	60	0	0.0	800	12	0	11	1	0	0	0	0
Tomato	1 cup	50	0	0.0	600	10	1	6	2	0	26	1	430
V-8	1 cup	45	0	0.0	640	9	2	7	2	0	40	1	470
healthy greens	1 cup	60	0	0.0	180	15	0	13	1	0	30	1	300

FRUITS

	Amount	Calories	Fat (g)	Saturated Fat (g)	Sodium (mg)	Carbohydrate (g)	Fiber (g)	Sugar (g)	Protein (g)	Vitamin D (mcg)	Calcium (mg)	Iron (mg)	Potassium (mg)
Apples													
dried	12 pcs	130	0	0.0	0	32	3	28	0	0	7	7	310
fresh	1 medium	80	0	0.0	0	22	4	15	0	0	11	0	195
Applesauce													
natural/unsweetened	½ cup	50	0	0.0	10	12	1	11	0	0	5	0	110
sweetened	½ cup	90	0	0.0	10	23	1	20	0	0	5	0	90
Apricots													
can													
heavy syrup	½ cup	100	0	0.0	5	25	1	21	0	0	0	0	181
light syrup	½ cup	70	0	0.0	10	17	1	15	1	0	0	0	175
dried	5	100	0	0.0	0	25	3	21	1	0	20	1	460
fresh	1	17	0	0.0	0	4	1	4	0	0	0	1	427
Avocado	⅓ medium	80	8	1.0	0	4	3	0	1	0	10	0	250
Banana chips, sweetened	¼ cup	200	11	10.0	0	27	1	12	0	0	0	0	350
Banana, fresh	1 medium	105	0	0.0	2	27	3	14	1	0	13	0	422
Blackberries, fresh	1 cup	60	1	0.0	1	12	6	6	1	0	52	1	233
Blueberries, fresh/frozen	1 cup	70	1	0.0	0	17	4	12	0	0	0	0	80
Boysenberries, fresh	1 cup	62	1	0.0	1	14	8	7	2	0	42	1	233
Cantaloupe, fresh	1 cup	53	0	0.0	25	13	1	12	1	0	14	0	417
Cherries													
maraschino	1 medium	5	0	0.0	0	2	0	2	0	0	3	0	1
red	½ cup	43	0	0.0	0	11	1	9	1	0	9	0	153
sweet, heavy syrup, can	⅓ cup	100	0	0.0	15	24	0	20	0	0	0	0	100
tart, juice packed, jar	5	10	0	0.0	4	2	0	2	0	0	3	0	30
Coconut, shredded													
dried													
sweetened	2 T	70	5	4.0	45	7	1	5	0	0	2	0	39
unsweetened	2½ T	100	10	9.0	5	4	2	1	1	0	4	0	80
fresh	1 cup	283	27	24.0	16	12	7	5	3	0	11	2	285

FRUITS	Amount	Calories	Fat (g)	Saturated Fat (g)	Sodium (mg)	Carbohydrate (g)	Fiber (g)	Sugar (g)	Protein (g)	Vitamin D (mcg)	Calcium (mg)	Iron (mg)	Potassium (mg)
Cranberries													
Craisins/sweetened, dried	¼ cup	100	0	0.0	0	33	10	12	0	0	4	0	20
fresh/frozen	1 cup	90	0	0.0	0	22	3	18	1	0	20	1	310
Currants, fresh	1 cup	63	0	0.0	1	15	5	8	1	0	37	1	308
Dates, dried	2	110	0	0.0	0	30	3	25	1	0	20	0	270
Figs													
dried	3	110	0	0.0	0	26	5	20	1	0	60	1	240
fresh	1 medium	111	1	0.0	1	29	4	24	1	0	53	1	348
Fruit cocktail, can													
100% juice	½ cup	60	0	0.0	5	15	1	12	1	0	8	0	170
heavy syrup	½ cup	100	0	0.0	5	25	1	21	0	0	0	0	100
Gooseberries, fresh	1 cup	70	1	0.0	2	15	6	0	1	0	40	0	270
Grapefruit													
light syrup, can	½ cup	90	0	0.0	0	21	1	17	1	0	20	3	164
whole, fresh	½ medium	52	0	0.0	0	13	2	8	1	0	27	0	166
Grapes, fresh	1 cup	52	0	0.0	2	14	1	12	1	0	8	0	144
Guava, fresh	1 medium	38	1	0.0	1	8	3	5	1	0	10	0	229
Honeydew melon, fresh	1 cup	61	0	0.0	31	15	1	13	1	0	10	0	388
Kiwifruit, fresh	1 medium	42	0	0.0	2	10	2	6	1	0	23	0	215
Kumquat, fresh	1 medium	13	0	0.0	2	3	1	2	0	0	13	0	35
Lemon, fresh	1	17	0	0.0	1	5	2	1	1	0	15	0	80
Lime, fresh	1	20	0	0.0	1	7	2	1	0	0	22	0	68
Loganberries, fresh	1 cup	80	1	0.0	2	19	0	11	2	0	38	1	213
Mandarin oranges, can	½ cup	80	0	0.0	0	19	2	17	1	0	30	0	140
Mangoes, fresh	½ cup	50	0	0.0	1	12	1	11	1	0	9	0	139
Melon balls, frozen	1 cup	40	0	0.0	15	10	0	8	2	0	40	0	242
Mixed fruit													
dried	¼ cup	110	0	0.0	95	27	4	18	1	0	16	1	330
no sugar added, frozen	1 cup	60	0	0.0	0	16	2	12	1	0	20	1	200
Mulberries, fresh	1 cup	60	2	0.0	14	14	2	11	2	0	54	3	218
Nectarine, fresh	1 medium	62	0	0.0	0	15	2	11	2	0	9	0	285
Orange, fresh	1 medium	69	0	0.0	0	18	3	12	1	0	60	0	232
Papayas, fresh	½ cup	31	0	0.0	6	8	1	6	0	0	15	0	132
Passion fruit, fresh	1 medium	18	0	0.0	5	4	2	2	0	0	2	0	63
Peaches													
can													
100% juice	½ cup	70	0	0.0	10	17	1	13	0	0	26	0	210
heavy syrup	½ cup	100	0	0.0	5	25	1	21	0	0	0	0	100
fresh	1 medium	60	0	0.0	0	14	2	13	1	0	9	0	292
Pears													
can													
100% juice	½ cup	60	0	0.0	5	15	2	11	0	0	26	0	115
heavy syrup	½ cup	100	0	0.0	5	25	2	20	0	0	0	0	60
fresh	1 medium	112	0	0.0	2	27	5	17	1	0	16	0	179

FRUITS

	Amount	Calories	Fat (g)	Saturated Fat (g)	Sodium (mg)	Carbohydrate (g)	Fiber (g)	Sugar (g)	Protein (g)	Vitamin D (mcg)	Calcium (mg)	Iron (mg)	Potassium (mg)
Persimmon, fresh	1 medium	32	0	0.0	0	8	0	8	0	0	7	1	78
Pineapple chunks													
can													
100% juice	2 slices	60	0	0.0	10	16	1	14	0	0	18	0	186
heavy syrup	½ cup	90	0	0.0	10	24	1	22	0	0	18	0	146
fresh	1 cup	83	0	0.0	2	22	2	16	1	0	21	1	180
Plantains, cooked	½ cup	170	7	1.0	150	29	2	13	1	0	3	1	447
Plum, fresh	1 medium	30	0	0.0	0	8	1	7	0	0	4	0	104
Pomegranate, fresh	½ medium	72	1	0.0	3	16	4	12	1	0	13	0	205
seeds	½ cup	100	1	0.0	0	20	5	14	2	0	0	0	188
Prickly pear, fresh	1 medium	61	1	0.0	8	14	5	9	1	0	83	0	328
Prunes, dried	6	110	0	0.0	5	26	2	13	1	0	0	1	330
Quince, fresh	1 medium	52	0	0.0	4	14	2	12	0	0	10	1	181
Raisins	¼ cup	140	0	0.0	10	33	1	26	1	0	20	1	310
Raspberries, fresh	1 cup	64	1	0.0	1	15	8	5	1	0	31	1	186
Rhubarb													
fresh	1 cup	11	0	0.0	2	2	1	1	1	0	44	0	147
sweetened, cooked	1 cup	278	0	0.0	2	75	5	69	1	0	348	1	230
Starfruit, fresh	1 medium	41	0	0.0	3	9	4	5	1	0	4	0	176
Strawberries													
fresh	1 cup	23	0	0.0	1	6	1	4	0	0	12	0	110
sweetened, frozen	23	50	0	0.0	0	13	3	6	1	0	20	1	200
Tangerine, fresh	1 medium	50	0	0.0	0	13	2	9	1	0	52	0	146
Tropical fruit, light, can	½ cup	90	0	0.0	0	21	1	20	0	0	0	0	140
Watermelon, fresh	1 cup	45	0	0.0	2	11	1	9	1	0	11	0	170

MEATS*

Beef & Veal

	Amount	Calories	Fat (g)	Saturated Fat (g)	Sodium (mg)	Carbohydrate (g)	Fiber (g)	Sugar (g)	Protein (g)	Vitamin D (mcg)	Calcium (mg)	Iron (mg)	Potassium (mg)
Bottom round, roasted	3 oz	190	11	4.0	29	0	0	0	22	0	5	2	179
Chuck roast, braised													
arm	3 oz	174	5	2.0	49	0	0	0	29	0	15	3	239
blade	3 oz	215	11	4.5	60	0	0	0	26	0	11	3	224
Corned brisket, roasted	3 oz	214	16	5.5	828	0	0	0	16	0	7	2	123
Eye of round, roasted	3 oz	177	8	3.0	32	0	0	0	24	0	6	2	193
Filet mignon, broiled	3 oz	185	8	3.5	49	0	0	0	26	0	12	3	303
Flank steak, broiled	3 oz	165	7	3.0	48	0	0	0	24	0	13	3	288
Ground													
extra lean, 5% fat, pan-browned	3 oz	164	6	3.0	72	0	0	0	22	0	8	3	390
lean													
10% fat	3 oz	196	10	4.0	74	0	0	2	24	0	14	3	368
15% fat	3 oz	218	13	5.0	78	0	0	0	24	0	19	3	346
regular, 20% fat	3 oz	231	15	5.5	77	0	0	0	23	0	24	2	323
London broil	3 oz	165	7	3.0	48	0	0	0	24	0	13	2	288

* Cooked w/o fat unless indicated.

MEATS

Beef & Veal

	Amount	Calories	Fat (g)	Saturated Fat (g)	Sodium (mg)	Carbohydrate (g)	Fiber (g)	Sugar (g)	Protein (g)	Vitamin D (mcg)	Calcium (mg)	Iron (mg)	Potassium (mg)
New York Strip, boneless	3 oz	125	6	2.0	37	0	0	0	18	0	12	2	242
Porterhouse steak	3 oz	173	7	3.0	57	0	0	0	25	0	17	3	248
Pot roast, chuck	3 oz	207	15	6.0	53	0	0	0	16	0	14	1	247
Prime rib	3 oz	349	30	12.5	55	0	0	0	19	0	11	2	275
Rib eye steak	3 oz	153	9	3.5	75	0	0	0	17	0	5	2	303
Round steak, top, grilled	3 oz	134	4	1.0	59	0	0	0	26	0	14	3	324
Rump roast	3 oz	204	10	3.5	37	0	0	0	28	0	7	2	229
Short ribs, bone in	3 oz	204	12	3.0	89	0	0	0	25	0	12	3	235
Sirloin steak, grilled	3 oz	154	6	2.5	53	0	0	0	24	0	15	2	315
Sirloin tips	3 oz	155	7	2.5	47	0	0	0	23	0	15	1	289
Stew meat	3 oz	164	6	2.5	55	0	0	0	28	0	15	3	268
T-bone steak	3 oz	210	14	5.0	57	0	0	0	21	0	4	3	257
Tenderloin, lean	3 oz	179	8	3.0	48	0	0	0	25	0	11	3	298
Top round	3 oz	160	5	2.0	36	0	0	0	27	0	0	2	234
Top sirloin	3 oz	171	11	4.0	44	0	0	0	17	0	20	1	268
Tri tip roast	3 oz	179	9	3.0	45	0	0	0	22	0	16	1	275
Veal													
chops													
breaded & fried	3 oz	190	13	5.0	370	10	2	2	12	0	26	1	207
grilled	3 oz	135	4	1.5	72	0	0	0	25	0	11	1	203
cutlets/loin chops, braised	3 oz	190	10	4.0	95	0	0	0	21	0	20	1	243
ground	3 oz	196	15	7.0	60	0	0	0	16	0	9	1	298
loin, braised	3 oz	241	15	5.5	68	0	0	0	26	0	24	1	238
patties, breaded & fried	3 oz	190	13	5.0	370	10	2	2	12	0	20	0	240
shoulder, roasted	3 oz	139	5	2.0	77	0	0	0	22	0	23	1	303
sirloin, braised	3 oz	214	11	4.5	67	0	0	0	27	0	15	4	273

Game

	Amount	Calories	Fat (g)	Saturated Fat (g)	Sodium (mg)	Carbohydrate (g)	Fiber (g)	Sugar (g)	Protein (g)	Vitamin D (mcg)	Calcium (mg)	Iron (mg)	Potassium (mg)
Beefalo, roasted	3 oz	160	5	2.5	70	0	0	0	26	0	20	3	390
Bison/buffalo, roasted	3 oz	122	2	1.0	49	0	0	0	24	0	7	3	307
Rabbit													
domestic, roasted	3 oz	168	7	2.0	40	0	0	0	25	0	16	2	326
wild, stewed	3 oz	147	3	1.0	38	0	0	0	28	0	15	4	292
Venison, roasted	3 oz	134	3	1.0	46	0	0	0	26	0	6	4	285

Lamb

	Amount	Calories	Fat (g)	Saturated Fat (g)	Sodium (mg)	Carbohydrate (g)	Fiber (g)	Sugar (g)	Protein (g)	Vitamin D (mcg)	Calcium (mg)	Iron (mg)	Potassium (mg)
Chops	3 oz	253	22	9.5	54	0	0	0	13	0	12	1	223
Leg	3 oz	183	10	4.5	55	0	0	0	22	0	12	2	291
Shoulder	3 oz	202	9	3.5	66	0	0	0	29	0	23	2	244

Pork

	Amount	Calories	Fat (g)	Saturated Fat (g)	Sodium (mg)	Carbohydrate (g)	Fiber (g)	Sugar (g)	Protein (g)	Vitamin D (mcg)	Calcium (mg)	Iron (mg)	Potassium (mg)
Chops													
broiled	3 oz	172	10	3.0	50	1	0	0	21	1	7	1	346
fried	3 oz	166	7	2.0	84	1	0	0	25	0	43	1	322
Ground, 96% lean	3 oz	157	5	1.5	75	0	0	0	27	0	17	1	353

MEATS

Pork	Amount	Calories	Fat (g)	Saturated Fat (g)	Sodium (mg)	Carbohydrate (g)	Fiber (g)	Sugar (g)	Protein (g)	Vitamin D (mcg)	Calcium (mg)	Iron (mg)	Potassium (mg)
Ham													
cured, lean	3 oz	90	3	1.0	882	0	0	0	16	0	3	1	271
hocks	2 oz	118	7	2.0	41	0	0	0	13	0	8	1	176
leg, fresh	3 oz	208	16	5.5	40	0	0	0	15	0	4	1	268
picnic/shoulder roast	3 oz	194	11	3.5	68	0	0	0	23	1	8	1	298
Loin	3 oz	196	11	4.0	71	0	0	0	23	1	28	1	298
Spareribs, lean & fat, braised	3 oz	338	26	9.5	79	0	0	0	25	2	40	2	272
Tenderloin, lean, broiled	3 oz	122	3	1.0	49	0	0	0	22	0	5	1	358
Processed & Luncheon Meats													
Bacon	1 oz	118	11	4.0	188	0	0	0	4	0	1	0	56
Bacon bits	1 T	25	2	1.0	210	0	0	0	3	0	7	0	10
imitation	1 T	33	2	0.5	124	2	1	0	2	0	65	1	10
Beef jerky	1 oz	90	1	0.0	330	1	0	0	20	0	6	2	179
Beef sticks/Slim Jim	3	110	8	3.0	390	4	0	0	5	0	30	1	110
Bologna													
beef/beef & pork	1 oz	87	7	2.5	272	2	0	2	4	0	24	0	89
turkey	1 oz	59	5	1.0	300	1	0	1	3	0	34	1	38
Braunschweiger	1 oz	93	8	2.5	277	1	0	0	4	0	3	3	56
Canadian bacon	1 slice	45	2	0.5	371	0	0	0	6	0	2	0	94
Corned beef, can	2 oz	142	9	3.5	509	0	0	0	15	0	7	1	77
hash, can	1 cup	372	23	10.0	934	21	3	1	20	0	43	2	390
Deviled ham spread	¼ cup	180	15	5.0	480	1	0	0	8	0	26	0	0
Ham													
deli, extra lean	1 slice	23	1	0.0	294	0	0	0	4	0	13	1	113
chopped, can	1 oz	68	5	2.0	363	0	0	0	5	0	2	0	81
Headcheese	1 oz	71	5	1.5	424	0	0	0	4	0	7	1	14
Hot dogs													
beef	1	180	20	5.0	820	4	2	0	10	0	20	1	121
bun length	1	340	31	12.0	1250	4	0	1	11	0	20	2	170
w/ cheese	1	190	16	6.0	627	4	0	2	7	0	234	1	198
chicken/pork	1	150	13	4.5	550	4	0	3	4	0	26	0	60
Liverwurst	1 oz	90	8	3.0	285	1	0	0	5	0	0	0	48
Mortadella	1 oz	76	7	2.5	248	0	0	0	5	0	0	0	46
Olive loaf	1 oz	67	5	2.0	274	3	0	0	3	0	31	0	85
Pastrami, beef	1 oz	42	2	1.0	306	0	0	0	6	0	3	1	60
Pepperoni	1 oz	138	12	4.0	493	0	0	0	6	0	6	1	78
Roast beef, deli	1 oz	33	1	0.5	242	0	0	0	5	0	1	1	183
Salami													
beef	1 oz	74	6	3.0	323	1	0	0	4	0	2	1	53
& pork	1 oz	95	7	3.0	493	1	0	0	6	0	4	0	90
Sandwich steaks, frozen	1 (2 oz)	120	10	4.0	35	0	0	0	8	0	0	0	169

MEATS

Processed & Luncheon Meats

	Amount	Calories	Fat (g)	Saturated Fat (g)	Sodium (mg)	Carbohydrate (g)	Fiber (g)	Sugar (g)	Protein (g)	Vitamin D (mcg)	Calcium (mg)	Iron (mg)	Potassium (mg)
Sausages													
bockwurst	1 (1.5 oz)	100	9	3.0	280	0	0	0	5	0	0	0	118
bratwurst	1 (2 oz)	196	17	4.0	560	1	0	0	8	0	5	1	187
breakfast	2 (1.5 oz)	150	13	4.0	374	1	0	1	9	0	0	1	157
chorizo	1 (2 oz)	258	22	8.0	700	1	0	0	14	1	5	1	226
Italian	1 (2 oz)	195	16	5.5	684	2	0	1	11	1	12	1	172
kielbasa	1 (2 oz)	110	8	2.5	520	1	0	0	8	0	39	1	213
knockwurst	1 (2 oz)	155	14	6.0	475	1	0	0	8	0	1	1	90
Polish	1 (2 oz)	185	16	6.0	497	1	0	0	8	0	6	1	134
smoked													
beef	1 (2 oz)	177	15	6.5	641	1	0	0	8	0	4	1	100
pork	1 (2 oz)	175	16	5.0	469	1	0	1	13	1	6	0	274
summer	1 (1 oz)	120	11	3.0	420	1	0	0	6	0	23	1	58
Vienna	1 (1 oz)	65	6	2.0	249	1	0	0	3	0	3	0	29
Spam, can	2 oz	100	10	0.0	790	1	0	0	7	0	0	0	229
lite	2 oz	110	8	3.0	580	1	0	0	9	0	0	0	258
reduced sodium	2 oz	180	16	6.0	580	1	0	1	7	0	0	0	140

Specialty & Organ Meats

	Amount	Calories	Fat (g)	Saturated Fat (g)	Sodium (mg)	Carbohydrate (g)	Fiber (g)	Sugar (g)	Protein (g)	Vitamin D (mcg)	Calcium (mg)	Iron (mg)	Potassium (mg)
Brains, beef, pan fried	3 oz	167	14	3.0	134	0	0	0	11	0	8	2	301
Chitterlings, pork, stewed	3 oz	198	17	8.0	15	0	0	0	11	0	21	1	12
Frog legs	3 oz	73	0	0.0	58	0	0	0	10	0	18	2	285
Hearts, beef	3 oz	140	4	1.0	50	0	0	0	24	0	4	5	186
Liver, beef, pan fried	3 oz	142	4	2.0	62	4	0	0	22	1	5	5	284
Oxtail, beef	3 oz	207	12	5.0	48	0	0	0	23	0	39	2	285
Pigs' feet, pickled	3 oz	80	6	2.0	620	0	0	0	7	0	20	0	11
Sweetbreads	3 oz	122	6	2.0	44	0	0	0	18	0	5	1	301
Tongue, beef	3 oz	241	19	7.0	55	0	0	0	16	0	4	2	156
Tripe, beef	3 oz	80	3	1.0	58	2	0	0	10	0	69	1	36

MILK & YOGURT

Milk & Alternatives

	Amount	Calories	Fat (g)	Saturated Fat (g)	Sodium (mg)	Carbohydrate (g)	Fiber (g)	Sugar (g)	Protein (g)	Vitamin D (mcg)	Calcium (mg)	Iron (mg)	Potassium (mg)
Acidophilus milk, low-fat	1 cup	105	3	1.5	95	13	0	12	8	3	307	0	388
Almond milk	1 cup	60	3	0.0	150	8	0	7	1	5	450	1	170
chocolate	1 cup	100	3	0.0	150	21	1	19	1	5	450	1	220
vanilla	1 cup	80	3	0.0	150	14	0	13	1	5	450	1	170
unsweetened	1 cup	30	3	0.0	170	1	0	0	1	5	450	1	160
Buttermilk													
dried	2 T	60	1	0.5	70	8	0	7	5	3	132	0	266
low-fat	1 cup	90	0	0.0	260	14	0	12	9	3	315	0	422
Carnation Breakfast Essentials	1 bottle	240	6	1.0	160	36	0	11	10	10	300	4	580
high protein	1 bottle	220	6	1.0	210	27	0	12	15	10	350	4	450
Chocolate milk													
low-fat	1 cup	150	3	1.5	200	22	0	21	8	3	260	1	470
ultra-filtered	1 cup	140	5	3.0	280	13	1	12	13	5	390	1	550

Milk & Alternatives	Amount	Calories	Fat (g)	Saturated Fat (g)	Sodium (mg)	Carbohydrate (g)	Fiber (g)	Sugar (g)	Protein (g)	Vitamin D (mcg)	Calcium (mg)	Iron (mg)	Potassium (mg)
Coconut milk	1 cup	70	5	4.0	10	9	1	7	0	3	130	0	40
can	⅓ cup	120	13	11.0	15	2	0	1	0	0	40	0	30
light	⅓ cup	40	4	3.5	15	1	0	0	0	0	40	0	20
unsweetened	1 cup	50	5	4.5	105	1	0	0	1	3	350	0	60
Condensed milk, sweetened, can													
fat-free	2 T	110	0	0.0	55	25	0	25	4	0	195	0	90
whole	2 T	130	3	2.0	35	22	0	22	3	0	130	0	90
DREAM rice drink	1 cup	120	3	0.0	80	24	0	11	0	0	20	0	40
vanilla	1 cup	130	3	0.0	80	28	0	13	0	0	20	0	50
Eggnog, nonalcoholic													
low-fat	1 cup	140	3	1.5	85	23	0	22	6	0	260	0	175
whole	½ cup	190	9	5.0	130	24	0	20	4	0	131	0	175
Evaporated milk, can													
low-fat	2 T	25	1	0.0	30	3	0	3	2	1	70	0	120
whole	2 T	40	2	1.0	25	3	0	3	2	1	78	0	94
Filled milk	2 T	120	3	1.5	45	21	0	21	3	0	130	0	42
Goat milk	1 cup	140	10	4.0	115	11	0	11	8	2	300	0	420
Human breast milk	½ cup	86	5	2.5	21	9	0	8	1	0	79	0	125
Kefir													
flavored, low-fat	1 cup	140	2	1.5	125	20	3	20	11	5	390	0	376
plain													
low-fat	1 cup	110	2	1.5	125	12	3	12	11	5	390	0	376
non-fat	1 cup	90	0	0.0	120	12	0	12	11	5	390	0	376
Lactaid milk													
1%	1 cup	110	3	1.5	125	13	0	12	8	3	300	0	410
2%	1 cup	130	5	3.0	125	13	0	12	8	3	300	0	410
fat-free	1 cup	90	0	0.0	125	13	0	12	8	3	310	0	420
whole	1 cup	160	8	5.0	125	12	0	12	8	3	300	0	400
Low-fat milk													
1%	1 cup	110	3	1.5	135	13	0	12	8	5	310	0	420
protein fortified	1 cup	100	3	1.5	120	6	0	6	13	5	390	0	420
2%	1 cup	130	5	3.0	135	13	0	12	8	5	320	0	420
Malted milk powder	3 T	90	2	1.0	100	16	0	12	2	0	50	0	130
Oat milk	1 cup	120	5	0.5	100	16	2	7	3	4	350	0	390
Ovaltine, low-fat, chocolate													
malt	1 cup	140	3	1.5	160	22	0	22	8	4	410	3	450
rich	1 cup	140	3	1.5	125	22	0	22	8	4	410	3	420
Powdered milk, dry													
nonfat	¼ cup	90	0	0.0	100	13	1	11	8	0	310	0	410
whole	¼ cup	140	8	4.5	105	11	0	10	8	3	480	0	370
Silk soy milk	1 cup	110	5	0.5	90	9	2	6	8	3	450	1	380
chocolate	1 cup	150	5	1.0	85	19	3	15	9	3	470	3	440
organic unsweetened	1 cup	80	5	0.5	80	4	2	0	7	3	300	1	300
vanilla	1 cup	100	4	0.5	85	11	1	9	6	3	470	1	300
Very	1 cup	130	4	0.5	90	18	1	16	6	3	470	1	300

MILK & YOGURT

Milk & Alternatives	Amount	Calories	Fat (g)	Saturated Fat (g)	Sodium (mg)	Carbohydrate (g)	Fiber (g)	Sugar (g)	Protein (g)	Vitamin D (mcg)	Calcium (mg)	Iron (mg)	Potassium (mg)
Skim/nonfat milk	1 cup	80	0	0.0	135	13	0	12	8	5	300	0	430
Strawberry milk, Nesquik, 1%	1 cup	160	3	1.5	120	26	0	26	8	3	300	0	360
Whole milk	1 cup	160	8	5.0	135	12	0	12	8	5	310	0	410
Yogurt & Alternatives													
Almond	1 cup	120	3	0.0	30	22	1	11	5	0	150	1	90
Silk, mixed berry acai	1 (5 oz)	180	11	1.0	75	19	3	14	5	3	130	1	210
Greek													
Chobani, mixed berry	1 (5 oz)	140	3	1.5	75	17	0	14	11	0	130	0	188
Chobani Less Sugar, Clingstone peach	1 (5 oz)	110	3	1.5	50	10	0	9	12	0	130	0	188
Stonyfield, vanilla	1 (7 oz)	170	5	3.5	55	18	0	15	14	1	150	0	180
Yoplait, Greek 100	1 (5 oz)	100	0	0.0	55	10	0	7	15	2	160	0	210
Light													
Yoplait, strawberry	1 (6 oz)	80	0	0.0	75	15	0	7	5	3	210	0	260
Low-fat													
Dannon, vanilla	1 (5 oz)	140	2	1.5	90	24	0	22	7	0	325	0	310
Original, flavored													
Dannon, creamy strawberry	1 (4 oz)	70	0	0.0	60	14	0	10	4	3	195	0	190
Dannon, fruit on the bottom strawberry	1 (5 oz)	130	2	1.0	90	25	0	21	5	2	195	0	282
Yoplait original, vanilla	1 (6 oz)	150	1	0.5	75	30	0	21	5	3	180	0	240
Plain, Dannon													
low-fat	1 (6 oz)	110	3	1.5	110	12	0	10	8	0	310	0	380
nonfat	1 (6 oz)	80	0	0.0	115	13	0	10	8	0	320	0	390
whole milk	1 (6 oz)	110	6	4.0	85	7	0	7	6	0	230	0	290
Soy													
Silk, peach mango	1 (5 oz)	120	4	0.0	85	17	2	12	6	2	200	1	370
Yogurt Drinks & Squeeze Yogurts													
Drinkable yogurt													
Activia probiotic yogurt drink, strawberry	7 oz	160	4	2.0	115	25	2	22	7	4	290	0	360
Chobani Greek yogurt, strawberry banana	7 oz	140	4	2.5	90	18	0	15	10	0	195	0	376
Stonyfield probiotic smoothie, wild berry	6 oz	110	2	1.0	85	17	0	15	6	2	210	0	280
Yogurt tubes													
Stonyfield, Cherry & Berry	1 tube	50	1	0.5	35	8	0	6	2	1	80	0	110
Yoplait GoGurt, Strawberry Splash & Cool Cotton Candy	3 tubes	150	0	0.0	75	30	0	23	6	3	440	0	240
Yoplait smoothies	7 oz	150	3	2.0	85	23	0	18	5	3	200	0	260

NUTS, SEEDS & NUT/SEED BUTTERS	Amount	Calories	Fat (g)	Saturated Fat (g)	Sodium (mg)	Carbohydrate (g)	Fiber (g)	Sugar (g)	Protein (g)	Vitamin D (mcg)	Calcium (mg)	Iron (mg)	Potassium (mg)
Almond butter	1 T	98	9	1.0	36	3	2	1	3	0	56	1	120
Almond paste	1 T	65	4	0.5	1	7	1	5	1	0	24	0	45
Almonds	23	160	14	1.0	1	6	3	1	6	0	74	1	202
Brazil nuts	8	264	27	6.5	1	5	3	1	6	0	64	1	264
Cashew butter	1 T	97	8	1.5	47	5	0	1	2	0	10	1	72
Cashews, salted	18	160	13	3.0	181	9	1	1	4	0	13	2	160
Chestnuts	3	59	1	0.0	0	13	1	3	1	0	7	0	142
Filberts/hazelnuts	20	188	18	1.0	0	5	3	1	4	0	34	1	204
Flax seeds	2 T	112	9	1.0	6	6	6	0	4	0	54	1	171
Macadamias	11	197	21	3.5	97	4	2	1	2	0	19	1	100
Mixed nuts, salted													
w/ peanuts	¼ cup	215	19	2.5	111	7	3	2	7	0	33	1	214
w/o peanuts	¼ cup	217	20	2.5	114	8	3	2	6	0	48	1	218
Nutella	2 T	200	11	3.5	15	22	1	21	3	0	40	2	151
Peanut butter													
chunky	2 T	190	17	2.5	117	6	2	3	8	0	14	6	238
creamy	2 T	195	17	3.0	114	5	2	1	8	0	14	1	250
natural	2 T	190	16	3.0	110	7	3	2	8	0	18	1	201
reduced fat	2 T	187	12	2.0	194	13	2	3	9	0	13	1	241
Peanuts													
Beer Nuts original peanuts	1 oz	160	10	2.5	110	9	2	0	7	0	16	1	185
dry roasted, salted	1 oz	170	15	2.5	91	4	3	1	8	0	17	0	206
honey roasted	1 oz	223	18	3.0	136	12	3	6	8	0	19	1	210
Pecans	20	104	11	1.0	0	2	1	1	1	0	10	0	62
Pine nuts	¼ cup	227	23	2.0	1	4	1	1	5	0	5	2	201
Pistachio nuts, salted	32	92	8	1.0	62	4	2	1	3	0	16	1	155
Poppy seeds	1 T	45	4	0.5	2	2	2	0	2	0	127	1	63
Pumpkin/squash seeds	2 T	103	9	2.0	3	3	1	0	5	0	9	1	141
Sesame butter/tahini	1 T	89	8	1.0	17	3	1	0	3	0	64	1	62
Sesame seeds	2 T	101	10	1.5	8	2	2	0	3	0	10	1	59
Soynut butter	2 T	170	11	1.5	140	10	3	3	7	0	60	0	324
Soy nuts, salted	3 T	160	9	1.5	55	11	6	1	12	0	40	1	508
Sunflower seeds, salted	2 T	104	9	1.0	83	4	2	0	3	0	13	1	151
Trail mix													
w/ chocolate chips	¼ cup	175	11	2.0	51	17	2	12	4	0	28	1	172
w/ fruit, tropical	¼ cup	158	9	1.0	47	18	2	13	4	0	22	1	183
w/ seeds	¼ cup	177	12	2.0	44	16	2	8	5	0	40	1	237
Walnuts, chopped	2 T	98	10	1.0	0	2	1	0	2	0	15	0	66

PASTA, RICE & OTHER GRAINS

Pasta*	Amount	Calories	Fat (g)	Saturated Fat (g)	Sodium (mg)	Carbohydrate (g)	Fiber (g)	Sugar (g)	Protein (g)	Vitamin D (mcg)	Calcium (mg)	Iron (mg)	Potassium (mg)
Cellophane noodles, dry	1 cup	176	0	0.0	4	44	2	9	0	0	30	0	0
Chow mein noodles, can	1 cup	292	18	3.0	212	29	1	0	6	0	12	1	50
Couscous	1 cup	178	0	0.0	302	37	2	0	6	0	13	1	93
Egg noodles	1 cup	221	3	1.0	264	40	2	1	8	0	19	2	61
Gnocchi, potato	1 cup	250	12	7.0	541	32	2	2	4	0	41	1	256
Macaroni/pasta	1 cup	308	1	0.0	36	63	4	1	11	0	29	4	239
whole wheat	1 cup	174	1	0.0	4	37	4	1	7	0	21	1	62
Pastina	1 cup	219	3	0.0	378	40	2	1	7	0	19	2	61
Pierogi, potato, frozen													
w/ cheese	4 (1.3 oz)	280	9	2.0	660	43	2	2	7	0	50	2	260
w/o cheese	4 (1.3 oz)	220	3	0	560	44	3	4	6	0	60	3	300
Ramen noodles w/ seasoning	1 cup	67	3	1.5	790	26	0	0	2	0	0	0	28
Ravioli w/o sauce													
beef	9 (2 in)	257	10	4.0	1053	24	1	0	17	0	43	3	193
cheese	9 (2 in)	232	8	4.0	875	29	1	0	10	0	132	2	165
Rice noodles	1 cup	187	0	0.0	438	42	2	0	3	0	7	0	7
Soba noodles	1 cup	113	0	0.0	68	24	1	1	6	0	5	1	40
Spaghetti	1 cup	207	2	0.0	329	42	5	1	8	0	18	2	133
Tortellini w/o sauce													
beef	1 cup	280	5	2.0	350	47	3	1	11	0	20	4	245
cheese	1 cup	354	8	4.0	234	54	2	1	16	0	166	1	32
Rice													
Basmati	1 cup	204	0	0.0	387	44	1	0	4	0	16	2	55
Brown	1 cup	238	2	0.5	394	50	3	0	5	0	6	1	168
instant	1 cup	360	4	0.0	0	78	4	0	8	0	0	0	140
Pilaf	1 cup	280	6	1.0	853	50	1	1	7	0	60	2	115
Rice-A-Roni, chicken	1 cup	250	7	1.5	800	41	1	1	5	0	10	2	90
lower sodium	1 cup	220	4	1.0	500	41	1	0	5	0	20	2	400
Risotto w/ cream sauce	1 cup	440	19	8.0	795	37	3	1	14	1	259	1	282
Spanish	1 cup	245	2	0.5	765	48	3	4	7	0	51	3	306
White	1 cup	204	0	0.0	387	44	1	0	4	0	16	2	55
instant	1 cup	340	0	0.0	0	76	0	0	8	0	0	2	30
Wild	1 cup	164	0	0.0	238	21	2	1	4	0	3	1	100
Other Grains													
Barley													
pearled	½ cup	97	0	0.0	2	22	3	0	2	0	9	3	280
whole	½ cup	104	0	0.0	159	24	3	0	2	0	9	1	79
Buckwheat/kasha	½ cup	78	0	0.0	123	17	2	1	3	0	6	1	75
Bulgur	½ cup	58	0	0.0	154	13	3	0	2	0	7	1	48
Millet	½ cup	101	1	0.0	143	1	1	0	3	0	3	1	53

* Cooked unless indicated.

PASTA, RICE & OTHER GRAINS

Other Grains	Amount	Calories	Fat (g)	Saturated Fat (g)	Sodium (mg)	Carbohydrate (g)	Fiber (g)	Sugar (g)	Protein (g)	Vitamin D (mcg)	Calcium (mg)	Iron (mg)	Potassium (mg)
Polenta													
fried, slice													
w/ oil	1 (4 oz)	199	14	2.0	300	16	0	1	2	0	0	2	57
w/o oil	1 (4 oz)	80	0	0.0	300	16	0	1	2	0	0	2	57
w/ water	1 cup	140	0	0.0	0	32	4	1	3	0	10	2	50
Quinoa, dry	¼ cup	157	3	0.5	4	27	3	1	6	0	20	2	239
Semolina, dry	1 T	38	0	0.0	0	8	0	0	1	0	2	0	19

POULTRY

Chicken	Amount	Calories	Fat (g)	Saturated Fat (g)	Sodium (mg)	Carbohydrate (g)	Fiber (g)	Sugar (g)	Protein (g)	Vitamin D (mcg)	Calcium (mg)	Iron (mg)	Potassium (mg)
Breasts													
BBQ w/ skin	3 oz	149	7	2.0	280	0	0	0	22	0	14	0	235
breaded & fried w/ skin	3 oz	221	11	3.0	234	8	0	0	21	0	11	1	207
deli	1 oz	50	2	0.5	93	0	0	0	7	0	5	0	78
fried													
w/ skin & flour	3 oz	222	9	2.0	76	2	0	0	32	0	16	1	259
w/o skin	3 oz	188	4	1.0	435	9	0	0	28	0	19	1	345
roasted													
w/ skin	3 oz	197	8	2.0	60	0	0	0	30	0	14	1	245
w/o skin	3 oz	165	4	1.0	63	0	0	0	31	0	15	1	256
Capon, roasted, w/ skin	3 oz	229	12	3.0	42	0	0	0	29	0	14	1	255
Cornish hens, roasted													
w/ skin	3 oz	220	16	4.5	54	0	0	0	19	0	11	1	208
w/o skin	3 oz	114	3	1.0	54	0	0	0	20	0	11	1	212
Giblets, fried	3 oz	277	13	4.0	96	4	0	0	33	0	18	10	330
Gizzards, simmered	3 oz	154	3	1.0	56	0	0	0	30	0	17	3	179
Hearts, simmered	3 oz	185	8	2.0	48	0	0	0	26	0	19	9	132
Hot dogs, chicken	1 (1.6 oz)	134	10	2.0	519	2	0	1	7	0	89	1	223
Legs													
breaded & fried w/ skin	3 oz	273	16	4.0	237	9	0	0	22	0	18	1	189
fried													
w/ skin & flour	3 oz	254	14	4.0	75	3	0	0	27	0	13	1	233
w/o skin	3 oz	247	13	2.5	82	0	0	0	24	0	21	1	233
roasted													
w/ skin	3 oz	184	9	2.5	74	0	0	0	24	0	12	1	264
w/o skin	3 oz	162	7	2.0	81	0	0	0	24	0	10	1	259
Livers, simmered	3 oz	167	7	2.0	76	1	0	0	24	0	11	12	263
Pâté, chicken liver, can	1 oz	201	13	4.0	109	7	0	0	13	0	10	9	95
Patties, breaded & fried	1 (3 oz)	220	9	2.0	300	16	1	1	18	0	0	1	222
Strips, breaded & fried	4 (1.6 oz)	511	28	5.5	1432	31	2	1	34	1	31	1	659

POULTRY

Chicken	Amount	Calories	Fat (g)	Saturated Fat (g)	Sodium (mg)	Carbohydrate (g)	Fiber (g)	Sugar (g)	Protein (g)	Vitamin D (mcg)	Calcium (mg)	Iron (mg)	Potassium (mg)
Thighs													
breaded & fried w/ skin	3 oz	277	17	4.5	288	9	1	0	22	0	18	1	192
fried													
w/ skin & flour	3 oz	262	15	4.0	88	3	0	0	27	0	14	1	237
w/o skin	3 oz	190	6	1.5	463	0	0	0	25	0	22	1	256
roasted													
w/ skin	3 oz	232	15	4.0	102	0	0	0	23	0	9	1	253
w/o skin	3 oz	179	8	2.5	106	0	0	0	25	0	9	1	269
Wings													
fried w/ skin & flour	1 (1 oz)	321	22	6.0	22	2	0	0	7	0	15	1	177
roasted w/ skin	1 (1 oz)	254	17	5.0	98	0	0	0	23	0	18	1	212
Game													
Duck, roasted													
w/ skin	3 oz	338	28	10.0	221	0	0	0	19	0	11	3	203
w/o skin	3 oz	200	11	4.0	227	0	0	0	23	0	12	3	251
Goose, roasted													
w/ skin	3 oz	305	21	7.0	70	0	0	0	25	0	13	3	329
w/o skin	3 oz	238	13	4.5	76	0	0	0	29	0	14	3	388
Ostrich													
ground	3 oz	165	8	2.0	72	0	0	0	20	0	7	3	291
tenderloin	3 oz	123	3	1.0	86	0	0	0	22	0	6	5	320
Pheasant, roasted													
w/ skin	3 oz	205	11	3.0	45	0	0	0	26	0	14	1	230
w/o skin	3 oz	151	4	1.5	42	0	0	0	27	0	3	0	223
Quail, roasted													
w/ skin	3 oz	218	14	4.0	60	0	0	0	22	0	13	4	183
w/o skin	3 oz	152	5	1.5	58	0	0	0	25	0	15	5	268
Turkey													
Bacon	2 slices (1 oz)	104	7	2.0	573	1	0	1	8	0	46	1	189
Breast, deli	1 oz	100	2	0.5	922	0	0	2	16	0	7	0	401
Dark meat, roasted													
w/ skin	3 oz	206	10	3.0	105	0	0	0	27	0	17	1	228
w/o skin	3 oz	173	6	2.0	104	0	0	0	28	0	17	1	227
Ground													
extra lean	3 oz	120	2	0.5	65	0	0	0	28	0	5	1	303
lean	3 oz	128	7	2.0	59	0	0	0	16	0	18	1	181
Ham, deli	1 oz	124	4	1.0	1038	3	0	0	20	0	5	1	299
Hot dogs	1 (1.6 oz)	140	12	3.0	560	1	0	1	7	0	89	1	223
Light meat, roasted													
w/ skin	3 oz	177	6	1.5	101	0	0	0	30	0	11	1	248
w/o skin	3 oz	147	2	0.5	99	0	0	0	30	0	9	1	249
Pastrami, deli	1 oz	41	2	1.0	302	0	0	0	6	0	3	1	59
Patties, breaded & fried	1 (3 oz)	241	15	4.0	680	13	0	0	12	0	13	2	259
Sausages	1 (2 oz)	93	6	1.5	470	0	0	0	11	0	11	0	103

RESTAURANT FAVORITES

Appetizers	Amount	Calories	Fat (g)	Saturated Fat (g)	Sodium (mg)	Carbohydrate (g)	Fiber (g)	Sugar (g)	Protein (g)	Vitamin D (mcg)	Calcium (mg)	Iron (mg)	Potassium (mg)
Breadsticks	1 medium	147	6	1.5	264	19	1	0	5	0	37	2	57
Bruschetta	1 (4 in)	73	3	0.5	113	9	1	1	2	0	21	1	80
Buffalo wings	4	353	27	9.0	1044	4	0	3	25	0	38	1	310
Clams casino	6	211	9	2.0	587	18	2	4	35	0	16	2	286
Crab cakes, fried	1 (4 oz)	290	19	4.0	893	20	0	1	9	0	88	1	243
Focaccia bread	1 slice (6 in)	284	9	1.0	640	41	2	2	10	0	40	4	130
Garlic bread	1 slice (4 in)	136	6	2.0	242	16	0	1	3	0	10	1	40
Jalapeño poppers	6	360	22	10.0	810	32	3	6	7	1	186	3	349
Mozzarella sticks	4	572	32	12.0	1516	44	4	4	26	0	588	1	190
Mushrooms													
fried	8	346	20	0.0	507	38	2	3	7	0	40	2	298
stuffed	3	211	11	3.0	480	20	2	3	4	1	8	2	292
Nachos, deluxe	1 order	1133	66	19.0	1881	87	8	6	52	0	702	3	908
Onion rings	5	175	10	1.5	288	20	1	2	2	0	36	0	76
Oysters Rockefeller	6	186	10	4.5	624	13	3	2	11	0	152	5	364
Pork dumplings, fried	1 (3.5 oz)	263	17	4.0	463	22	1	6	7	0	31	3	214
Potato skins	6	416	26	9.0	876	34	3	2	13	0	296	1	792
Shrimp cocktail w/ sauce	5	141	2	0.5	585	12	1	5	2	0	80	1	251
Spring rolls w/ meat	1 (2.5 oz)	111	3	0.5	389	17	1	4	6	0	35	1	219
Wontons w/ meat	1 (0.7 oz)	190	11	2.5	464	14	0	3	9	0	29	1	299
Desserts													
Apple pie à la mode	1 (6 oz)	418	20	9.0	366	56	2	14	5	0	100	1	211
Caramel apple bar	1 (4 oz)	395	22	14.0	210	51	3	39	2	0	35	1	131
Carrot cake w/ icing	1 (4 oz)	428	27	9.0	234	46	2	34	4	0	33	1	122
Cheesecake	1 (3 oz)	321	23	10.0	438	26	0	22	6	0	51	1	90
Chocolate chip cookie	1 (2 oz)	419	19	6.0	290	65	2	32	3	0	13	3	106
Chocolate mousse cake	1 (3 oz)	299	20	10.0	130	30	2	21	3	0	60	1	110
Chocolate peanut butter pie	1 (6 oz)	650	49	25.0	330	43	3	30	9	0	40	2	118
Crème brûlée	¾ cup	215	5	3.0	146	35	0	35	8	2	227	0	295
Fortune cookie	1	30	0	0.0	2	7	0	4	0	0	1	0	3
Fudge brownie sundae	1 (8 oz)	706	42	23.0	229	84	4	65	8	0	193	1	485
Key lime pie	1 (4.5 oz)	352	17	13.0	242	45	1	34	5	0	138	1	188
Smoothie	1 (16 fl oz)	272	5	2.0	121	50	5	36	10	3	350	1	778
Tiramisu	1 (5 oz)	354	24	14.0	155	30	0	19	6	1	66	1	156
Entrées													
American													
Baked potato w/ broccoli & cheese	1 (11 oz)	444	20	12.0	734	56	6	3	13	0	227	3	1420
BBQ beef sandwich	1 (6.5 oz)	600	35	11.0	1310	50	2	20	26	0	200	4	601
BBQ pork sandwich	1 (6.5 oz)	209	4	1.0	582	30	1	16	12	0	57	1	244
BBQ ribs	8 oz	776	50	18.0	879	29	1	23	48	1	102	4	691
Chicken fried steak	8 oz	612	35	12.0	887	27	1	0	48	1	61	5	488
Eggs Benedict	2 eggs	878	67	35.0	1526	27	2	4	43	4	189	5	1014
Filet mignon	8 oz	734	56	22.0	129	0	0	0	54	1	20	7	749
Fried shrimp	12 large	432	24	4.0	914	22	1	2	31	1	161	2	289

RESTAURANT FAVORITES

Entrées	Amount	Calories	Fat (g)	Saturated Fat (g)	Sodium (mg)	Carbohydrate (g)	Fiber (g)	Sugar (g)	Protein (g)	Vitamin D (mcg)	Calcium (mg)	Iron (mg)	Potassium (mg)
Grilled salmon	8 oz	468	28	5.5	138	0	0	0	50	26	260	1	872
King crab legs	9 oz	248	4	0.0	2735	0	0	0	50	0	150	2	668
Lobster Newburg	2 cups	1186	98	54.0	2320	20	0	12	57	5	542	2	986
Prime rib	12 oz	1160	92	37.0	216	0	0	0	76	0	34	8	1100
Shrimp Creole w/ rice	2 cups	598	18	3.0	2120	58	4	5	50	0	374	2	554
Shrimp jambalaya	2 cups	768	36	9.0	2524	73	2	4	35	0	90	3	831
Stuffed shrimp	2 cups	488	25	6.0	1510	17	1	1	46	1	222	2	554
T-bone steak	10 oz	453	21	8.0	99	0	0	0	63	0	59	5	743
Turkey & cheese bagel	1 (11 oz)	478	14	7.0	1636	61	2	4	26	1	309	2	418
Asian													
Beef & broccoli	2 cups	682	46	8.0	1906	23	6	6	46	0	148	5	1332
Cashew chicken	2 cups	947	48	9.0	1774	41	4	13	88	0	113	6	1689
Chicken curry	2 cups	508	31	7.5	1804	31	7	12	31	0	96	4	1344
Egg rolls, meatless	1 (2.5 oz)	172	9	1.5	296	19	2	4	4	0	30	1	134
Kung pao chicken	2 cups	418	23	4.0	1302	22	5	10	32	0	65	2	706
Pork chow mein w/ noodles	2 cups	630	28	9.0	1430	49	7	7	46	1	88	6	950
Shrimp & snow peas	2 cups	488	19	3.5	1223	19	4	6	60	0	243	5	1005
Stir-fry chicken & fried rice	2 cups	686	15	2.5	1422	109	4	2	29	0	48	2	396
Sushi w/ fish & vegetables	1 cup	140	1	0.0	642	28	2	3	4	0	9	0	71
Sushi rolls w/ rice													
fish	1 small	29	0	0.0	103	5	0	0	2	0	1	0	36
vegetarian	1 small	20	0	0.0	79	4	0	0	0	0	1	0	15
Sweet & sour pork w/ rice	2 cups	898	35	6.5	1634	96	4	36	49	1	137	5	1098
Tofu & vegetable stir-fry	2 cups	293	14	2.0	445	34	10	2	15	0	279	7	524
Italian/Mediterranean													
Calzone w/ pepperoni	1 (6 oz)	1450	74	24.5	1840	131	6	3	62	1	746	10	670
Chicken cacciatore	2 cups	850	52	12.5	1500	34	5	8	64	0	204	5	1416
Chicken cordon bleu	1 cup	294	13	4.5	846	13	1	1	32	0	136	2	357
Chicken Marsala	8 oz	346	15	4.0	1330	5	0	1	49	0	64	1	571
Chicken/veal parmigiana	8 oz	395	19	6.0	941	19	2	4	37	0	268	2	517
Fettuccine Alfredo	2 cups	1186	73	44.0	884	106	6	4	28	1	290	4	268
Gyro	½ pita	326	9	0.5	92	9	1	1	6	0	23	1	102
Linguine w/ pesto sauce	2 cups	735	57	9.0	771	43	4	2	17	0	207	4	329
Moussaka	2 cups	390	22	8.0	730	19	6	12	29	1	236	4	914
Pasta carbonara	2 cups	764	25	8.0	724	100	6	2	33	1	285	5	290
Pasta marinara	2 cups	520	6	1.0	1010	99	9	15	18	0	85	5	880
Seafood Alfredo	2 cups	1033	47	16.0	1399	104	4	17	45	2	180	3	307
Shrimp scampi	2 cups	538	33	5.0	262	5	0	0	53	0	224	2	430
Spanakopita	8 oz	305	23	7.0	573	17	2	2	8	1	200	3	344
Stuffed grape leaves	4	372	27	4.0	372	31	7	6	5	0	199	3	340
Veal scallopini	8 oz	670	49	13.5	1042	4	1	2	52	1	109	2	754
Vegetarian lasagna	2 cups	930	47	25.0	1916	73	6	12	56	1	1344	4	1030

RESTAURANT FAVORITES

Entrées	Amount	Calories	Fat (g)	Saturated Fat (g)	Sodium (mg)	Carbohydrate (g)	Fiber (g)	Sugar (g)	Protein (g)	Vitamin D (mcg)	Calcium (mg)	Iron (mg)	Potassium (mg)
Mexican & Tex-Mex													
Chimichangas, beef & cheese	1 (6.5 oz)	454	21	7.0	1172	49	5	5	16	0	225	4	424
Enchiladas													
cheese	2 (6 in)	420	28	12.0	538	28	5	5	17	0	466	1	372
seafood	2 (6 in)	734	36	20.0	1174	56	3	9	38	0	500	4	576
Fajitas w/ tortillas													
chicken	1 (9 oz)	370	17	5.5	980	34	3	6	22	0	129	3	455
steak	1 (9 oz)	380	16	6.0	807	34	3	6	24	0	131	3	513
Huevos rancheros	1 order	280	15	4.0	988	21	4	5	16	2	113	3	516
Quesadillas	1 (2 oz)	486	25	11.5	959	46	3	4	18	0	453	3	155
Rice & beans	2 cups	558	14	2.0	786	86	13	1	22	0	184	9	1112
Salads*													
Caesar	3 cups	481	40	8.0	1152	23	6	5	10	0	250	3	613
Chicken Caesar	4 cups	618	34	8.0	952	16	4	4	58	0	200	4	860
Greek	14 oz	448	38	14.0	925	19	4	11	13	0	325	2	595
Niçoise	12 oz	398	19	3.0	455	39	9	3	23	4	122	6	1277
Oriental chicken	9 oz	197	17	2.0	207	9	2	3	4	0	45	1	220
Tossed w/ gorgonzola	4 cups	398	29	6.0	325	33	4	26	7	0	138	1	293
Side Dishes													
Garlic mashed potatoes	1 cup	252	10	6.0	1599	34	3	3	9	0	190	1	643
Grilled vegetables	1½ cups	78	5	0.5	84	8	2	0	1	0	21	0	398
Oven roasted potatoes	1½ cups	224	0	0.0	381	51	4	4	5	0	12	1	933
Polenta	½ cup	70	0	0.0	85	15	1	0	1	0	5	1	25
Ratatouille	1 cup	140	10	1.5	327	12	4	7	2	0	45	1	471
Risotto	½ cup	281	15	9.0	851	29	1	0	7	0	112	1	72
Soft pretzels	1 large	493	6	2.0	1110	99	2	0	12	0	33	5	123
Soups													
Borscht	1 cup	93	4	2.5	348	11	2	7	3	0	56	1	299
Cheese	1 cup	166	7	5.0	926	20	3	11	5	1	201	0	241
Chicken chili	1 cup	143	2	0.0	578	18	5	3	15	0	50	2	417
Chilled fruit	1 cup	68	0	0.0	19	17	2	14	1	0	22	1	257
Clam chowder	1 cup	134	3	2.0	1000	19	3	4	7	0	67	3	384
Egg drop	1 cup	66	2	0.5	903	11	1	0	3	0	17	1	54
French onion, w/ cheese toast	1 cup	369	16	7.5	1030	39	2	6	17	0	328	3	374
Gazpacho	1 cup	95	6	1.0	625	10	3	6	2	0	34	1	508
Hot & sour	1 cup	95	3	0.5	917	11	1	1	6	0	46	2	134
Minestrone	1 cup	143	3	0.5	611	23	4	3	8	0	63	3	479
Seafood stew	1 cup	225	9	2.0	506	5	1	1	31	7	75	2	638
Shrimp gumbo	1 cup	149	5	2.0	922	11	2	4	16	0	161	3	471
Tomato Florentine	1 cup	140	2	0.0	1600	26	2	9	5	0	100	2	504
Vichyssoise	1 cup	62	2	1.0	324	9	1	3	2	1	68	0	153
Wonton	1 cup	77	1	0.0	978	13	0	1	5	0	12	1	77

* Dressing included.

SALADS

	Amount	Calories	Fat (g)	Saturated Fat (g)	Sodium (mg)	Carbohydrate (g)	Fiber (g)	Sugar (g)	Protein (g)	Vitamin D (mcg)	Calcium (mg)	Iron (mg)	Potassium (mg)
Caesar w/ dressing	1 cup	160	13	3.0	384	8	2	2	3	0	83	1	204
Carrot-raisin	½ cup	208	15	2.5	176	17	2	11	1	0	30	1	309
Chef													
w/ dressing	1 cup	312	23	7.5	924	9	2	5	17	1	150	2	566
w/o dressing	1 cup	178	11	5.5	496	3	2	4	17	1	28	1	306
Chicken w/ mayonnaise	½ cup	236	18	3.0	351	3	0	2	16	0	14	0	199
Coleslaw													
w/ mayonnaise	½ cup	98	7	1.0	178	9	1	8	1	0	35	0	165
w/ vinaigrette	½ cup	41	2	0.0	14	7	1	6	1	0	36	0	179
Cucumber													
creamy w/ mayonnaise	½ cup	59	4	3.0	13	5	1	2	1	0	35	0	124
w/ vinegar	½ cup	26	0	0.0	188	6	0	4	0	0	11	0	98
Egg w/ mayonnaise	½ cup	286	26	5.0	420	1	0	1	11	2	47	1	117
Fruit, fresh	½ cup	40	0	0.0	3	10	1	7	1	0	7	0	143
Gelatin w/ fruit	½ cup	73	0	0.0	30	18	1	9	1	0	10	2	125
Ham	½ cup	273	20	6.0	1360	13	0	0	11	1	10	1	152
Lobster	½ cup	170	14	2.0	459	1	0	1	9	0	56	1	170
Macaroni w/ mayonnaise	½ cup	163	4	1.0	214	27	1	3	4	0	8	1	52
Pasta primavera	½ cup	152	4	1.0	311	26	2	2	4	0	45	1	184
Potato													
German-style	½ cup	95	3	1.0	158	15	2	1	3	0	15	1	390
w/ mayonnaise	½ cup	231	15	2.0	245	22	2	2	2	0	14	0	359
& eggs	½ cup	216	13	2.0	453	22	2	7	3	0	21	1	333
Seafood													
w/ mayonnaise	½ cup	191	16	2.5	579	0	0	1	10	0	67	1	166
w/ pasta, vinaigrette	½ cup	126	7	1.0	524	11	1	1	5	1	5	1	132
Shrimp w/ mayonnaise	½ cup	204	10	1.5	299	1	0	2	7	0	28	1	53
Spinach w/o dressing	1 cup	60	4	0.0	146	2	1	0	5	0	61	2	342
Tabbouleh	1 cup	202	16	2.0	792	15	3	2	3	0	32	1	246
Taco													
w/ salsa	1 (16 oz)	170	9	3.0	363	15	3	1	7	0	95	2	229
& shell	1 (19 oz)	400	22	7.0	720	39	5	3	11	0	166	4	290
Three bean w/ oil	½ cup	81	4	0.5	200	10	3	3	3	0	20	1	158
Tortellini, cheese	½ cup	189	14	3.0	561	14	2	1	5	0	95	1	87
Tossed w/o dressing	1 cup	28	0	0.0	24	7	2	3	1	0	41	1	219
Tuna w/ mayonnaise	½ cup	233	19	3.0	493	3	0	2	12	1	24	1	184
Waldorf w/ dressing	½ cup	118	10	1.0	59	8	1	6	1	0	11	0	99

SALAD DRESSINGS*

SALAD DRESSINGS*	Amount	Calories	Fat (g)	Saturated Fat (g)	Sodium (mg)	Carbohydrate (g)	Fiber (g)	Sugar (g)	Protein (g)	Vitamin D (mcg)	Calcium (mg)	Iron (mg)	Potassium (mg)
Blue cheese	1 T	74	8	1.5	98	1	0	1	0	0	6	0	14
fat-free	1 T	18	0	0.0	135	4	0	1	0	0	8	0	32
light	1 T	15	1	0.5	144	0	0	0	1	0	14	0	1
Buttermilk	1 T	63	7	1.0	132	1	0	1	0	0	4	0	9
Caesar	1 T	80	9	1.5	178	0	0	0	0	0	7	0	4
fat-free	1 T	18	0	0.0	177	4	0	1	0	0	5	0	7
light	1 T	16	0	0.0	172	3	0	2	0	0	4	0	4
Catalina	1 T	65	6	1.0	103	3	0	3	0	0	4	0	17
fat-free	1 T	40	0	0.0	300	10	0	6	0	0	1	0	13
Chipotle ranch	1 T	150	7	1.0	130	1	0	1	0	0	0	0	0
Creamy parmesan	1 T	70	8	1.0	135	1	0	1	1	0	4	0	5
French	1 T	73	7	1.0	134	3	0	3	0	0	4	0	11
fat-free	1 T	132	0	0.0	853	32	0	16	0	0	5	1	84
light	1 T	36	2	0.0	136	5	0	3	0	0	2	0	17
Green Goddess	1 T	65	7	1.0	133	1	0	1	0	0	5	0	9
Honey mustard	1 T	72	6	1.0	80	4	0	2	0	0	2	0	3
Italian	1 T	35	3	0.5	146	2	0	2	0	0	2	0	12
creamy	1 T	63	7	1.0	132	1	0	1	0	0	4	0	9
fat-free	1 T	7	0	0.0	158	1	0	1	0	0	4	0	14
light	1 T	14	1	0.0	125	1	0	1	0	0	2	0	13
Oil & vinegar	1 T	43	4	0.5	243	2	0	1	0	0	1	0	7
Peppercorn parmesan	1 T	60	6	1.0	135	1	0	1	1	0	2	0	9
Ranch	1 T	65	7	1.0	135	1	0	1	0	0	4	0	10
fat-free	1 T	17	0	0.0	126	4	0	1	0	0	7	0	16
light	1 T	30	3	1.0	155	2	0	1	0	0	7	0	14
Russian	1 T	54	4	0.5	173	5	0	3	0	0	2	0	27
light	1 T	23	1	0.0	139	4	0	4	0	0	3	0	25
Sesame	1 T	66	7	1.0	150	1	0	1	0	0	3	0	24
Thousand Island	1 T	60	5	1.0	150	2	0	2	0	0	3	0	17
fat-free	1 T	21	0	0.0	126	5	1	3	0	0	2	0	20
light	1 T	30	2	0.0	146	4	0	3	0	0	4	0	31
Vinaigrette													
balsamic	1 T	45	4	1.0	155	2	0	2	0	0	0	0	0
raspberry, light	1 T	30	1	0.0	240	5	0	5	0	0	0	0	0
red wine	1 T	60	5	0.5	210	6	0	5	0	0	0	0	0
fat-free	1 T	15	0	0.0	115	4	0	3	0	0	0	0	0
light	1 T	23	2	0.5	160	2	0	1	0	0	0	0	0
Western	1 T	170	12	2.0	250	13	0	12	0	0	4	0	10
fat-free	1 T	25	0	0.0	140	6	0	1	0	0	1	0	13

* For mayonnaise/Miracle Whip, see Fats, Oils, Cream & Gravy.

SOUPS

Canned & Prepared

	Amount	Calories	Fat (g)	Saturated Fat (g)	Sodium (mg)	Carbohydrate (g)	Fiber (g)	Sugar (g)	Protein (g)	Vitamin D (mcg)	Calcium (mg)	Iron (mg)	Potassium (mg)
Bean													
w/ bacon	1 cup	172	6	1.5	896	23	8	4	8	0	84	2	496
w/ franks	1 cup	280	8	2.0	960	38	8	14	12	0	80	2	560
Beef barley w/ veg	1 cup	127	2	1.0	725	19	2	3	7	0	27	1	295
Beef broth	1 cup	17	1	0.5	893	0	0	0	3	0	14	0	130
reduced sodium	1 cup	14	0	0.0	540	0	0	0	3	0	7	0	48
Beef consommé	1 cup	7	0	0.0	372	0	0	0	1	0	6	0	54
Beef noodle	1 cup	171	6	1.5	793	11	1	1	18	0	34	2	320
Black bean	1 cup	114	2	0.5	1200	19	8	8	6	0	47	2	309
Cheddar cheese	1 cup	166	7	4.5	926	20	3	11	5	1	201	0	241
Chicken alphabet	1 cup	140	3	1.0	960	24	2	2	6	0	0	0	860
Chicken & dumplings	1 cup	99	3	1.5	737	11	2	1	7	0	27	1	282
Chicken & rice	1 cup	82	2	0.5	783	14	1	0	2	0	53	0	41
Chicken & stars	1 cup	140	2	0.5	790	10	0	0	3	0	10	0	60
Chicken broth	1 cup	14	1	0.0	890	1	0	1	2	0	10	0	43
reduced sodium	1 cup	17	0	0.0	554	1	0	1	3	0	19	1	204
Chicken gumbo	1 cup	56	1	0.5	954	8	2	2	3	0	24	1	76
Chicken noodle	1 cup	58	2	0.5	834	7	1	0	3	0	12	1	58
Chili beef w/ beans	1 cup	272	9	3.0	1140	33	8	5	15	0	84	3	671
Chunky, Campbell's													
chicken & sausage gumbo	1 cup	140	4	1.5	850	21	2	3	6	0	40	1	240
chicken corn chowder	1 cup	190	9	2.0	850	20	2	4	6	0	30	1	320
classic chicken noodle	1 cup	120	3	1.0	790	14	1	2	9	0	20	1	510
creamy chicken & dumplings	1 cup	170	10	2.0	800	14	1	2	7	0	30	1	150
hearty beef & barley	1 cup	150	2	0.5	790	23	4	4	9	0	30	1	350
New England clam chowder	1 cup	180	10	1.5	790	16	2	1	6	0	30	1	250
savory chicken w/ white & wild rice	1 cup	110	0	0.0	790	19	1	1	6	0	30	1	250
savory vegetable	1 cup	90	1	0.0	770	19	3	5	3	0	50	1	430
sirloin burger w/ country vegetables	1 cup	130	4	1.5	790	18	3	4	6	0	30	1	360
steak & potato	1 cup	120	3	1.0	790	17	1	0	6	0	10	1	300
Clam chowder													
Manhattan	1 cup	134	3	2.0	1000	19	3	4	7	0	67	3	384
New England	1 cup	151	5	2.5	682	19	1	7	8	1	176	3	466
Corn chowder	1 cup	91	5	2.0	312	8	1	4	4	1	92	1	219
Cream of asparagus	1 cup	149	7	2.5	880	17	1	7	6	1	184	1	365
Cream of broccoli	1 cup	68	4	1.5	353	6	1	4	3	1	80	0	174
Cream of celery	1 cup	151	8	3.0	687	15	1	8	6	1	196	1	315
Cream of chicken	1 cup	120	4	2.0	880	13	1	6	7	1	162	1	252
Cream of mushroom	1 cup	161	9	2.5	903	15	1	7	6	2	171	0	275
condensed	1 cup	158	10	2.0	1382	14	2	0	2	0	24	0	128
low-fat	1 cup	120	4	1.0	1500	18	2	0	2	0	20	0	100
low-fat	1 cup	140	5	1.0	820	20	0	4	2	0	20	0	960
reduced sodium	1 cup	126	5	2.0	523	16	1	9	6	1	171	1	657
Cream of potato	1 cup	154	5	2.5	796	22	1	8	6	1	176	0	399
Cream of shrimp	1 cup	151	8	5.0	878	14	0	7	7	1	171	1	236

SOUPS

Canned & Prepared	Amount	Calories	Fat (g)	Saturated Fat (g)	Sodium (mg)	Carbohydrate (g)	Fiber (g)	Sugar (g)	Protein (g)	Vitamin D (mcg)	Calcium (mg)	Iron (mg)	Potassium (mg)
Double Noodle, Campbell's	1 cup	100	2	0.5	790	17	1	0	3	0	10	1	40
Escarole	1 cup	74	2	1.0	446	7	2	4	7	1	179	3	698
French onion	1 cup	140	3	0.0	1580	24	2	10	4	0	60	0	320
Gazpacho	1 cup	95	6	1.0	625	10	3	6	2	0	34	1	508
Green pea	1 cup	320	6	2.5	1740	52	10	17	17	0	54	4	372
Healthy Request, Campbell's													
cream of mushroom	1 cup	140	5	1.0	820	20	0	4	2	0	20	0	960
chicken noodle	1 cup	120	4	1.0	820	16	0	0	6	0	20	1	1060
tomato	1 cup	140	0	0.0	820	32	2	16	4	0	20	1	1200
vegetable beef	1 cup	160	1	0.0	820	28	4	4	10	0	40	1	1400
Hot & sour	1 cup	95	3	0.5	917	11	1	1	6	0	46	2	134
Italian-style wedding	1 cup	120	4	1.5	690	15	1	2	6	0	0	0	320
Lentil	1 cup	159	4	0.5	464	22	8	3	10	0	30	3	342
Lobster bisque	1 cup	129	6	3.5	600	4	1	3	13	0	131	1	362
Matzo ball	1 cup	145	5	1.0	831	19	1	2	6	1	34	1	154
Minestrone	1 cup	82	2	0.5	629	11	1	2	4	0	39	1	308
Mushroom	1 cup	95	6	1.0	830	8	1	0	2	0	17	0	76
Oyster stew	1 cup	194	12	7.0	786	10	0	9	10	2	260	4	394
Pasta e fagioli	1 cup	228	6	1.5	531	33	6	2	12	0	134	3	423
Pepper pot	1 cup	47	2	1.5	174	3	0	1	3	0	18	0	180
Scotch broth	1 cup	97	4	1.0	156	7	1	2	7	0	10	1	189
Seafood chowder	1 cup	273	15	9.0	339	15	2	2	20	1	44	1	622
Split pea w/ ham	1 cup	195	4	1.5	762	28	4	5	12	0	35	2	321
Tomato													
bisque	1 cup	220	5	3.0	1740	42	2	30	2	0	40	1	520
creamy, ready to serve	1 cup	83	5	3.5	208	8	2	4	1	0	12	0	154
reduced sodium	1 cup	57	1	0.5	33	9	1	7	2	1	66	1	185
regular													
w/ milk	1 cup	58	1	0.5	211	10	1	7	2	1	66	0	352
w/ water	1 cup	32	0	0.0	186	8	1	4	1	0	8	0	275
& rice	1 cup	116	3	0.5	788	21	2	7	2	0	27	1	319
Turkey noodle	1 cup	58	2	0.5	834	7	1	0	3	0	12	1	58
Vegetable													
non-vegetarian	1 cup	94	1	0.0	643	19	3	4	3	0	43	1	434
vegetarian	1 cup	72	2	0.5	629	12	1	4	2	0	24	1	207
Vegetable beef	1 cup	141	4	2.5	923	16	2	7	10	1	171	1	365
Vegetable broth	1 cup	12	0	0.0	710	2	0	1	1	0	7	0	46
Wild rice w/ chicken	1 cup	143	5	1.0	848	13	1	2	12	0	28	1	219
Dehydrated/Boxed													
Beef noodle	½ cup	190	7	3.5	790	26	1	1	4	0	0	2	85
Bouillon, dry													
regular	1 cube	10	1	0.0	966	1	0	1	1	0	15	0	15
beef	1 cube	6	0	0.0	864	1	0	1	1	0	2	0	15
chicken	1 cube	10	0	0.0	1150	1	0	0	1	0	9	0	18
vegetable	1 cup	13	0	0.0	269	2	0	0	0	0	2	0	24

SOUPS

Dehydrated/Boxed	Amount	Calories	Fat (g)	Saturated Fat (g)	Sodium (mg)	Carbohydrate (g)	Fiber (g)	Sugar (g)	Protein (g)	Vitamin D (mcg)	Calcium (mg)	Iron (mg)	Potassium (mg)
sodium-free													
beef	1 tsp	10	0	0.0	0	2	0	1	0	0	0	0	380
chicken	1 tsp	10	0	0.0	0	2	0	1	0	0	0	0	380
Chicken noodle	1 cup	56	1	0.5	561	9	0	1	2	0	4	0	32
Chicken rice	1 cup	58	1	0.5	931	9	1	0	2	0	7	0	11
Cup-a-Soup													
chicken noodle	1 cup	80	2	0.0	640	12	0	0	3	0	0	1	0
cream of chicken	1 cup	70	2	1.5	640	13	0	0	0	0	0	0	0
Cup Noodles													
beef	1 (14 oz)	290	11	5.0	1150	41	2	2	7	0	0	3	180
chicken	1 (14 oz)	290	11	5.0	1160	41	2	2	6	0	0	3	260
Leek	1 cup	60	1	0.0	690	12	0	0	1	0	0	0	150
Minestrone	1 cup	90	1	0.0	560	20	3	3	4	0	30	1	300
Miso	1 cup	79	4	0.5	1460	8	1	2	8	0	38	1	127
Onion	1 cup	30	0	0.0	851	7	1	0	1	0	22	0	76
Ramen noodle													
beef	1 cup	190	7	3.5	790	26	1	0	5	0	0	2	85
chicken	1 cup	190	7	3.5	790	26	1	0	5	0	0	2	90
shrimp	1 cup	190	7	3.5	860	26	1	0	5	0	0	2	90
Tomato	1 cup	101	2	1.0	943	19	1	10	2	0	77	0	294
Vegetable	1 cup	101	6	1.5	893	12	1	4	2	0	38	1	94
Vegetable beef	1 cup	110	1	0.0	790	22	3	2	4	0	40	1	182

VEGETABLES*

	Amount	Calories	Fat (g)	Saturated Fat (g)	Sodium (mg)	Carbohydrate (g)	Fiber (g)	Sugar (g)	Protein (g)	Vitamin D (mcg)	Calcium (mg)	Iron (mg)	Potassium (mg)
Alfalfa sprouts, raw	½ cup	4	0	0.0	1	0	0	0	1	0	5	0	13
Artichokes													
boiled/steamed	1 medium	64	0	0.0	72	14	7	1	3	0	25	1	343
hearts, marinated	½ cup	58	4	0.0	244	7	2	0	2	0	7	0	120
Asparagus, cooked	½ cup	44	2	0.5	114	4	2	2	2	0	23	2	194
Bamboo shoots, raw	½ cup	21	0	0.0	3	4	2	2	2	0	10	0	405
Bean sprouts, raw	½ cup	14	0	0.0	3	3	1	2	1	0	6	0	67
Beets, pickled	½ cup	55	0	0.0	177	14	1	9	1	0	9	0	98
Bok choy, cooked	½ cup	12	0	0.0	160	2	1	1	1	0	93	1	223
Broccoli													
cooked	½ cup	49	3	0.0	120	5	2	1	2	0	38	1	255
w/ cheese sauce	½ cup	90	5	3.0	260	7	2	1	5	0	132	1	241
florets, raw	½ cup	10	0	0.0	10	2	1	1	1	0	21	0	142
Brussels sprouts, cooked	½ cup	35	0	0.0	114	7	3	2	3	0	34	1	313
Cabbage													
cooked													
Chinese	½ cup	12	0	0.0	160	2	1	1	1	0	93	1	223
green	½ cup	40	2	0.0	105	5	2	3	1	0	31	0	133
red, raw	½ cup	14	0	0.0	12	3	1	2	1	0	20	0	110

* For dried beans, peas, and lentils, see Vegetarian Foods & Legumes.

VEGETABLES

	Amount	Calories	Fat (g)	Saturated Fat (g)	Sodium (mg)	Carbohydrate (g)	Fiber (g)	Sugar (g)	Protein (g)	Vitamin D (mcg)	Calcium (mg)	Iron (mg)	Potassium (mg)
Carrots													
cooked	½ cup	49	0	0.0	221	11	3	6	1	0	39	0	382
raw	1 large	30	0	0.0	50	7	2	3	1	0	24	0	230
Cauliflower													
cooked	½ cup	42	3	0.0	118	4	2	2	2	0	18	0	242
w/ cheese sauce	½ cup	85	6	1.5	310	7	1	3	3	1	247	0	149
raw	½ cup	14	0	0.0	17	3	1	1	1	0	12	0	165
Celery													
cooked	½ cup	30	2	0.5	166	2	1	1	1	0	33	0	210
raw	1 medium	6	0	0.0	32	1	1	1	0	0	16	0	104
Chinese-style, frozen	½ cup	40	1	0.0	10	8	2	4	1	0	40	0	320
Chives, raw	1 T	1	0	0.0	0	0	0	0	0	0	3	0	9
Corn, cooked													
cream-style, can	½ cup	92	1	0.0	365	23	2	4	2	0	4	1	168
on the cob	1 (4 oz)	86	1	0.0	15	29	3	3	3	0	2	1	270
w/ butter sauce, frozen	½ cup	91	1	0.0	394	20	1	6	2	0	0	4	0
whole kernel													
can	½ cup	55	1	0.0	168	12	2	4	2	0	2	0	108
frozen	½ cup	80	1	0.0	3	18	2	2	3	0	4	0	195
Cucumbers, raw													
w/ skin	½ large	23	0	0.0	3	5	1	3	1	0	24	0	221
w/o skin	½ large	14	0	0.0	3	3	1	2	1	0	20	0	191
Eggplant, cooked	½ cup	13	0	0.0	61	3	2	2	1	0	5	0	117
Endive, raw	1 cup	9	0	0.0	11	2	2	0	1	0	7	0	39
Green beans, cooked													
French	½ cup	20	0	0.0	380	3	1	1	1	0	40	0	100
snap	½ cup	22	0	0.0	150	5	2	2	1	0	28	0	91
Green onions, raw	¼ cup	8	0	0.0	4	2	1	1	0	0	18	0	69
Greens, cooked													
beet	½ cup	35	2	0.5	275	3	3	0	2	0	92	2	595
collard	½ cup	22	0	0.0	93	4	3	0	2	0	162	0	148
dandelion	½ cup	39	2	0.5	116	5	2	0	2	0	107	1	228
mustard	½ cup	20	0	0.0	102	4	2	1	2	0	86	1	289
turnip	½ cup	15	0	0.0	73	2	2	0	1	0	69	0	101
Hominy, cooked	½ cup	75	2	1.0	428	12	2	1	1	0	9	1	8
Jicama													
cooked	½ cup	25	0	0.0	3	6	3	1	1	0	7	0	89
raw	½ cup	25	0	0.0	3	6	3	1	0	0	8	0	98
Kale, cooked	½ cup	25	1	0.0	118	3	3	1	2	0	177	1	243
Kohlrabi, cooked	½ cup	43	2	0.5	125	5	3	2	1	0	21	0	300
Leeks, raw	¼ cup	14	0	0.0	5	3	0	1	0	0	13	0	41
Lettuce, raw	1 cup	5	0	0.0	7	1	0	0	0	0	9	0	59
Mixed vegetables, frozen	½ cup	83	3	0.5	135	12	4	3	3	0	22	1	152

VEGETABLES

	Amount	Calories	Fat (g)	Saturated Fat (g)	Sodium (mg)	Carbohydrate (g)	Fiber (g)	Sugar (g)	Protein (g)	Vitamin D (mcg)	Calcium (mg)	Iron (mg)	Potassium (mg)
Mushrooms													
can	½ cup	38	2	0.5	338	4	2	2	1	0	9	1	101
fried	5 medium	216	13	2.0	317	21	1	1	5	0	25	2	186
raw	½ cup	8	0	0.0	2	1	0	1	1	0	1	0	112
Okra, cooked	½ cup	28	0	0.0	106	6	3	1	2	0	71	1	257
Onions, raw	½ cup	32	0	0.0	3	7	1	3	1	0	18	0	117
Parsley, raw	¼ cup	5	0	0.0	8	1	1	0	0	0	21	1	83
Parsnips, cooked	½ cup	73	2	0.5	106	13	3	4	1	0	29	0	285
Pea pods, cooked	½ cup	35	0	0.0	100	6	2	3	2	0	36	2	167
Peas, green, cooked	½ cup	89	3	0.5	101	12	5	5	5	0	21	1	203
Peppers, raw													
bell, green/red/yellow	½ cup	15	0	0.0	2	3	1	2	1	0	8	0	131
chile, green, diced	½ cup	30	0	0.0	5	7	1	4	2	0	14	1	255
jalapeño	1 medium	5	0	0.0	1	1	0	1	0	0	2	0	43
Pimientos, can	¼ cup	11	0	0.0	7	2	1	1	1	0	3	1	76
Potatoes, cooked													
au gratin, box	½ cup	164	9	6.0	530	14	2	0	6	0	146	1	485
baked w/ skin	1 (4 oz)	214	0	0.0	416	49	3	4	4	0	12	1	895
blintz, frozen													
w/ cheese	1 (2.2 oz)	130	5	1.5	301	14	0	7	6	0	81	1	82
w/ fruit	1 (2.2 oz)	122	4	1.0	133	17	0	12	4	1	38	1	81
boiled w/o skin	1 (4 oz)	108	0	0.0	301	25	3	1	2	0	10	0	410
French fries, frozen	14 medium	45	3	0.5	74	6	0	0	1	0	2	0	87
hash browns, frozen	½ cup	174	9	1.0	319	23	3	0	2	0	14	0	393
knish, frozen	1 (2 oz)	213	12	2.5	223	21	1	0	5	1	13	1	95
mashed w/ margarine & milk	½ cup	119	4	1.0	350	18	2	1	2	0	22	0	343
O'Brien, frozen	½ cup	171	12	1.5	382	16	2	2	2	0	11	1	346
pancakes, homemade	1 medium (2.5 oz)	126	8	1.5	283	14	2	1	3	0	16	1	314
scalloped, box	½ cup	210	12	6.5	520	17	1	3	9	1	231	0	303
steak fries	7 medium	138	4	0.5	347	25	2	0	2	0	9	1	427
tots, frozen	10	189	12	2.0	337	20	2	0	2	0	10	0	194
twice baked w/ cheese	1 (5 oz)	146	6	3.5	442	18	2	2	5	1	274	1	473
Pumpkin, can	½ cup	69	3	1.0	18	10	3	4	1	0	32	2	245
Radishes, raw	10 medium	8	0	0.0	20	2	1	1	0	0	13	0	116
Rutabagas, cooked	½ cup	55	3	0.5	126	8	2	4	1	0	39	0	278
Salad greens, raw	1 cup	6	0	0.0	13	1	0	0	1	0	16	0	95
Sauerkraut, can	½ cup	14	0	0.0	470	3	4	1	1	0	21	1	121
Scallions, raw	1 T	2	0	0.0	1	0	0	0	0	0	4	0	17
Shallots, raw	1 T	7	0	0.0	1	2	0	1	0	0	4	0	33
Spinach													
cooked	½ cup	52	4	0.5	206	4	2	0	3	0	105	3	590
creamed	½ cup	86	6	3.5	431	7	2	1	2	0	82	2	409
raw	1 cup	6	0	0.0	20	1	1	0	1	0	25	1	140

VEGETABLES

	Amount	Calories	Fat (g)	Saturated Fat (g)	Sodium (mg)	Carbohydrate (g)	Fiber (g)	Sugar (g)	Protein (g)	Vitamin D (mcg)	Calcium (mg)	Iron (mg)	Potassium (mg)
Squash													
acorn, cooked	½ cup	58	0	0.0	4	15	5	2	1	0	45	1	448
butternut, cooked	½ cup	41	0	0.0	4	11	3	2	1	0	42	1	291
spaghetti, cooked	½ cup	21	0	0.0	14	5	1	2	0	0	16	0	91
summer													
cooked	½ cup	47	3	0.5	128	4	1	3	1	0	19	0	255
raw	½ cup	11	0	0.0	1	2	1	2	1	0	12	0	128
winter, cooked	½ cup	42	0	0.0	132	10	3	4	1	0	25	0	270
zucchini													
cooked	½ cup	19	0	0.0	128	4	1	3	1	0	20	0	255
raw	½ cup	11	0	0.0	5	2	1	2	1	0	10	0	162
Succotash, cooked	½ cup	81	0	0.0	132	17	3	2	4	0	15	1	235
Sweet potatoes													
baked w/ skin	1 (4 oz)	135	0	0.0	285	31	5	10	3	0	57	1	710
candied, frozen	½ cup	223	4	1.0	178	47	2	36	1	0	25	1	206
mashed w/o fat	½ cup	129	0	0.0	96	30	2	7	3	0	38	2	268
Swiss chard, cooked	½ cup	18	0	0.0	363	4	2	1	2	0	51	2	481
Tomatoes													
cherry, raw	6 medium	18	0	0.0	5	4	1	3	1	0	10	0	237
paste, can	½ cup	108	1	0.0	47	25	5	16	6	0	47	4	325
puree, can	½ cup	48	0	0.0	253	11	2	6	2	0	23	2	550
stewed, can	½ cup	33	0	0.0	282	8	1	4	1	0	43	2	264
sun-dried	½ cup	71	1	0.0	29	15	3	10	4	0	30	3	940
whole													
can	½ cup	21	2	0.5	67	2	1	1	0	0	18	0	103
raw	1 medium	23	0	0.0	6	5	2	3	1	0	13	0	296
Turnips, cooked	½ cup	42	2	0.5	161	5	2	3	1	0	26	0	159
Water chestnuts, can	½ cup	35	0	0.0	6	9	2	3	1	0	5	1	145
Watercress, raw	½ cup	2	0	0.0	7	0	0	0	0	0	20	0	56
Wax beans, cooked	½ cup	36	2	0.5	95	5	2	1	1	0	35	1	89
Yams, cooked	½ cup	92	0	0.0	246	21	3	6	2	0	38	1	475

VEGETARIAN FOODS & LEGUMES

	Amount	Calories	Fat (g)	Saturated Fat (g)	Sodium (mg)	Carbohydrate (g)	Fiber (g)	Sugar (g)	Protein (g)	Vitamin D (mcg)	Calcium (mg)	Iron (mg)	Potassium (mg)
Aduki/adzuki beans													
dry, cooked	½ cup	147	0	0.0	9	29	8	0	9	0	32	2	612
sweetened, can	½ cup	351	0	0.0	323	82	4	27	6	0	33	2	176
Bacon, vegetarian	2 slices	60	5	0.5	220	2	0	0	2	0	4	0	10
Baked beans, vegetarian, can	½ cup	150	0	0.0	570	30	5	13	7	0	50	2	390
Beyond Meat meatless products													
beef crumbles	½ cup	90	3	0.0	140	2	0	0	14	0	40	5	190
burger/ground beef	1 patty (4 oz)	230	14	5.0	390	7	2	0	20	0	100	4	330
chicken tenders	2 pcs	210	12	2.0	450	15	2	1	13	0	20	1	250

VEGETARIAN FOODS & LEGUMES	Amount	Calories	Fat (g)	Saturated Fat (g)	Sodium (mg)	Carbohydrate (g)	Fiber (g)	Sugar (g)	Protein (g)	Vitamin D (mcg)	Calcium (mg)	Iron (mg)	Potassium (mg)
meatballs	5	290	21	7.0	500	9	3	0	19	0	110	5	460
sausage	2 links	130	9	3.0	240	3	2	0	8	0	50	2	220
Black beans													
can	½ cup	121	0	0.0	313	22	9	0	8	0	46	3	408
dry, cooked	½ cup	114	0	0.0	204	20	8	0	8	0	23	2	306
Black-eyed peas/cowpeas													
can	½ cup	93	1	0.0	352	16	4	3	6	0	24	1	207
dry, cooked	½ cup	100	1	0.0	218	17	3	3	7	0	22	3	321
Black turtle beans													
can	½ cup	109	0	0.0	461	20	8	0	7	0	42	2	370
dry, cooked	½ cup	120	0	0.0	221	23	8	0	8	0	51	3	401
Boca meatless products													
burger	1 (2.6 oz)	80	1	0.0	110	7	1	0	11	0	70	0	0
Chik'N Nuggets	4 (3 oz)	180	8	1.0	520	13	3	0	14	0	52	2	0
Chik'N Patties	1 (2.5 oz)	140	6	1.0	460	11	2	0	11	0	26	2	0
crumbles	½ cup	60	0	0.0	190	5	0	1	11	0	52	2	0
Broad/fava beans													
can	½ cup	91	0	0.0	580	16	5	0	7	0	33	1	310
dry, cooked	½ cup	94	0	0.0	205	17	5	2	6	0	31	1	228
Butter beans, can	½ cup	29	2	1.0	213	3	1	1	1	0	26	1	69
Cannellini beans, can	½ cup	90	0	0.0	310	16	8	1	6	0	70	2	370
Chickpeas/garbanzo beans													
can	½ cup	132	3	0.5	295	20	7	4	7	0	52	2	216
dry, cooked	½ cup	135	2	0.0	200	22	6	4	7	0	40	2	239
Chili, vegetarian, can	1 cup	126	1	0.0	453	11	3	1	10	0	18	2	161
Chili beans, can	½ cup	120	1	0.0	410	21	8	1	7	0	60	2	380
Cranberry/Roman beans													
can	½ cup	108	0	0.0	432	20	8	0	7	0	44	2	338
dry, cooked	½ cup	121	0	0.0	210	22	8	0	8	0	44	2	343
Crowder peas, can	½ cup	131	1	0.0	378	24	6	4	8	0	23	2	371
Falafel patties	1 (0.6 oz)	333	18	2.5	294	5	0	0	13	0	54	3	585
Gardenburger burger	1 (3.4 oz)	150	5	2.0	550	22	3	0	7	0	110	1	160
Great Northern beans													
can	½ cup	150	1	0.0	485	28	6	2	10	0	70	2	460
dry, cooked	½ cup	105	0	0.0	211	19	6	0	7	0	60	2	346
Ground meat alternative	¾ cup	120	2	0.0	360	7	5	1	18	0	80	2	560
Hot dogs													
tofu	1 (1.5 oz)	60	3	0.0	270	0	1	0	7	0	20	1	50
veggie	1 (1.5 oz)	60	1	0.0	370	5	0	2	9	0	10	1	30
Hummus	½ cup	312	21	3.0	578	24	7	3	10	0	136	4	301
Kidney beans													
can	½ cup	122	1	0.0	280	22	7	3	8	0	43	2	390
dry, cooked	½ cup	113	0	0.0	211	20	7	0	8	0	25	3	357

VEGETARIAN FOODS & LEGUMES

	Amount	Calories	Fat (g)	Saturated Fat (g)	Sodium (mg)	Carbohydrate (g)	Fiber (g)	Sugar (g)	Protein (g)	Vitamin D (mcg)	Calcium (mg)	Iron (mg)	Potassium (mg)
Lentils, cooked	½ cup	113	0	0.0	236	19	8	2	9	0	19	3	366
Lima beans													
baby, frozen	½ cup	108	0	0.0	43	21	5	1	6	0	29	2	371
can	½ cup	113	3	0.5	346	17	5	1	5	0	28	2	271
dry, cooked	½ cup	105	0	0.0	215	20	5	1	6	0	27	2	485
Miso, brown	1 T	34	1	0.0	644	4	1	1	2	0	10	0	36
Morningstar Farms													
burger													
garden veggie	1 (2.4 oz)	100	3	0.0	280	10	5	2	10	0	40	1	250
spicy black bean	1 (2.4 oz)	110	5	0.5	320	13	4	1	9	0	50	2	250
Veggie Grillers original	1 (2.3 oz)	130	5	0.5	390	8	4	1	16	0	60	1	120
Chik'N Nuggets	4 (3 oz)	190	8	1.0	300	18	4	2	13	0	30	2	200
Mung beans, dry, cooked	½ cup	144	6	1.0	202	16	7	2	6	0	23	1	229
Natto	½ cup	186	10	1.5	6	11	5	4	17	0	191	8	640
Navy beans													
can	½ cup	148	1	0.0	440	27	7	0	10	0	62	2	378
dry, cooked	½ cup	128	1	0.0	216	24	10	0	8	0	63	2	354
Pigeon peas													
can	½ cup	100	1	0.0	290	17	4	2	5	0	31	2	391
dry, cooked	½ cup	110	1	0.5	257	20	4	2	6	0	41	2	453
Pink beans, dry, cooked	½ cup	182	6	1.0	202	24	5	0	8	0	45	2	437
Pinto beans													
can	½ cup	124	1	0.0	284	23	7	2	7	0	70	2	413
dry, cooked	½ cup	123	1	0.0	204	22	8	0	8	0	39	2	373
Red beans, dry, cooked	½ cup	113	0	0.0	211	20	7	0	8	0	25	3	357
Refried beans, can	½ cup	185	2	0.5	955	30	10	1	12	0	78	4	765
fat-free	½ cup	91	1	0.0	404	16	5	1	6	0	39	2	398
Sausages, vegetarian													
ground	2 oz	80	3	0.0	320	5	3	1	9	0	42	2	218
links	2 (1.6 oz)	70	3	0.0	300	3	1	0	9	0	10	3	40
patties	1 (1.3 oz)	80	3	0.0	230	5	2	1	9	0	30	1	110
Seitan													
chicken-style	5 oz	110	2	0.0	770	4	2	1	20	0	40	1	66
stir-fry strips	⅓ cup	120	2	0.0	380	5	1	2	21	0	20	0	100
traditional	3 oz	90	1	0.0	380	3	1	0	18	0	40	1	60
Soy meal, defatted	½ cup	206	1	0.0	2	22	11	13	30	0	149	8	1520
Soy protein													
concentrate	1 oz	93	0	0.0	1	7	2	6	18	0	103	3	624
isolate	1 oz	95	1	0.0	284	0	0	0	25	0	51	4	23
Soybeans													
green, cooked	½ cup	127	6	0.5	225	10	4	2	11	0	131	2	485
mature													
cooked	½ cup	148	8	1.0	1	7	5	2	16	0	86	4	443
roasted, salted	¼ cup	202	11	1.5	70	13	8	2	17	0	59	2	633

	Amount	Calories	Fat (g)	Saturated Fat (g)	Sodium (mg)	Carbohydrate (g)	Fiber (g)	Sugar (g)	Protein (g)	Vitamin D (mcg)	Calcium (mg)	Iron (mg)	Potassium (mg)
Split peas, dry, cooked	½ cup	114	0	0.0	233	20	8	3	8	0	14	1	355
Tempeh													
flax	4 oz	160	7	1.0	10	9	7	1	15	0	80	3	260
soy	4 oz	140	5	1.0	10	10	7	0	16	0	60	2	280
wild rice	3 oz	170	5	1.0	10	18	7	1	14	0	60	2	290
Tofurky													
deli slices, smoked ham	5 (1.8 oz)	100	4	0.0	320	4	1	1	13	0	20	1	430
sausage, Italian	1 link (3.5 oz)	260	15	1.5	440	9	2	2	24	0	52	3	705
Tofu													
firm	1 slice (3 oz)	71	4	0.5	28	1	1	0	9	0	125	1	70
lite	1 slice (3 oz)	45	2	0.0	65	1	0	0	8	0	150	1	48
flavored, baked	1 slice (3 oz)	90	5	1.0	250	3	1	1	8	0	10	1	120
silken	1 slice (3 oz)	50	2	0.0	25	1	1	0	6	0	37	1	167
lite	1 slice (3 oz)	30	1	0.0	50	0	0	0	6	0	37	1	56
soft	1 slice (3 oz)	50	2	0.5	20	2	1	0	5	0	66	1	110
TVP (textured vegetable protein)	¼ cup	90	0	0.0	5	9	5	2	12	0	62	2	643
White (cannellini) beans, dry, cooked	½ cup	125	0	0.0	217	22	6	0	9	0	81	3	500
Winged beans, dry, cooked	½ cup	127	5	0.5	214	13	2	0	9	0	122	4	241
Yeast													
brewer's buds/flakes	3 T	117	3	0.0	18	15	10	0	15	0	11	1	345
nutritional flakes	3 T	60	0	0.0	2	12	4	0	7	0	6	1	264

RESTAURANT & FAST FOOD CHAINS

A&W

Entrées

	Amount	Calories	Fat (g)	Saturated Fat (g)	Sodium (mg)	Carbohydrate (g)	Fiber (g)	Sugar (g)	Protein (g)	Vitamin D (mcg)	Calcium (mg)	Iron (mg)	Potassium (mg)
Burger patty	1	130	9	3.5	80	0	0	0	13	n/a	12	1	n/a
Cheeseburger	1	400	16	6.0	990	42	0	10	22	n/a	117	4	n/a
Chicken sandwich													
hand-breaded	1	440	15	2.5	1150	42	0	7	33	n/a	15	3	n/a
grilled	1	410	12	1.5	930	38	0	7	19	n/a	15	3	n/a
Chicken club sandwich													
crispy	1	540	25	5.0	1510	52	2	12	26	n/a	8	3	n/a
hand-breaded	1	490	20	5.0	1390	42	0	7	36	n/a	103	3	n/a
grilled	1	470	17	4.0	1170	39	0	7	22	n/a	103	3	n/a
Chicken tenders													
freezer-to-fryer	3 pcs	370	18	2.5	1190	29	2	8	21	n/a	0	2	n/a
hand-breaded	3 pcs	260	9	2.5	1100	5	1	0	40	n/a	0	2	n/a
Coney dog	1	320	19	7.0	960	26	0	4	12	n/a	61	0	n/a
footlong	1	630	37	15.0	1810	48	0	7	25	n/a	96	2	n/a
Coney cheese dog	1	360	22	8.0	1160	29	0	4	13	n/a	75	0	n/a
footlong	1	700	42	17.0	2230	54	2	7	26	n/a	125	2	n/a
Corn dog nuggets	5 pcs	270	13	2.5	330	30	6	6	8	n/a	87	2	n/a
Fish sandwich	1	440	21	4.5	810	61	1	9	12	n/a	114	2	n/a
Hamburger	1	350	11	3.5	650	41	0	9	20	n/a	28	4	n/a

RESTAURANT & FAST FOOD CHAINS

A&W

	Amount	Calories	Fat (g)	Saturated Fat (g)	Sodium (mg)	Carbohydrate (g)	Fiber (g)	Sugar (g)	Protein (g)	Vitamin D (mcg)	Calcium (mg)	Iron (mg)	Potassium (mg)
Hot dog	1	310	18	6.0	860	28	0	6	10	n/a	56	0	n/a
footlong	1	610	34	14.0	1610	52	1	12	21	n/a	96	2	n/a
Mushroom onion melt													
burger single	1	400	17	6.0	960	38	0	7	23	n/a	129	4	n/a
chicken													
hand-breaded	1	430	14	4.0	1610	42	0	7	36	n/a	117	3	n/a
grilled	1	410	11	3.0	1300	38	0	7	23	n/a	117	3	n/a
Texas toast single	1	380	18	6.0	1060	34	0	3	23	n/a	210	4	n/a
Original bacon cheeseburger single	1	460	23	7.0	840	40	1	8	23	n/a	118	4	n/a
Papa Burger single	1	450	22	7.0	890	42	1	10	22	n/a	118	4	n/a
Pork tenderloin sandwich	1	520	17	2.5	1180	65	3	7	21	n/a	44	4	n/a
Shrimp	16 pcs	480	26	6.0	1010	45	3	1	18	n/a	125	3	n/a
Sides													
Cheese curds	1 order	570	40	21.0	1220	27	2	3	27	n/a	80	10	n/a
Coleslaw	1 order	100	8	1.5	200	7	2	5	1	n/a	42	0	n/a
Fries	1 order	310	13	3.0	460	45	4	0	3	n/a	0	0	n/a
cheese	1 order	390	17	4.5	880	50	1	0	5	n/a	28	0	n/a
chili	1 order	380	16	4.5	840	49	1	2	7	n/a	15	1	n/a
chili cheese	1 order	410	18	5.0	1040	51	1	2	8	n/a	29	1	n/a
Onion rings	1 order	280	4	0.0	930	53	2	5	6	n/a	0	6	n/a
Sauces													
BBQ	1 oz	40	0	0.0	370	10	0	9	0	n/a	0	0	n/a
Buttermilk ranch	1 oz	130	14	2.5	220	1	0	1	0	n/a	0	0	n/a
Honey mustard	1 oz	45	0	0.0	160	10	0	9	0	n/a	0	0	n/a
Spicy Papa	1 oz	130	12	2.0	340	6	0	5	0	n/a	0	0	n/a
Desserts													
Cones													
chocolate	1 (5.5 oz)	290	7	4.5	210	51	1	40	6	n/a	223	0	n/a
root beer	1 (5.5 oz)	260	8	4.5	210	41	0	32	6	n/a	245	0	n/a
vanilla	1 (5.5 oz)	270	8	5.0	220	42	0	33	7	n/a	260	0	n/a
Floats													
orange	regular	330	5	3.0	1010	71	0	67	4	n/a	165	0	n/a
root beer	regular	340	5	3.0	190	68	0	66	4	n/a	165	0	n/a
diet	regular	160	5	3.0	200	24	0	21	4	n/a	165	0	n/a
Freezes													
orange	regular	500	12	7.0	1050	94	0	87	10	n/a	377	0	n/a
root beer	regular	520	12	7.0	350	92	0	86	10	n/a	377	0	n/a
diet	regular	360	12	7.0	360	54	0	48	10	n/a	377	0	n/a
Shakes													
chocolate	regular	770	23	14.0	540	129	0	109	17	n/a	615	0	n/a
strawberry	regular	730	22	14.0	510	115	0	98	16	n/a	615	0	n/a
vanilla	regular	690	22	14.0	510	110	0	94	16	n/a	615	0	n/a

RESTAURANT & FAST FOOD CHAINS

A&W	Amount	Calories	Fat (g)	Saturated Fat (g)	Sodium (mg)	Carbohydrate (g)	Fiber (g)	Sugar (g)	Protein (g)	Vitamin D (mcg)	Calcium (mg)	Iron (mg)	Potassium (mg)
Polar Swirls													
cookie dough	16 oz	740	26	15.0	500	111	0	88	17	n/a	580	1	n/a
M&M's	16 oz	900	32	19.0	500	137	2	122	19	n/a	657	1	n/a
Oreo	16 oz	750	20	11.0	620	114	0	90	17	n/a	585	2	n/a
Reese's	16 oz	780	32	16.0	620	109	2	97	20	n/a	610	1	n/a
Root beer	regular	290	0	0.0	135	78	0	75	0	n/a	30	0	n/a
diet	regular	0	0	0.0	180	0	0	0	0	n/a	0	0	n/a
Sundaes													
chocolate	1	360	11	8.0	240	61	0	50	7	n/a	259	0	n/a
hot caramel	1	380	11	7.0	270	65	0	51	7	n/a	259	0	n/a
strawberry	1	340	11	7.0	220	54	0	44	7	n/a	259	0	n/a

Applebee's

Appetizers

	Amount	Calories	Fat (g)	Saturated Fat (g)	Sodium (mg)	Carbohydrate (g)	Fiber (g)	Sugar (g)	Protein (g)	Vitamin D (mcg)	Calcium (mg)	Iron (mg)	Potassium (mg)
Brew Pub loaded waffle fries	1 order	1520	104	30.0	4290	107	9	6	38	n/a	n/a	n/a	n/a
Brew Pub pretzels & beer cheese dip	1 order	1160	49	15.0	3580	146	6	17	34	n/a	n/a	n/a	n/a
Chicken quesadilla	1 order	1120	69	31.0	2820	78	5	7	45	n/a	n/a	n/a	n/a
Chicken wonton tacos	1 order	600	26	5.0	1530	58	3	27	32	n/a	n/a	n/a	n/a
Crispy cheese bites	1 order	1660	126	47.0	3110	48	4	7	58	n/a	n/a	n/a	n/a
Crunchy onion rings	1 order	1320	60	11.0	3160	180	11	50	15	n/a	n/a	n/a	n/a
Mozzarella sticks	1 order	860	43	18.0	2520	76	7	11	41	n/a	n/a	n/a	n/a
Neighborhood Nachos													
beef	1 order	1940	130	55.0	4440	120	12	13	76	n/a	n/a	n/a	n/a
chicken	1 order	1830	117	49.0	4910	118	11	12	79	n/a	n/a	n/a	n/a
Spinach & artichoke dip	1 order	980	61	14.0	2670	89	9	8	21	n/a	n/a	n/a	n/a
The Classic Combo	1 order	2230	127	38.0	5920	189	16	15	83	n/a	n/a	n/a	n/a
White queso dip & chips	1 order	920	53	20.0	2630	83	5	6	27	n/a	n/a	n/a	n/a
Wings													
boneless	1 order	630	31	6.0	1550	50	4	0	40	n/a	n/a	n/a	n/a
double crunch bone-in	1 order	580	35	9.0	1940	5	2	0	60	n/a	n/a	n/a	n/a
dressings													
bleu cheese	1 order	200	22	4.0	260	0	0	0	1	n/a	n/a	n/a	n/a
ranch	1 order	160	16	3.0	300	2	0	1	0	n/a	n/a	n/a	n/a
sauces													
Buffalo hot, classic	1 order	210	22	8.0	2700	3	0	0	0	n/a	n/a	n/a	n/a
Buffalo hot, extra	1 order	220	22	8.0	2700	3	0	0	0	n/a	n/a	n/a	n/a
garlic Parmesan	1 order	390	41	9.0	690	5	0	0	2	n/a	n/a	n/a	n/a
honey BBQ	1 order	190	0	0.0	820	48	3	40	0	n/a	n/a	n/a	n/a
honey pepper	1 order	230	0	0.0	190	59	0	51	0	n/a	n/a	n/a	n/a
sweet Asian chile	1 order	260	3	0.0	1440	56	1	46	3	n/a	n/a	n/a	n/a

RESTAURANT & FAST FOOD CHAINS

	Amount	Calories	Fat (g)	Saturated Fat (g)	Sodium (mg)	Carbohydrate (g)	Fiber (g)	Sugar (g)	Protein (g)	Vitamin D (mcg)	Calcium (mg)	Iron (mg)	Potassium (mg)
Bowls													
Southwest chicken	1	830	29	5.0	2210	90	10	6	54	n/a	n/a	n/a	n/a
Tex-Mex shrimp	1	710	27	4.5	2070	91	10	6	30	n/a	n/a	n/a	n/a
Burgers*													
Bourbon Street mushroom Swiss burger	1	1610	111	33.0	2830	99	7	12	57	n/a	n/a	n/a	n/a
Classic bacon cheeseburger	1	1330	83	28.0	2690	92	8	8	56	n/a	n/a	n/a	n/a
Classic burger	1	1120	66	20.0	1880	90	7	7	43	n/a	n/a	n/a	n/a
Classic cheeseburger	1	1220	74	25.0	2340	91	8	8	48	n/a	n/a	n/a	n/a
Impossible cheeseburger	1	1050	56	18.0	2600	101	13	9	37	n/a	n/a	n/a	n/a
Neighborhood double burger	1	1400	95	29.0	2850	91	8	7	48	n/a	n/a	n/a	n/a
Quesadilla burger	1	1590	105	40.0	3420	94	8	5	68	n/a	n/a	n/a	n/a
Whisky bacon burger	1	1630	102	35.0	2890	117	8	19	63	n/a	n/a	n/a	n/a
Add-ons													
bacon	1 order	110	9	3.0	350	0	0	0	8	n/a	n/a	n/a	n/a
burger patty	1	400	31	13.0	300	0	0	0	30	n/a	n/a	n/a	n/a
Substitutions													
chicken breast patty	1	190	3	1.0	770	0	0	0	40	n/a	n/a	n/a	n/a
Bourbon Street burger	1	190	3	1.0	690	0	0	0	40	n/a	n/a	n/a	n/a
quesadilla burger	1	190	3	1.0	1050	1	0	0	41	n/a	n/a	n/a	n/a
Impossible burger patty	1	230	13	6.0	560	9	5	0	19	n/a	n/a	n/a	n/a
Bourbon Street burger	1	230	13	6.0	480	9	6	0	19	n/a	n/a	n/a	n/a
quesadilla burger	1	230	13	6.0	840	10	6	0	19	n/a	n/a	n/a	n/a
Lettuce cup	1	5	0	0.0	0	1	0	0	0	n/a	n/a	n/a	n/a
Chicken**													
Bourbon Street chicken & shrimp	1 order	790	43	9.0	2510	47	6	7	55	n/a	n/a	n/a	n/a
Chicken tenders													
	plate	1080	62	11.0	2360	95	7	10	37	n/a	n/a	n/a	n/a
	platter	1410	80	14.0	2990	123	9	22	50	n/a	n/a	n/a	n/a
Fiesta lime chicken	1 order	1170	60	14.0	3580	98	6	8	60	n/a	n/a	n/a	n/a
Grilled chicken breast	1 order	550	22	8.0	1730	43	6	5	48	n/a	n/a	n/a	n/a
Pasta***													
Breadsticks w/ Alfredo sauce	1 order	1500	89	42.0	2540	139	6	19	38	n/a	n/a	n/a	n/a
Classic broccoli blackened shrimp Alfredo	1 order	1290	75	43.0	2770	103	8	12	54	n/a	n/a	n/a	n/a
Classic broccoli chicken Alfredo	1 order	1390	76	44.0	2730	102	8	12	78	n/a	n/a	n/a	n/a
Four-cheese mac & cheese w/ honey pepper chicken tenders	1 order	1350	54	19.0	3210	160	7	44	55	n/a	n/a	n/a	n/a
Three-cheese chicken penne	1 order	1320	69	39.0	2620	99	6	11	76	n/a	n/a	n/a	n/a

* Side of classic fries included.
** Fixed sides included.
*** Breadstick included (except for Breadsticks w/ Alfredo sauce).

Applebee's

	Amount	Calories	Fat (g)	Saturated Fat (g)	Sodium (mg)	Carbohydrate (g)	Fiber (g)	Sugar (g)	Protein (g)	Vitamin D (mcg)	Calcium (mg)	Iron (mg)	Potassium (mg)
Sandwiches & More													
Bacon ranch chicken sandwich													
w/ crispy chicken	1	1260	72	15.0	3090	110	7	8	45	n/a	n/a	n/a	n/a
w/ grilled chicken	1	1120	58	13.0	2900	91	7	8	61	n/a	n/a	n/a	n/a
Chicken fajita rollup	1	1390	75	27.0	4090	116	9	6	62	n/a	n/a	n/a	n/a
Clubhouse Grille	1	1450	80	21.0	3670	128	9	21	56	n/a	n/a	n/a	n/a
Sweet & spicy chicken sandwich	1	1350	62	12.0	3520	159	9	49	40	n/a	n/a	n/a	n/a
The Prime Rib Dipper	1	1380	72	22.0	4050	123	9	14	64	n/a	n/a	n/a	n/a
*Seafood**													
Blackened Cajun salmon	1 order	600	28	9.0	1790	47	7	5	43	n/a	n/a	n/a	n/a
Double crunch shrimp	1 order	1150	50	9.0	3940	143	12	32	33	n/a	n/a	n/a	n/a
Hand battered fish & chips	1 order	1470	95	21.0	3200	115	10	21	42	n/a	n/a	n/a	n/a
*Steaks & Ribs**													
Applebee's riblets													
plate	1 order	910	52	15.0	1390	55	5	2	57	n/a	n/a	n/a	n/a
add honey BBQ sauce	1 order	190	0	0.0	820	48	3	40	0	n/a	n/a	n/a	n/a
add sweet Asian chile	1 order	260	3	0.0	1440	56	1	46	3	n/a	n/a	n/a	n/a
platter	1 order	1350	80	24.0	1810	71	7	16	89	n/a	n/a	n/a	n/a
add honey BBQ sauce	1 order	320	0	0.0	1360	79	5	66	2	n/a	n/a	n/a	n/a
add sweet Asian chile	1 order	430	5	1.0	2410	93	2	76	5	n/a	n/a	n/a	n/a
Bourbon Street steak	1 order	820	47	11.0	1940	48	5	7	52	n/a	n/a	n/a	n/a
Double-glazed baby-back ribs	1 order	1440	91	30.0	1870	68	7	13	88	n/a	n/a	n/a	n/a
add honey BBQ sauce	1 order	130	0	0.0	550	32	2	26	0	n/a	n/a	n/a	n/a
add sweet Asian chile	1 order	170	2	0.0	960	37	0	31	2	n/a	n/a	n/a	n/a
half rack	1 order	850	51	16.0	1340	53	5	0	47	n/a	n/a	n/a	n/a
add honey BBQ sauce	1 order	60	0	0.0	270	16	0	13	0	n/a	n/a	n/a	n/a
add sweet Asian chile	1 order	90	1	0.0	480	19	0	15	0	n/a	n/a	n/a	n/a
Ribeye	12 oz	850	45	19.0	2010	44	7	6	71	n/a	n/a	n/a	n/a
Shrimp 'n Parmesan sirloin	1 order	900	51	26.0	2800	49	7	7	66	n/a	n/a	n/a	n/a
Top sirloin													
	6 oz	550	23	9.0	1800	43	6	5	44	n/a	n/a	n/a	n/a
	8 oz	620	26	11.0	1980	45	6	5	53	n/a	n/a	n/a	n/a
*Salads***													
Caesar													
w/ blackened shrimp	1	860	58	11.0	2100	57	8	9	31	n/a	n/a	n/a	n/a
w/ grilled chicken	1	970	60	12.0	2060	55	7	9	55	n/a	n/a	n/a	n/a
Crispy chicken tender	1	1200	79	20.0	1960	83	7	27	44	n/a	n/a	n/a	n/a
Grilled chicken	1	1000	61	17.0	1840	57	6	27	60	n/a	n/a	n/a	n/a
Oriental chicken	1	1560	103	17.0	1620	120	12	44	40	n/a	n/a	n/a	n/a
grilled	1	1430	89	14.0	2020	104	11	52	56	n/a	n/a	n/a	n/a
Strawberry balsamic chicken	1	850	49	8.0	1790	56	10	20	52	n/a	n/a	n/a	n/a

* Fixed sides included.
** Breadstick and dressing included.

RESTAURANT & FAST FOOD CHAINS

Applebee's

	Amount	Calories	Fat (g)	Saturated Fat (g)	Sodium (mg)	Carbohydrate (g)	Fiber (g)	Sugar (g)	Protein (g)	Vitamin D (mcg)	Calcium (mg)	Iron (mg)	Potassium (mg)
Side Salads													
Caesar	1	230	18	3.5	410	13	2	3	5	n/a	n/a	n/a	n/a
House	1	130	7	2.5	220	14	2	4	6	n/a	n/a	n/a	n/a
dressings													
bleu cheese	1 order	200	22	4.0	260	0	0	0	1	n/a	n/a	n/a	n/a
Caesar	1 order	200	21	3.5	340	2	0	0	0	n/a	n/a	n/a	n/a
Dijon honey mustard	1 order	200	18	2.5	250	10	0	10	0	n/a	n/a	n/a	n/a
fat free Italian	1 order	20	0	0.0	380	5	0	3	0	n/a	n/a	n/a	n/a
honey French	1 order	210	17	2.5	330	15	0	14	0	n/a	n/a	n/a	n/a
lemon olive oil vinaigrette	1 order	150	16	2.5	370	1	0	0	0	n/a	n/a	n/a	n/a
Mexi-ranch	1 order	140	14	2.5	530	3	0	2	0	n/a	n/a	n/a	n/a
oriental	1 order	250	22	3.5	80	13	0	13	0	n/a	n/a	n/a	n/a
ranch	1 order	160	16	3.0	300	2	0	1	0	n/a	n/a	n/a	n/a
Thousand Island	1 order	230	22	3.5	370	7	0	7	0	n/a	n/a	n/a	n/a
Soups													
Chicken tortilla	1	280	15	4.0	930	26	2	3	11	n/a	n/a	n/a	n/a
French onion	1	370	22	12.0	1250	26	2	9	16	n/a	n/a	n/a	n/a
Tomato basil	1	210	12	6.0	1270	22	2	8	5	n/a	n/a	n/a	n/a
Sides													
Baked potato	1	530	31	17.0	1120	59	4	4	9	n/a	n/a	n/a	n/a
loaded	1	590	35	19.0	1270	59	4	4	12	n/a	n/a	n/a	n/a
Breadstick	1	180	7	1.5	250	25	1	3	4	n/a	n/a	n/a	n/a
Crunchy onion rings	1 order	560	30	6.0	1170	66	4	5	7	n/a	n/a	n/a	n/a
Four-cheese mac & cheese w/ applewood-smoked bacon	1 order	390	18	9.0	1120	38	2	4	17	n/a	n/a	n/a	n/a
Fries													
classic	1 order	400	18	3.5	1000	53	5	0	6	n/a	n/a	n/a	n/a
basket	1	640	30	5.0	1580	84	8	0	10	n/a	n/a	n/a	n/a
waffle	1 order	480	24	4.5	1350	58	5	0	7	n/a	n/a	n/a	n/a
basket	1	770	39	7.0	2150	93	8	0	11	n/a	n/a	n/a	n/a
Garlicky green beans	1 order	150	12	2.5	420	8	3	2	2	n/a	n/a	n/a	n/a
Garlic mashed potatoes	1 order	260	11	2.5	720	37	4	3	5	n/a	n/a	n/a	n/a
loaded	1 order	430	26	11.0	900	40	4	5	10	n/a	n/a	n/a	n/a
Homestyle cheesy broccoli	1 order	210	17	10.0	710	8	3	3	9	n/a	n/a	n/a	n/a
Signature cole slaw	1 order	140	8	1.5	190	15	2	12	0	n/a	n/a	n/a	n/a
Steamed broccoli	1 order	100	8	5.0	240	5	2	2	3	n/a	n/a	n/a	n/a
Desserts													
Brownie bite	1	330	15	8.0	190	48	2	35	4	n/a	n/a	n/a	n/a
Cinnabon mini swirls	1 order	1620	62	23.0	1060	248	8	155	22	n/a	n/a	n/a	n/a
Sizzlin' butter pecan blondie	1	1040	59	30.0	910	116	2	71	13	n/a	n/a	n/a	n/a
Sugar dusted donut dippers	1 order	1520	54	20.0	840	247	4	178	17	n/a	n/a	n/a	n/a
Triple chocolate meltdown	1	850	37	14.0	650	125	5	89	13	n/a	n/a	n/a	n/a

RESTAURANT & FAST FOOD CHAINS

Applebee's

	Amount	Calories	Fat (g)	Saturated Fat (g)	Sodium (mg)	Carbohydrate (g)	Fiber (g)	Sugar (g)	Protein (g)	Vitamin D (mcg)	Calcium (mg)	Iron (mg)	Potassium (mg)
Fruit Smoothies													
Mango	1	260	0	0.0	0	65	0	55	0	n/a	n/a	n/a	n/a
Piña colada	1	430	8	6.0	45	89	2	84	0	n/a	n/a	n/a	n/a
Strawberry banana	1	280	0	0.0	10	71	2	69	0	n/a	n/a	n/a	n/a
Swirl													
strawberry colada	1	470	8	6.0	55	98	2	93	0	n/a	n/a	n/a	n/a
strawberry mango	1	290	0	0.0	10	74	0	64	0	n/a	n/a	n/a	n/a
Milkshakes													
Chocolate	1	900	37	24.0	340	127	2	99	16	n/a	n/a	n/a	n/a
Oreo cookie	1	870	43	25.0	430	108	1	74	16	n/a	n/a	n/a	n/a
Strawberry	1	810	36	23.0	330	107	1	83	14	n/a	n/a	n/a	n/a
Vanilla	1	710	36	23.0	310	83	0	61	14	n/a	n/a	n/a	n/a
Flavored Lemonade													
Blackberry	1	190	0	0.0	55	49	0	47	0	n/a	n/a	n/a	n/a
Blue raspberry	1	180	0	0.0	60	47	0	45	0	n/a	n/a	n/a	n/a
Dragon fruit	1	190	0	0.0	60	49	0	47	0	n/a	n/a	n/a	n/a
Kiwi	1	190	0	0.0	60	48	0	46	0	n/a	n/a	n/a	n/a
Mango	1	190	0	0.0	60	50	0	48	0	n/a	n/a	n/a	n/a
Passion fruit	1	190	0	0.0	60	50	0	48	0	n/a	n/a	n/a	n/a
Peach	1	190	0	0.0	60	50	0	48	0	n/a	n/a	n/a	n/a
Pomegranate	1	190	0	0.0	55	48	0	46	0	n/a	n/a	n/a	n/a
Raspberry	1	190	0	0.0	60	49	0	47	0	n/a	n/a	n/a	n/a
Strawberry	1	190	0	0.0	60	49	0	47	0	n/a	n/a	n/a	n/a
Iced Tea													
Blackberry	1	50	0	0.0	10	13	0	12	0	n/a	n/a	n/a	n/a
Dragon fruit	1	50	0	0.0	10	14	0	12	0	n/a	n/a	n/a	n/a
Kiwi	1	60	0	0.0	10	12	0	11	0	n/a	n/a	n/a	n/a
Mango	1	60	0	0.0	10	14	0	13	0	n/a	n/a	n/a	n/a
Passion fruit	1	60	0	0.0	10	14	0	13	0	n/a	n/a	n/a	n/a
Peach	1	60	0	0.0	10	14	0	13	0	n/a	n/a	n/a	n/a
Pomegranate	1	50	0	0.0	10	13	0	11	0	n/a	n/a	n/a	n/a
Raspberry	1	50	0	0.0	10	13	0	12	0	n/a	n/a	n/a	n/a
Regular brewed	1	0	0	0.0	5	2	0	0	0	n/a	n/a	n/a	n/a
Strawberry	1	50	0	0.0	10	13	0	11	0	n/a	n/a	n/a	n/a
Sweet	1	90	0	0.0	10	23	0	22	0	n/a	n/a	n/a	n/a
Cocktails													
Blue Aloha Mana Margarita	1	260	0	0.0	350	38	0	30	0	n/a	n/a	n/a	n/a
Blue Hawaiian Long Island Iced Tea	1	230	0	0.0	15	29	0	24	0	n/a	n/a	n/a	n/a
Captain Morgan Bahama Mama	1	280	0	0.0	10	41	1	39	1	n/a	n/a	n/a	n/a
Crown Whiskey Sour	1	180	0	0.0	35	20	0	19	0	n/a	n/a	n/a	n/a

RESTAURANT & FAST FOOD CHAINS

Applebee's	Amount	Calories	Fat (g)	Saturated Fat (g)	Sodium (mg)	Carbohydrate (g)	Fiber (g)	Sugar (g)	Protein (g)	Vitamin D (mcg)	Calcium (mg)	Iron (mg)	Potassium (mg)
Margarita	1	300	0	0.0	320	40	1	31	0	n/a	n/a	n/a	n/a
Patron	1	310	0	0.0	320	44	1	38	0	n/a	n/a	n/a	n/a
Strawberry	1	360	0	0.0	20	54	1	44	0	n/a	n/a	n/a	n/a
People's Pineapple Margarita	1	170	0	0.0	25	19	0	17	0	n/a	n/a	n/a	n/a
Red Sangria	1	230	0	0.0	10	36	1	30	0	n/a	n/a	n/a	n/a
Shark Bowl	1	600	0	0.0	30	119	0	111	0	n/a	n/a	n/a	n/a
Tito's Bay Breeze	1	150	0	0.0	0	12	0	11	0	n/a	n/a	n/a	n/a
Top-Shelf Long Island Iced Tea	1	220	0	0.0	15	23	0	19	0	n/a	n/a	n/a	n/a
White Peach Sangria (Barefoot)	1	270	0	0.0	20	47	1	41	1	n/a	n/a	n/a	n/a

Arby's

Chicken

	Amount	Calories	Fat (g)	Saturated Fat (g)	Sodium (mg)	Carbohydrate (g)	Fiber (g)	Sugar (g)	Protein (g)	Vitamin D (mcg)	Calcium (mg)	Iron (mg)	Potassium (mg)
Bacon & Swiss	1	610	30	9.0	1580	51	4	9	35	n/a	n/a	n/a	n/a
Buffalo	1	500	23	5.0	1960	48	4	7	24	n/a	n/a	n/a	n/a
Classic	1	510	25	5.0	1230	48	4	7	24	n/a	n/a	n/a	n/a
Nuggets	9 pcs	470	23	7.0	1360	28	2	2	38	n/a	n/a	n/a	n/a
Tenders	5 pcs	610	30	4.5	1990	47	3	0	39	n/a	n/a	n/a	n/a
sauces													
tangy barbeque	1 order	45	0	0.0	360	10	0	8	0	n/a	n/a	n/a	n/a
Buffalo	1 order	10	1	0.0	720	2	0	0	0	n/a	n/a	n/a	n/a
honey mustard	1 order	130	13	2.0	160	5	0	4	0	n/a	n/a	n/a	n/a
ranch	1 order	100	10	2.0	135	1	0	1	1	n/a	n/a	n/a	n/a

Market Fresh

Gyros	Amount	Calories	Fat (g)	Saturated Fat (g)	Sodium (mg)	Carbohydrate (g)	Fiber (g)	Sugar (g)	Protein (g)	Vitamin D (mcg)	Calcium (mg)	Iron (mg)	Potassium (mg)
Greek	1	700	44	13.0	1370	55	4	6	23	n/a	n/a	n/a	n/a
roast beef	1	540	29	7.0	1300	48	3	5	24	n/a	n/a	n/a	n/a
Reuben	1	680	31	8.0	2420	62	4	5	37	n/a	n/a	n/a	n/a
Turkey, ranch & bacon sandwich	1	810	35	10.0	2520	79	5	15	46	n/a	n/a	n/a	n/a
Wraps													
Buffalo chicken	1	790	45	9.0	2490	61	5	7	39	n/a	n/a	n/a	n/a
crispy chicken club	1	880	49	14.0	1870	64	5	12	48	n/a	n/a	n/a	n/a

Roast Beef

	Amount	Calories	Fat (g)	Saturated Fat (g)	Sodium (mg)	Carbohydrate (g)	Fiber (g)	Sugar (g)	Protein (g)	Vitamin D (mcg)	Calcium (mg)	Iron (mg)	Potassium (mg)
Beef 'n Cheddar	1	450	20	6.0	1280	45	2	9	23	n/a	n/a	n/a	n/a
double	1	630	32	11.0	2100	48	2	9	39	n/a	n/a	n/a	n/a
half pound	1	740	39	14.0	2530	48	2	9	49	n/a	n/a	n/a	n/a
French Dip 'n Swiss/Au Jus	1	530	21	10.0	2540	50	2	3	34	n/a	n/a	n/a	n/a
Roast beef	1	360	14	5.0	970	37	2	5	23	n/a	n/a	n/a	n/a
double	1	510	24	9.0	1610	38	2	5	38	n/a	n/a	n/a	n/a
half pound	1	610	30	12.0	2040	38	2	5	48	n/a	n/a	n/a	n/a
Smokehouse brisket	1	560	29	11.0	1140	42	3	3	36	n/a	n/a	n/a	n/a
Sauces													
Arby's	1 order	15	0	0.0	180	3	0	2	0	n/a	n/a	n/a	n/a
Horsey	1 order	60	5	1.0	150	3	0	2	0	n/a	n/a	n/a	n/a

RESTAURANT & FAST FOOD CHAINS

Arby's

	Amount	Calories	Fat (g)	Saturated Fat (g)	Sodium (mg)	Carbohydrate (g)	Fiber (g)	Sugar (g)	Protein (g)	Vitamin D (mcg)	Calcium (mg)	Iron (mg)	Potassium (mg)
Sliders													
Buffalo chicken	1	260	12	2.0	910	26	1	3	10	n/a	n/a	n/a	n/a
Chicken	1	230	9	2.0	620	25	1	2	11	n/a	n/a	n/a	n/a
Jalapeño Roast Beef 'n Cheese	1	180	7	3.0	490	16	1	2	10	n/a	n/a	n/a	n/a
Roast beef	1	170	7	3.0	490	16	1	2	10	n/a	n/a	n/a	n/a
Sides													
Fries													
crinkle	medium	390	19	2.5	460	49	0	0	5	n/a	n/a	n/a	n/a
curly	medium	410	22	3.0	940	49	5	0	5	n/a	n/a	n/a	n/a
add cheddar cheese sauce	1 order	50	35	3.5	370	4	0	0	1	n/a	n/a	n/a	n/a
add ketchup	1 order	10	0	0.0	85	3	0	2	0	n/a	n/a	n/a	n/a
Jalapeño Bites	8 pcs	470	27	10.0	1060	50	3	4	8	n/a	n/a	n/a	n/a
add Bronco Berry Sauce	1 order	60	0	0.0	25	15	0	15	0	n/a	n/a	n/a	n/a
Mozzarella sticks	6 pcs	650	35	14.0	2110	56	3	4	29	n/a	n/a	n/a	n/a
add marinara sauce	1 order	20	0	0.0	170	4	1	3	1	n/a	n/a	n/a	n/a
Desserts													
Shakes													
chocolate	regular	540	17	11.0	320	86	1	76	12	n/a	n/a	n/a	n/a
Jamocha	regular	540	10	10.0	320	80	1	74	12	n/a	n/a	n/a	n/a
orange cream	regular	549	16	10.0	284	90	1	82	11	n/a	n/a	n/a	n/a
vanilla	regular	480	17	11.0	300	70	0	64	12	n/a	n/a	n/a	n/a
Cookies													
salted caramel & chocolate	1	430	18	10.0	360	63	1	33	4	n/a	n/a	n/a	n/a
Reese's peanut butter cup	1	460	25	11.0	400	54	2	36	7	n/a	n/a	n/a	n/a
Turnovers													
apple	1	430	18	9.0	210	65	2	39	4	n/a	n/a	n/a	n/a
cherry	1	390	13	6.0	200	65	2	40	4	n/a	n/a	n/a	n/a
Boston Market													
Meals (w/o sides or bread)													
Dark chicken (2 drumsticks, 1 thigh)													
creamy garlic	1 order	350	20	7.0	1120	5	0	2	39	n/a	130	3	n/a
honey balsamic basil	1 order	460	30	6.0	850	11	0	7	38	n/a	104	2	n/a
Parmesan rotisserie	1 order	400	21	7.0	1340	12	0	2	41	n/a	130	1	n/a
roasted garlic	1 order	450	27	12.0	1330	13	0	2	40	n/a	130	2	n/a
rotisserie	1 order	300	16	5.0	780	0	0	0	37	n/a	52	1	n/a
sesame	1 order	430	23	6.0	1230	18	0	0	38	n/a	78	2	n/a
Meatloaf	1 order	470	33	14.0	910	17	2	5	26	n/a	52	3	n/a
Quarter white chicken													
creamy garlic	1 order	320	14	5.0	930	5	0	1	45	n/a	130	1	n/a
honey balsamic basil	1 order	430	24	4.5	660	11	0	7	44	n/a	104	2	n/a
Parmesan rotisserie	1 order	370	15	6.0	1150	12	0	2	46	n/a	130	1	n/a

RESTAURANT & FAST FOOD CHAINS

Boston Market	Amount	Calories	Fat (g)	Saturated Fat (g)	Sodium (mg)	Carbohydrate (g)	Fiber (g)	Sugar (g)	Protein (g)	Vitamin D (mcg)	Calcium (mg)	Iron (mg)	Potassium (mg)
roasted garlic	1 order	420	22	10.0	1140	12	0	2	45	n/a	130	1	n/a
rotisserie	1 order	270	11	3.5	590	0	0	0	43	n/a	52	1	n/a
skinless	1 order	210	5	1.5	480	1	0	1	40	n/a	52	1	n/a
sesame	1 order	400	17	4.0	1040	18	0	3	43	n/a	78	1	n/a
Rotisserie chicken pot pie	1 order	750	42	19.0	1780	64	3	10	28	n/a	195	5	n/a
Rotisserie prime rib	1 order	630	47	12.0	770	0	1	1	55	n/a	26	12	n/a
Turkey breast	1 order	160	5	2.0	440	0	0	0	30	n/a	26	2	n/a
Turkey pot pie	1 order	710	38	18.0	1670	64	3	10	28	n/a	130	4	n/a
Market Bowls													
BBQ chicken	1 order	580	21	8.0	1290	76	6	17	20	n/a	52	3	n/a
Cheeseburger mac & cheese	1 order	510	23	12.0	1790	54	2	20	22	n/a	520	2	n/a
Home style meatloaf	1 order	680	36	14.0	1460	61	7	17	25	n/a	104	5	n/a
Rotisserie chicken	1 order	510	18	7.0	1020	51	8	10	34	n/a	26	5	n/a
Rotisserie turkey breast	1 order	330	13	2.5	870	28	0	5	25	n/a	78	3	n/a
Southwest chicken & cilantro lime rice	1 order	520	15	2.5	790	58	1	3	26	n/a	130	5	n/a
Vegetarian	1 order	470	14	5.0	640	64	4	5	9	n/a	195	3	n/a
Ribs													
½ order baby back ribs	1 order	1020	60	21.0	2170	260	0	29	70	n/a	130	5	n/a
w/ ¼ rotisserie chicken	1 order	1280	71	24.0	2760	51	0	29	113	n/a	195	6	n/a
Full order baby back ribs	1 order	1870	117	40.0	4130	70	0	46	138	n/a	195	6	n/a
Sandwiches													
Chicken avocado club	1	1110	66	19.0	2130	75	7	4	56	n/a	390	6	n/a
Chicken salad carver	1	870	51	10.0	1430	63	7	5	38	n/a	130	5	n/a
Roasted turkey carver	1	970	55	16.0	1930	73	5	4	46	n/a	390	6	n/a
Rotisserie chicken carver	1	980	53	15.0	1880	73	5	4	52	n/a	390	6	n/a
Southwest chicken carver	1	1110	65	19.0	2330	76	7	5	17	n/a	390	5	n/a
Salads & Soups													
Caesar side salad	1	310	24	6.0	870	16	2	3	9	n/a	260	2	n/a
House side salad	1	200	16	3.0	350	10	2	3	4	n/a	104	1	n/a
Southwest Cobb salad	1	760	53	10.0	1390	30	8	10	43	n/a	130	5	n/a
Chicken noodle soup	1	240	9	3.0	1100	20	2	3	16	n/a	26	2	n/a
Sides													
Bacon Brussels sprouts	1 order	240	15	2.5	530	20	6	6	7	n/a	52	1	n/a
Cinnamon apples	1 order	250	5	4.0	270	55	4	49	0	n/a	26	1	n/a
Cornbread	1 order	160	3	1.5	220	31	0	12	2	n/a	26	1	n/a
Creamed spinach	1 order	240	17	11.0	640	12	3	3	11	n/a	325	4	n/a
Fresh steamed vegetables	1 order	60	4	0.0	40	7	3	3	2	n/a	52	1	n/a
Fresh vegetable stuffing	1 order	220	10	1.0	520	28	1	5	4	n/a	52	2	n/a
Garlic dill new potatoes	1 order	100	2	0.5	75	20	2	2	2	n/a	26	1	n/a
Macaroni & cheese	1 order	310	10	6.0	1270	41	1	10	14	n/a	325	2	n/a
Mashed potatoes	1 order	270	11	5.0	620	37	4	2	5	n/a	26	2	n/a

RESTAURANT & FAST FOOD CHAINS

Boston Market	Amount	Calories	Fat (g)	Saturated Fat (g)	Sodium (mg)	Carbohydrate (g)	Fiber (g)	Sugar (g)	Protein (g)	Vitamin D (mcg)	Calcium (mg)	Iron (mg)	Potassium (mg)
Steamed broccoli	1 order	60	0	0.0	260	6	4	2	4	n/a	52	1	n/a
Sweet corn	1 order	160	7	2.0	135	20	5	10	3	n/a	0	1	n/a
Sweet potato casserole	1 order	460	12	3.0	220	87	4	56	3	n/a	52	2	n/a
Sauces													
Beef gravy	1 order	10	0	0.0	180	2	0	0	0	n/a	0	0	n/a
Horseradish	1 order	60	3	0.0	115	6	0	0	0	n/a	0	0	n/a
Zesty barbecue, mild	1 order	40	0	0.0	230	10	0	9	0	n/a	0	0	n/a
Desserts													
Cake													
carrot	1 slice	730	35	13.0	520	99	1	79	5	n/a	52	1	n/a
chocolate	1 slice	570	33	11.0	360	66	3	46	5	n/a	52	1	n/a
Chocolate chip fudge brownie	1	340	14	3.5	180	53	3	39	5	n/a	26	4	n/a
Chocolate chunk cookie	1	370	18	9.0	200	53	2	32	4	n/a	26	4	n/a
Pie													
apple	1 slice	550	32	15.0	290	66	3	47	4	n/a	26	2	n/a
pecan	1 slice	720	42	15.0	550	80	2	76	7	n/a	26	3	n/a
Burger King													
Breakfast													
Bacon, egg & cheese													
biscuit	1	452	30	14.0	1585	33	1	4	17	n/a	n/a	n/a	n/a
Croissan'wich	1	412	25	12.0	1035	31	1	5	18	n/a	n/a	n/a	n/a
Bacon, sausage, egg & cheese													
biscuit	1	715	53	24.0	2389	35	1	4	29	n/a	n/a	n/a	n/a
Croissan'wich	1	675	48	22.0	1839	33	1	6	29	n/a	n/a	n/a	n/a
Egg & cheese													
biscuit	1	412	27	13.0	1415	33	1	4	14	n/a	n/a	n/a	n/a
Croissan'wich	1	372	22	11.0	875	31	1	5	15	n/a	n/a	n/a	n/a
Burritos													
Egg-Normous	1	830	46	17.0	2055	69	4	4	35	n/a	n/a	n/a	n/a
Jr.	1	462	30	11.0	1295	30	2	3	18	n/a	n/a	n/a	n/a
French toast sticks	3 pcs	350	12	2.0	220	57	1	27	4	n/a	n/a	n/a	n/a
Fully loaded													
biscuit	1	640	45	20.0	2340	34	1	4	31	n/a	n/a	n/a	n/a
Croissan'wich	1	714	49	22.0	2236	34	1	6	35	n/a	n/a	n/a	n/a
Ham, egg & cheese													
biscuit	1	452	27	13.0	1825	34	1	4	21	n/a	n/a	n/a	n/a
Croissan'wich	1	412	23	11.0	1275	32	1	6	21	n/a	n/a	n/a	n/a
Hash browns	medium	540	34	7.0	1480	54	5	0	4	n/a	n/a	n/a	n/a
Pancake platter	1	235	7	2.0	250	42	0	23	2	n/a	n/a	n/a	n/a
w/ sausage	1	413	23	8.0	625	42	0	23	9	n/a	n/a	n/a	n/a

RESTAURANT & FAST FOOD CHAINS

Burger King

	Amount	Calories	Fat (g)	Saturated Fat (g)	Sodium (mg)	Carbohydrate (g)	Fiber (g)	Sugar (g)	Protein (g)	Vitamin D (mcg)	Calcium (mg)	Iron (mg)	Potassium (mg)
Sausage biscuit	1	430	30	13.0	1150	30	1	2	11	n/a	n/a	n/a	n/a
Sausage, egg & cheese													
biscuit	1	592	43	19.0	1795	33	1	4	22	n/a	n/a	n/a	n/a
double	1	853	66	29.0	2526	34	1	4	33	n/a	n/a	n/a	n/a
Croissan'wich	1	552	38	17.0	1245	31	1	5	22	n/a	n/a	n/a	n/a
double	1	883	66	29.0	2196	33	1	5	39	n/a	n/a	n/a	n/a
Burgers													
Bacon King	1	1200	81	32.0	2270	58	3	16	66	n/a	n/a	n/a	n/a
Big King	1	490	30	12.0	990	34	2	9	26	n/a	n/a	n/a	n/a
Cheeseburger	1	290	13	6.0	780	31	1	7	15	n/a	n/a	n/a	n/a
bacon	1	340	16	7.0	940	31	1	7	18	n/a	n/a	n/a	n/a
double	1	440	24	11.0	970	32	1	8	27	n/a	n/a	n/a	n/a
double	1	400	21	9.0	810	32	1	8	24	n/a	n/a	n/a	n/a
Hamburger	1	250	10	4.0	560	29	1	7	13	n/a	n/a	n/a	n/a
King, single													
Impossible	1	550	22	11.0	2000	57	5	11	29	n/a	n/a	n/a	n/a
quarter pound	1	590	29	13.0	1820	50	2	11	32	n/a	n/a	n/a	n/a
Rodeo	1	340	13	4.5	500	41	2	10	16	n/a	n/a	n/a	n/a
cheeseburger	1	380	17	7.0	700	42	2	10	17	n/a	n/a	n/a	n/a
Whopper	1	670	41	12.0	1170	54	3	14	32	n/a	n/a	n/a	n/a
w/ bacon	1	750	49	13.0	1430	55	3	14	38	n/a	n/a	n/a	n/a
w/ cheese	1	770	51	15.0	1610	58	3	15	37	n/a	n/a	n/a	n/a
w/ bacon & cheese	1	820	53	18.0	1850	58	3	16	41	n/a	n/a	n/a	n/a
double	1	920	60	20.0	1240	54	3	14	53	n/a	n/a	n/a	n/a
w/ bacon	1	1010	68	21.0	1500	56	3	14	59	n/a	n/a	n/a	n/a
w/ cheese	1	1040	70	24.0	1580	58	3	15	58	n/a	n/a	n/a	n/a
w/ bacon & cheese	1	1090	75	25.0	1830	59	3	15	62	n/a	n/a	n/a	n/a
triple	1	1170	80	27.0	1300	56	3	14	72	n/a	n/a	n/a	n/a
w/ bacon	1	1260	87	29.0	1560	56	4	14	79	n/a	n/a	n/a	n/a
w/ cheese	1	1300	90	33.0	1940	59	4	15	78	n/a	n/a	n/a	n/a
w/ bacon & cheese	1	1350	94	33.0	1990	60	4	15	83	n/a	n/a	n/a	n/a
Impossible	1	630	34	10.0	1350	62	6	14	29	n/a	n/a	n/a	n/a
Whopper Jr.	1	330	19	5.0	560	30	2	7	15	n/a	n/a	n/a	n/a
w/ bacon	1	380	24	7.0	730	30	2	7	19	n/a	n/a	n/a	n/a
w/ cheese	1	380	24	8.0	780	31	2	9	17	n/a	n/a	n/a	n/a
w/ bacon & cheese	1	420	27	9.0	950	32	2	9	20	n/a	n/a	n/a	n/a
BBQ bacon	1	390	24	7.0	730	32	2	9	18	n/a	n/a	n/a	n/a
Chicken & More													
Big Fish	1	570	30	5.0	1270	58	3	8	19	n/a	n/a	n/a	n/a
Chicken fries	9 pcs	260	13	3.0	780	20	1	0	15	n/a	n/a	n/a	n/a
Chicken Jr.	1	440	27	5.0	700	39	2	5	13	n/a	n/a	n/a	n/a
Chicken nuggets	8 pcs	390	25	5.0	990	23	2	0	18	n/a	n/a	n/a	n/a
fiery	8 pcs	530	39	7.0	1220	26	2	2	19	n/a	n/a	n/a	n/a
Original chicken sandwich	1	680	39	7.0	1380	63	3	8	23	n/a	n/a	n/a	n/a

RESTAURANT & FAST FOOD CHAINS

Burger King	Amount	Calories	Fat (g)	Saturated Fat (g)	Sodium (mg)	Carbohydrate (g)	Fiber (g)	Sugar (g)	Protein (g)	Vitamin D (mcg)	Calcium (mg)	Iron (mg)	Potassium (mg)
Royal Crispy Chicken	1	600	33	5.0	1330	54	4	10	31	n/a	n/a	n/a	n/a
bacon & Swiss	1	740	45	11.0	1920	56	4	11	39	n/a	n/a	n/a	n/a
Italian	1	530	21	5.0	1640	57	9	8	33	n/a	n/a	n/a	n/a
spicy	1	760	49	8.0	1580	58	4	12	31	n/a	n/a	n/a	n/a
Sides													
Classic fries	medium	370	16	2.0	270	54	4	1	5	n/a	n/a	n/a	n/a
Onion rings	medium	360	16	2.5	640	48	5	5	4	n/a	n/a	n/a	n/a
Mozzarella sticks	4 pcs	330	14	5.0	820	37	2	5	13	n/a	n/a	n/a	n/a
Desserts													
Chocolate chip cookies	2	162	8	4.0	112	23	1	14	2	n/a	n/a	n/a	n/a
Hershey's sundae pie	1 order	310	18	12.0	230	32	1	22	3	n/a	n/a	n/a	n/a
Soft serve													
cone	1	200	5	3.5	150	33	0	22	5	n/a	n/a	n/a	n/a
cup	1	180	6	2.6	160	29	0	22	4	n/a	n/a	n/a	n/a
Shakes													
chocolate	1	590	14	9.0	420	103	1	84	13	n/a	n/a	n/a	n/a
Oreo	1	670	17	10.0	470	116	2	91	13	n/a	n/a	n/a	n/a
classic Oreo	1	640	17	10.0	460	109	1	86	13	n/a	n/a	n/a	n/a
vanilla	1	560	14	9.0	400	96	0	79	12	n/a	n/a	n/a	n/a
Chick-fil-A													
Breakfast													
Bacon, egg & cheese													
biscuit	1	420	23	11.0	1290	38	2	5	16	n/a	n/a	n/a	n/a
muffin	1	310	13	6.0	800	30	2	2	17	n/a	n/a	n/a	n/a
Buttered biscuit	1	290	15	6.0	760	37	2	4	4	n/a	n/a	n/a	n/a
Chick-n-Minis	4 pcs	360	13	4.0	1060	41	2	8	20	n/a	n/a	n/a	n/a
Chicken biscuit	1	460	23	8.0	1510	45	2	6	19	n/a	n/a	n/a	n/a
spicy	1	450	22	8.0	1570	44	2	5	19	n/a	n/a	n/a	n/a
Chicken, egg & cheese													
biscuit	1	550	28	12.0	1870	48	3	7	27	n/a	n/a	n/a	n/a
muffin	1	420	19	6.0	1350	37	1	4	27	n/a	n/a	n/a	n/a
Egg white grill	1	300	8	4.0	1020	31	2	2	28	n/a	n/a	n/a	n/a
English muffin	1	140	2	0.0	220	29	0	1	5	n/a	n/a	n/a	n/a
Greek yogurt parfait													
w/ cookie crumbs	1	240	8	3.5	85	31	1	26	12	n/a	n/a	n/a	n/a
w/ granola	1	270	9	3.5	80	36	1	26	13	n/a	n/a	n/a	n/a
Hash brown scramble													
bowl	1	470	30	9.0	1350	19	2	2	29	n/a	n/a	n/a	n/a
burrito	1	700	40	12.0	1770	51	3	2	34	n/a	n/a	n/a	n/a
Hash browns	large	420	29	4.0	700	35	4	0	4	n/a	n/a	n/a	n/a
Sausage, egg & cheese													
biscuit	1	620	42	18.0	1510	38	2	4	22	n/a	n/a	n/a	n/a
muffin	1	500	33	12.0	1030	30	1	2	23	n/a	n/a	n/a	n/a
Yeast mini rolls	4	240	8	2.5	450	36	2	7	6	n/a	n/a	n/a	n/a

RESTAURANT & FAST FOOD CHAINS

	Amount	Calories	Fat (g)	Saturated Fat (g)	Sodium (mg)	Carbohydrate (g)	Fiber (g)	Sugar (g)	Protein (g)	Vitamin D (mcg)	Calcium (mg)	Iron (mg)	Potassium (mg)
Entrées													
Chick-n-Strips	3 pcs	310	14	2.5	870	16	0	2	29	n/a	n/a	n/a	n/a
Chicken sandwich	1	420	18	3.5	1460	41	1	6	29	n/a	n/a	n/a	n/a
deluxe w/ American cheese	1	490	22	6.0	1700	43	1	7	32	n/a	n/a	n/a	n/a
grilled	1	390	12	2.0	770	44	3	12	28	n/a	n/a	n/a	n/a
club w/ Colby Jack cheese	1	520	22	8.0	1130	45	3	12	38	n/a	n/a	n/a	n/a
spicy	1	450	19	4.0	1730	45	1	6	28	n/a	n/a	n/a	n/a
deluxe w/ pepper Jack cheese	1	520	25	7.0	1790	46	2	7	31	n/a	n/a	n/a	n/a
Cool Wrap	1	660	45	9.0	1420	32	14	5	43	n/a	n/a	n/a	n/a
Nuggets	8 pcs	250	11	2.5	1210	11	0	1	27	n/a	n/a	n/a	n/a
grilled	8 pcs	130	3	0.5	440	1	0	1	25	n/a	n/a	n/a	n/a
Salads (w/ dressing)													
Cobb w/ nuggets	1	850	61	13.0	2220	34	5	10	42	n/a	n/a	n/a	n/a
Market w/ grilled filet	1	540	31	6.0	1010	41	4	26	28	n/a	n/a	n/a	n/a
Spicy southwest w/ spicy grilled filet	1	690	49	10.0	1570	29	8	8	33	n/a	n/a	n/a	n/a
Sides													
Chicken noodle soup	1 cup	170	4	1.0	1220	25	1	1	10	n/a	n/a	n/a	n/a
Chicken tortilla soup	1 cup	340	11	3.0	1070	38	17	4	24	n/a	n/a	n/a	n/a
Fruit cup	medium	60	0	0.0	0	15	2	11	1	n/a	n/a	n/a	n/a
Kale crunch	1	170	12	1.5	250	13	4	8	4	n/a	n/a	n/a	n/a
Mac & cheese	medium	450	29	16.0	1190	28	3	3	20	n/a	n/a	n/a	n/a
Side salad w/ avocado lime ranch dressing	1	470	42	8.0	700	14	4	5	6	n/a	n/a	n/a	n/a
Waffle potato chips	1 pkt	220	13	3.5	250	25	2	0	3	n/a	n/a	n/a	n/a
Waffle potato fries	medium	420	24	4.0	240	45	5	1	5	n/a	n/a	n/a	n/a
Drinks													
Frosted coffee	1	250	6	4.0	120	43	0	39	6	n/a	n/a	n/a	n/a
Lemonade	medium	220	0	0.0	10	58	0	55	0	n/a	n/a	n/a	n/a
diet	medium	50	0	0.0	10	14	0	10	0	n/a	n/a	n/a	n/a
frosted	1	330	6	4.0	120	65	0	63	6	n/a	n/a	n/a	n/a
Desserts													
Chocolate chunk cookie	1	370	17	9.0	230	49	3	26	5	n/a	n/a	n/a	n/a
Chocolate fudge brownie	1	380	21	7.0	150	48	2	36	4	n/a	n/a	n/a	n/a
Icedream													
cone	1	180	4	2.5	90	32	0	25	4	n/a	n/a	n/a	n/a
cup	1	140	4	2.5	75	24	0	24	4	n/a	n/a	n/a	n/a
Milkshakes													
chocolate	1	590	22	14.0	360	90	1	87	12	n/a	n/a	n/a	n/a
cookies & cream	1	630	26	15.0	440	90	1	84	13	n/a	n/a	n/a	n/a
strawberry	1	570	19	12.0	380	92	1	87	11	n/a	n/a	n/a	n/a
vanilla	1	580	23	15.0	390	82	1	80	13	n/a	n/a	n/a	n/a

Chili's

	Amount	Calories	Fat (g)	Saturated Fat (g)	Sodium (mg)	Carbohydrate (g)	Fiber (g)	Sugar (g)	Protein (g)	Vitamin D (mcg)	Calcium (mg)	Iron (mg)	Potassium (mg)
Appetizers													
Bone-in wings													
Buffalo	1 order	890	65	11.0	2770	3	1	1	73	n/a	n/a	n/a	n/a
honey chipotle	1 order	1060	54	9.0	2460	74	1	53	73	n/a	n/a	n/a	n/a
house BBQ	1 order	860	55	10.0	2210	18	1	16	74	n/a	n/a	n/a	n/a
Boneless wings													
Buffalo	1 order	1060	71	12.0	3810	57	4	2	49	n/a	n/a	n/a	n/a
honey chipotle	1 order	1190	57	10.0	2960	125	4	53	48	n/a	n/a	n/a	n/a
house BBQ	1 order	1090	60	10.0	3580	88	5	29	50	n/a	n/a	n/a	n/a
Chips													
w/ fresh guacamole	1 order	1140	66	10.0	2350	128	18	7	16	n/a	n/a	n/a	n/a
w/ salsa	1 order	910	45	7.0	1920	113	8	5	13	n/a	n/a	n/a	n/a
w/ skillet queso	1 order	1340	77	26.0	4560	129	10	13	35	n/a	n/a	n/a	n/a
white queso	1 order	1160	80	20.0	3310	128	9	12	31	n/a	n/a	n/a	n/a
Fried mozzarella	1 order	920	55	27.0	2950	59	6	8	48	n/a	n/a	n/a	n/a
Quesadillas													
brisket	1 order	1670	129	44.0	2920	76	4	17	64	n/a	n/a	n/a	n/a
chicken bacon ranch	1 order	1670	125	40.0	2950	69	4	10	70	n/a	n/a	n/a	n/a
Southwestern eggrolls	1 order	800	41	10.0	2170	82	8	9	28	n/a	n/a	n/a	n/a
Texas cheese fries	1 order	1800	122	51.0	4130	99	8	4	77	n/a	n/a	n/a	n/a
w/ chili	1 order	2140	141	58.0	5520	112	9	8	94	n/a	n/a	n/a	n/a
Baby Back Ribs (w/o sides)													
Dry rub half rack	1	780	54	20.0	2960	23	2	19	50	n/a	n/a	n/a	n/a
Honey chipotle BBQ half rack	1	760	53	20.0	900	23	0	17	49	n/a	n/a	n/a	n/a
House BBQ half rack	1	720	53	20.0	1090	11	1	9	49	n/a	n/a	n/a	n/a
Big Mouth Burgers (w/o fries)													
Alex's Santa Fe	1	920	61	23.0	1130	49	6	11	49	n/a	n/a	n/a	n/a
Bacon Rancher	1	1710	123	50.0	2660	48	3	14	100	n/a	n/a	n/a	n/a
BBQ brisket	1	1130	74	30.0	2020	52	3	18	64	n/a	n/a	n/a	n/a
Big Mouth Bites	4	1290	80	28.0	2670	77	5	20	65	n/a	n/a	n/a	n/a
Just Bacon	1	1020	69	26.0	1330	47	3	12	53	n/a	n/a	n/a	n/a
Mushroom Swiss	1	990	68	25.0	1000	47	4	12	50	n/a	n/a	n/a	n/a
Oldtimer w/ cheese	1	850	53	22.0	1220	46	4	11	48	n/a	n/a	n/a	n/a
Secret Sauce	1	970	65	24.0	1180	50	3	17	46	n/a	n/a	n/a	n/a
Add-ons													
applewood smoked bacon	1 order	70	6	2.0	210	0	0	0	5	n/a	n/a	n/a	n/a
avocado slices	1 order	80	7	1.0	0	4	3	0	1	n/a	n/a	n/a	n/a
The Original Chili	1 order	110	6	2.5	460	4	0	1	6	n/a	n/a	n/a	n/a
patties													
black bean	1	180	6	1.0	450	26	9	3	15	n/a	n/a	n/a	n/a
classic beef	1	470	37	16.0	330	0	0	0	36	n/a	n/a	n/a	n/a
sautéed mushrooms	1 order	60	5	1.5	150	3	1	1	1	n/a	n/a	n/a	n/a

RESTAURANT & FAST FOOD CHAINS

Chili's

	Amount	Calories	Fat (g)	Saturated Fat (g)	Sodium (mg)	Carbohydrate (g)	Fiber (g)	Sugar (g)	Protein (g)	Vitamin D (mcg)	Calcium (mg)	Iron (mg)	Potassium (mg)
Cajun Pasta													
w/ grilled chicken	1 order	1280	63	27.0	3820	111	8	6	70	n/a	n/a	n/a	n/a
w/ shrimp	1 order	1170	57	25.0	3690	109	8	5	54	n/a	n/a	n/a	n/a
Ultimate	1 order	1310	62	26.0	3690	109	8	5	78	n/a	n/a	n/a	n/a
Chicken Crispers													
Honey chipotle	5 pcs	1260	64	11.0	4330	118	3	53	57	n/a	n/a	n/a	n/a
Regular	5 pcs	990	64	11.0	3320	47	3	1	57	n/a	n/a	n/a	n/a
Sauces													
Buffalo	1 order	35	3	0.0	1380	2	0	1	0	n/a	n/a	n/a	n/a
Buffalo ranch	1 order	180	19	3.0	570	2	0	1	1	n/a	n/a	n/a	n/a
house BBQ	1 order	80	1	0.0	790	16	1	14	1	n/a	n/a	n/a	n/a
honey mustard	1 order	200	18	3.0	330	10	0	10	1	n/a	n/a	n/a	n/a
ranch	1 order	170	18	3.0	290	2	0	2	1	n/a	n/a	n/a	n/a
Sweet Chili Zing	1 order	120	0	0.0	930	28	1	26	1	n/a	n/a	n/a	n/a
Sides													
fries	1 order	420	17	2.5	660	60	5	0	6	n/a	n/a	n/a	n/a
white cheddar mac & cheese	1 order	270	16	8.0	850	22	1	0	10	n/a	n/a	n/a	n/a
Fajitas													
Grilled chicken	1 order	470	18	4.0	2090	22	3	10	58	n/a	n/a	n/a	n/a
Grilled steak	1 order	580	29	8.0	2200	25	3	11	57	n/a	n/a	n/a	n/a
Shrimp	1 order	310	15	3.5	2640	21	3	10	25	n/a	n/a	n/a	n/a
Toppings	1 order	250	20	12.0	490	4	0	2	14	n/a	n/a	n/a	n/a
grilled chicken	1 order	150	4	1.0	530	1	0	0	28	n/a	n/a	n/a	n/a
grilled steak	1 order	200	9	3.0	590	2	0	1	27	n/a	n/a	n/a	n/a
guacamole	1 order	50	5	0.5	95	3	2	0	1	n/a	n/a	n/a	n/a
jalepeño-cheddar sausage	1 order	250	21	9.0	890	3	1	0	14	n/a	n/a	n/a	n/a
peppers & onions	1 order	180	11	2.5	1020	20	3	9	3	n/a	n/a	n/a	n/a
seared shrimp	1 order	60	2	0.0	810	1	0	0	11	n/a	n/a	n/a	n/a
Tortillas													
corn	4	250	3	0.5	0	51	5	1	5	n/a	n/a	n/a	n/a
flour	4	360	10	4.5	430	58	4	4	9	n/a	n/a	n/a	n/a
Sides													
beans	1 order	120	1	0.0	710	20	6	2	7	n/a	n/a	n/a	n/a
rice	1 order	160	5	1.0	480	27	1	1	3	n/a	n/a	n/a	n/a
Guiltless Grill													
Ancho salmon	1 order	630	32	6.0	1810	41	5	3	48	n/a	n/a	n/a	n/a
Margarita grilled chicken	1 order	630	16	3.0	2280	68	7	9	52	n/a	n/a	n/a	n/a
Quesadillas													
Brisket	1 order	1670	129	44.0	2920	76	4	17	54	n/a	n/a	n/a	n/a
Chicken bacon ranch	1 order	1670	125	40.0	2950	69	4	10	70	n/a	n/a	n/a	n/a

RESTAURANT & FAST FOOD CHAINS

Chili's

Sandwiches (w/o fries)	Amount	Calories	Fat (g)	Saturated Fat (g)	Sodium (mg)	Carbohydrate (g)	Fiber (g)	Sugar (g)	Protein (g)	Vitamin D (mcg)	Calcium (mg)	Iron (mg)	Potassium (mg)
Bacon avocado grilled chicken	1	1150	62	16.0	2220	74	8	15	78	n/a	n/a	n/a	n/a
Big Mouth crispy chicken	1	1040	56	10.0	2530	90	6	20	45	n/a	n/a	n/a	n/a
Buffalo chicken ranch	1	980	51	9.0	4290	84	6	13	46	n/a	n/a	n/a	n/a
Chili's Philly	1	1070	54	20.0	3790	80	6	20	66	n/a	n/a	n/a	n/a
Smokehouse Combos													
Crispers													
honey chipotle w/ ranch	1 order	900	56	10.0	2790	66	2	28	35	n/a	n/a	n/a	n/a
w/o sauce	1 order	590	38	7.0	1990	28	2	1	34	n/a	n/a	n/a	n/a
Jalapeño-cheddar smoked sausage	1 order	250	21	9.0	890	3	1	0	14	n/a	n/a	n/a	n/a
Quesadillas													
brisket	1 order	730	54	20.0	1240	35	2	6	25	n/a	n/a	n/a	n/a
chicken	1 order	730	52	17.0	1260	32	2	3	34	n/a	n/a	n/a	n/a
Ribs													
dry rub	1 order	780	54	20.0	2960	23	2	19	50	n/a	n/a	n/a	n/a
honey chipotle BBQ	1 order	760	53	20.0	900	23	0	17	49	n/a	n/a	n/a	n/a
house BBQ	1 order	720	53	20.0	1090	11	1	9	49	n/a	n/a	n/a	n/a
Sides													
corn	1 order	390	28	5.0	270	30	3	12	6	n/a	n/a	n/a	n/a
fries	1 order	420	17	2.5	660	60	5	0	6	n/a	n/a	n/a	n/a
garlic toast	1 order	140	7	1.5	380	17	1	1	3	n/a	n/a	n/a	n/a
Steaks (w/o sides)													
Classic ribeye	1 order	620	39	17.0	1440	0	0	0	67	n/a	n/a	n/a	n/a
Classic sirloin													
	6 oz	250	12	4.5	630	1	0	0	34	n/a	n/a	n/a	n/a
w/ avocado		360	18	4.5	1010	12	6	3	39	n/a	n/a	n/a	n/a
	10 oz	390	18	6.0	950	2	0	1	54	n/a	n/a	n/a	n/a
w/ avocado		510	26	7.0	1310	13	6	3	60	n/a	n/a	n/a	n/a
Add seared shrimp	1 order	60	2	0.0	810	1	0	0	11	n/a	n/a	n/a	n/a
Salads													
Caesar side	1	410	34	9.0	690	13	2	2	13	n/a	n/a	n/a	n/a
House side w/o dressing	1	140	7	3.0	280	15	2	4	6	n/a	n/a	n/a	n/a
add ancho salmon	1 order	370	21	3.5	880	4	0	1	41	n/a	n/a	n/a	n/a
add shrimp	1 order	60	2	0.0	810	1	0	0	11	n/a	n/a	n/a	n/a
Sante Fe													
w/ grilled chicken	1	560	39	7.0	650	24	7	6	30	n/a	n/a	n/a	n/a
w/ crispers	1	810	60	10.0	1980	43	8	7	28	n/a	n/a	n/a	n/a
Quesadilla explosion w/ grilled chicken	1	1160	78	24.0	1510	67	6	16	53	n/a	n/a	n/a	n/a
Dressings													
avocado ranch	1.5 oz	140	14	2.5	240	3	1	1	1	n/a	n/a	n/a	n/a
bleu cheese	1.5 oz	250	27	5.0	260	1	0	1	1	n/a	n/a	n/a	n/a

RESTAURANT & FAST FOOD CHAINS

Chili's	Amount	Calories	Fat (g)	Saturated Fat (g)	Sodium (mg)	Carbohydrate (g)	Fiber (g)	Sugar (g)	Protein (g)	Vitamin D (mcg)	Calcium (mg)	Iron (mg)	Potassium (mg)
Caesar	1.5 oz	220	23	4.0	250	2	0	1	2	n/a	n/a	n/a	n/a
citrus balsamic vinaigrette	1.5 oz	250	25	4.0	230	5	0	5	0	n/a	n/a	n/a	n/a
honey mustard	1.5 oz	200	18	3.0	330	10	0	10	1	n/a	n/a	n/a	n/a
ranch	1.5 oz	170	18	3.0	290	2	0	2	1	n/a	n/a	n/a	n/a
Santa Fe	1.5 oz	210	22	3.5	530	2	0	2	1	n/a	n/a	n/a	n/a
Thousand Island	1.5 oz	200	19	3.0	370	6	0	6	0	n/a	n/a	n/a	n/a
Soups & Chili													
Chicken enchilada	1 order	410	26	9.0	1490	24	3	3	20	n/a	n/a	n/a	n/a
Loaded baked potato	1 order	430	30	19.0	1280	25	2	7	17	n/a	n/a	n/a	n/a
The Original Chili	1 order	600	35	13.0	2000	28	2	5	27	n/a	n/a	n/a	n/a
Sides													
Asparagus	1 order	35	1	0.0	135	5	3	2	3	n/a	n/a	n/a	n/a
Black beans	1 order	120	1	0.0	710	20	6	2	7	n/a	n/a	n/a	n/a
Homestyle fries	1 order	420	17	2.5	660	60	5	0	6	n/a	n/a	n/a	n/a
Loaded mashed potatoes	1 order	350	20	6.0	820	33	3	3	10	n/a	n/a	n/a	n/a
Mexican rice	1 order	160	5	1.0	480	27	1	1	3	n/a	n/a	n/a	n/a
Roasted street corn	1 order	390	28	5.0	270	30	3	12	6	n/a	n/a	n/a	n/a
Steamed broccoli	1 order	40	0	0.0	250	8	4	2	3	n/a	n/a	n/a	n/a
Sweet corn on the cob	1 order	180	6	1.0	360	29	3	11	4	n/a	n/a	n/a	n/a
White cheddar mac & cheese	1 order	270	16	8.0	850	22	1	0	10	n/a	n/a	n/a	n/a
Desserts													
Cheesecake	1 order	720	43	23.0	430	73	1	60	11	n/a	n/a	n/a	n/a
Molten chocolate cake	1 order	1170	59	30.0	1030	155	5	109	12	n/a	n/a	n/a	n/a
mini	1 order	670	31	14.0	700	95	0	65	7	n/a	n/a	n/a	n/a
Skillet chocolate chip cookie	1 order	1230	52	25.0	1020	174	3	103	13	n/a	n/a	n/a	n/a
Chipotle													
Meals													
Bases													
burrito, flour	1	320	9	0.5	600	50	3	0	8	n/a	n/a	n/a	n/a
taco													
crispy corn	1	70	3	0.0	0	10	1	0	1	n/a	n/a	n/a	n/a
flour	1	80	3	0.0	160	13	0	0	2	n/a	n/a	n/a	n/a
Toppings													
barbacoa	1 order	170	7	2.5	530	2	1	0	24	n/a	n/a	n/a	n/a
beans													
black	1 order	130	1.5	0.0	210	22	7	2	8	n/a	n/a	n/a	n/a
pinto	1 order	130	1.5	0.0	210	21	8	1	8	n/a	n/a	n/a	n/a
carnitas	1 order	210	12	7.0	450	0	0	0	23	n/a	n/a	n/a	n/a
chicken	1 order	180	7	3.0	310	0	0	0	32	n/a	n/a	n/a	n/a
cheese	1 order	110	8	5.0	190	1	0	0	6	n/a	n/a	n/a	n/a
chipotle-honey vinaigrette	1 order	220	16	2.5	850	18	1	12	1	n/a	n/a	n/a	n/a

RESTAURANT & FAST FOOD CHAINS

Chipotle	Amount	Calories	Fat (g)	Saturated Fat (g)	Sodium (mg)	Carbohydrate (g)	Fiber (g)	Sugar (g)	Protein (g)	Vitamin D (mcg)	Calcium (mg)	Iron (mg)	Potassium (mg)
cilantro-lime rice													
brown	1 order	210	6	1.0	190	36	2	0	4	n/a	n/a	n/a	n/a
white	1 order	210	4	0.5	350	40	1	0	4	n/a	n/a	n/a	n/a
fajita vegetables	1 order	20	0	0.0	150	5	1	2	1	n/a	n/a	n/a	n/a
lettuce													
romaine	1 order	5	0	0.0	0	1	1	0	0	n/a	n/a	n/a	n/a
supergreens blend	1 order	15	0	0.0	15	3	2	1	1	n/a	n/a	n/a	n/a
quesadilla cheese	1 order	330	24	15.0	570	3	0	0	18	n/a	n/a	n/a	n/a
salsa													
fresh tomato	1 order	25	0	0.0	550	4	1	1	0	n/a	n/a	n/a	n/a
roasted chili-corn	1 order	80	2	0.0	330	16	3	4	3	n/a	n/a	n/a	n/a
tomatillo green-chili	1 order	15	0	0.0	260	4	0	2	0	n/a	n/a	n/a	n/a
tomatillo red-chili	1 order	30	0	0.0	500	4	1	0	0	n/a	n/a	n/a	n/a
sofritas	1 order	150	10	1.5	560	9	3	5	8	n/a	n/a	n/a	n/a
sour cream	1 order	110	9	7.0	30	2	0	2	2	n/a	n/a	n/a	n/a
steak	1 order	150	6	2.5	330	1	1	0	21	n/a	n/a	n/a	n/a
Sides													
Chips	regular	540	25	3.5	390	73	7	1	7	n/a	n/a	n/a	n/a
Guacamole	side (4 oz)	230	22	3.5	370	8	6	1	2	n/a	n/a	n/a	n/a
Queso blanco	side (4 oz)	240	18	12.0	400	7	0	2	10	n/a	n/a	n/a	n/a

Dairy Queen

Burgers	Amount	Calories	Fat (g)	Saturated Fat (g)	Sodium (mg)	Carbohydrate (g)	Fiber (g)	Sugar (g)	Protein (g)	Vitamin D (mcg)	Calcium (mg)	Iron (mg)	Potassium (mg)
Backyard Bacon Ranch Stackburger	1	820	51	19.0	1900	53	1	15	38	n/a	n/a	n/a	n/a
triple	1	1020	67	27.0	2310	54	1	15	50	n/a	n/a	n/a	n/a
FlameThrower Stackburger	1	720	49	19.0	1430	37	2	7	34	n/a	n/a	n/a	n/a
triple	1	910	65	27.0	1820	38	2	7	46	n/a	n/a	n/a	n/a
Hamburger	1	320	13	5.0	870	38	1	7	15	n/a	n/a	n/a	n/a
Original cheeseburger	1	370	18	8.0	1120	37	1	8	17	n/a	n/a	n/a	n/a
double	1	570	34	15.0	1530	38	1	8	29	n/a	n/a	n/a	n/a
triple	1	760	50	23.0	1940	39	1	9	40	n/a	n/a	n/a	n/a
Two Cheese Deluxe Stackburger	1	620	39	16.0	1510	39	2	9	29	n/a	n/a	n/a	n/a
triple	1	820	55	24.0	1930	40	2	9	41	n/a	n/a	n/a	n/a
bacon	1	720	47	19.0	1890	39	2	9	37	n/a	n/a	n/a	n/a
triple	1	920	63	26.0	2300	40	2	9	49	n/a	n/a	n/a	n/a
Chicken													
Chicken strip basket	4 pcs	1020	48	8.0	2120	111	6	3	35	n/a	n/a	n/a	n/a
honey BBQ sauced & tossed	4 pcs	1140	48	8.0	2640	142	7	32	35	n/a	n/a	n/a	n/a
Chicken strip sandwiches													
original	1	550	26	4.5	990	62	3	6	18	n/a	n/a	n/a	n/a
spicy	1	530	23	4.0	1060	63	3	8	18	n/a	n/a	n/a	n/a
Rotisserie-style chicken bites	regular	150	6	2.0	440	1	0	0	25	n/a	n/a	n/a	n/a

Dairy Queen

	Amount	Calories	Fat (g)	Saturated Fat (g)	Sodium (mg)	Carbohydrate (g)	Fiber (g)	Sugar (g)	Protein (g)	Vitamin D (mcg)	Calcium (mg)	Iron (mg)	Potassium (mg)
Hot Dogs													
Chili cheese dog	1	420	26	11.0	1070	28	1	4	18	n/a	n/a	n/a	n/a
Hot dog	1	330	19	8.0	820	25	1	3	12	n/a	n/a	n/a	n/a
Salads													
Crispy chicken strips salad bowl	1	430	22	7.0	1030	35	4	5	24	n/a	n/a	n/a	n/a
Rotisserie-style chicken bites salad bowl	1	310	15	6.0	850	8	2	4	37	n/a	n/a	n/a	n/a
Side salad	1	20	0	0.0	10	4	1	3	1	n/a	n/a	n/a	n/a
Sides													
Cheese curds	regular	500	34	19.0	990	26	0	1	24	n/a	n/a	n/a	n/a
Fries	regular	280	13	2.0	590	36	3	0	5	n/a	n/a	n/a	n/a
Onion rings	regular	290	13	2.0	680	39	2	3	5	n/a	n/a	n/a	n/a
Pretzel sticks w/ zesty queso	1 order	330	9	3.0	2060	52	2	7	9	n/a	n/a	n/a	n/a
Dressings & Sauces													
Dressings													
honey mustard	1 order	130	9	1.5	330	12	0	0	0	n/a	n/a	n/a	n/a
Dijon	1 order	180	16	2.5	230	· 7	0	7	0	n/a	n/a	n/a	n/a
Italian													
fat-free	1 order	25	0	0.0	380	4	0	3	1	n/a	n/a	n/a	n/a
light	1 order	15	1	0.0	730	2	0	2	0	n/a	n/a	n/a	n/a
Sauces													
BBQ	1 order	90	0	0.0	430	21	1	16	1	n/a	n/a	n/a	n/a
country gravy	1 order	70	5	1.5	360	6	0	1	0	n/a	n/a	n/a	n/a
honey mustard	1 order	240	20	3.0	450	15	0	14	1	n/a	n/a	n/a	n/a
house-made Hidden Valley Ranch	1 order	220	22	4.0	370	3	0	2	1	n/a	n/a	n/a	n/a
wild Buffalo	1 order	90	10	1.0	1000	1	0	0	0	n/a	n/a	n/a	n/a
zesty queso	1 order	110	10	3.0	570	3	0	1	2	n/a	n/a	n/a	n/a
Blizzards													
Butterfinger	mini	350	12	7.0	150	52	1	41	9	n/a	n/a	n/a	n/a
	medium	730	26	15.0	330	107	2	81	18	n/a	n/a	n/a	n/a
Choco Brownie Extreme	mini	400	17	10.0	180	56	2	45	9	n/a	n/a	n/a	n/a
	medium	810	36	21.0	370	111	4	87	16	n/a	n/a	n/a	n/a
Chocolate chip cookie dough	mini	420	16	9.0	220	61	1	46	8	n/a	n/a	n/a	n/a
	medium	1030	41	24.0	570	151	2	111	17	n/a	n/a	n/a	n/a
Heath	mini	370	15	9.0	180	53	0	46	8	n/a	n/a	n/a	n/a
	medium	860	37	23.0	440	119	1	106	16	n/a	n/a	n/a	n/a
M&M's	mini	370	12	8.0	125	58	1	50	8	n/a	n/a	n/a	n/a
	medium	800	27	17.0	250	124	2	107	16	n/a	n/a	n/a	n/a
Oreo	mini	380	14	7.0	180	56	0	44	8	n/a	n/a	n/a	n/a
	medium	790	31	15.0	400	117	1	88	14	n/a	n/a	n/a	n/a
Reese's	mini	360	14	7.0	170	50	1	43	9	n/a	n/a	n/a	n/a
	medium	750	31	16.0	380	102	2	88	19	n/a	n/a	n/a	n/a

RESTAURANT & FAST FOOD CHAINS

	Amount	Calories	Fat (g)	Saturated Fat (g)	Sodium (mg)	Carbohydrate (g)	Fiber (g)	Sugar (g)	Protein (g)	Vitamin D (mcg)	Calcium (mg)	Iron (mg)	Potassium (mg)
Royal New York Cheesecake Strawberry	mini	450	18	8.0	220	65	1	53	8	n/a	n/a	n/a	n/a
	medium	1040	46	21.0	530	140	2	112	19	n/a	n/a	n/a	n/a
Royal Ultimate Choco Brownie	mini	480	21	13.0	220	68	2	55	9	n/a	n/a	n/a	n/a
	medium	1040	45	29.0	480	146	5	117	19	n/a	n/a	n/a	n/a
Snickers	mini	350	12	7.0	150	53	0	45	8	n/a	n/a	n/a	n/a
	medium	800	28	15.0	340	120	1	102	19	n/a	n/a	n/a	n/a
Turtle pecan cluster	mini	430	22	14.0	160	51	1	42	8	n/a	n/a	n/a	n/a
	medium	1020	52	29.0	390	123	3	99	18	n/a	n/a	n/a	n/a
Cakes & Treatzzas													
Blizzard cakes (10 in)													
Oreo	⅛ cake	864	37	26.0	391	120	2	92	14	n/a	n/a	n/a	n/a
Signature all-occasion	⅛ cake	730	30	22.5	394	111	4	81	15	n/a	n/a	n/a	n/a
Treatzza pizzas													
choco brownie	⅛ pizza	190	10	6.0	95	26	1	18	3	n/a	n/a	n/a	n/a
Heath	⅛ pizza	190	9	6.0	90	26	1	19	2	n/a	n/a	n/a	n/a
M&M's	⅛ pizza	200	9	7.0	85	28	1	20	3	n/a	n/a	n/a	n/a
Reese's peanut butter cup	⅛ pizza	200	10	6.0	110	24	1	17	3	n/a	n/a	n/a	n/a
Cones													
Chocolate	medium	340	10	6.0	130	52	0	35	8	n/a	n/a	n/a	n/a
Dipped													
butterscotch	medium	460	21	17.0	150	59	0	45	8	n/a	n/a	n/a	n/a
cherry	medium	460	22	18.0	140	58	0	44	8	n/a	n/a	n/a	n/a
chocolate	medium	460	22	17.0	140	58	1	43	9	n/a	n/a	n/a	n/a
Vanilla	medium	320	10	6.0	130	50	0	36	8	n/a	n/a	n/a	n/a
Frozen Drinks													
Misty Freeze	medium	450	12	8.0	160	77	0	68	10	n/a	n/a	n/a	n/a
Misty Slush	medium	260	0	0.0	40	65	0	64	0	n/a	n/a	n/a	n/a
Moolatté													
caramel	medium	620	18	13.0	240	103	0	87	10	n/a	n/a	n/a	n/a
mocha	medium	620	23	14.0	240	94	2	82	11	n/a	n/a	n/a	n/a
vanilla	medium	560	17	12.0	190	93	0	84	9	n/a	n/a	n/a	n/a
Shakes													
banana	medium	590	22	16.0	240	83	1	68	16	n/a	n/a	n/a	n/a
caramel	medium	750	25	17.0	330	115	0	93	17	n/a	n/a	n/a	n/a
chocolate	medium	710	23	16.0	290	110	1	96	16	n/a	n/a	n/a	n/a
hot fudge	medium	750	30	23.0	330	105	1	85	17	n/a	n/a	n/a	n/a
peanut butter	medium	930	53	20.0	590	91	3	69	22	n/a	n/a	n/a	n/a
strawberry	medium	630	23	16.0	260	92	1	80	16	n/a	n/a	n/a	n/a
vanilla	medium	660	23	16.0	260	97	0	85	16	n/a	n/a	n/a	n/a
add Make It a Malt	medium	80	1	0.5	80	18	1	12	1	n/a	n/a	n/a	n/a
Smoothies													
mango pineapple	medium	330	0	0.0	135	77	1	74	6	n/a	n/a	n/a	n/a
strawberry banana	medium	350	0	0.0	140	83	3	75	6	n/a	n/a	n/a	n/a
tripleberry	medium	370	0	0.0	135	87	2	84	6	n/a	n/a	n/a	n/a

RESTAURANT & FAST FOOD CHAINS

	Amount	Calories	Fat (g)	Saturated Fat (g)	Sodium (mg)	Carbohydrate (g)	Fiber (g)	Sugar (g)	Protein (g)	Vitamin D (mcg)	Calcium (mg)	Iron (mg)	Potassium (mg)
Dairy Queen													
Sundaes													
Caramel	medium	430	11	7.0	190	73	0	58	9	n/a	n/a	n/a	n/a
Chocolate	medium	400	10	6.0	160	70	1	60	8	n/a	n/a	n/a	n/a
Hot fudge	medium	430	15	11.0	190	66	1	52	9	n/a	n/a	n/a	n/a
Peanut butter	medium	560	32	10.0	380	56	2	40	13	n/a	n/a	n/a	n/a
Pineapple	medium	330	10	6.0	120	54	1	47	8	n/a	n/a	n/a	n/a
Strawberry	medium	340	10	6.0	135	56	1	49	8	n/a	n/a	n/a	n/a
Add DQ sprinkles	1 order	35	2	1.0	0	6	0	3	0	n/a	n/a	n/a	n/a
Other Treats													
Banana split	1	520	14	9.0	150	94	4	74	9	n/a	n/a	n/a	n/a
Brownie & Oreo Cupfection	1	720	23	9.0	330	122	2	96	10	n/a	n/a	n/a	n/a
Buster bar	1	442	27	16.0	193	43	3	34	11	n/a	n/a	n/a	n/a
Dilly bar	1	202	12	10.0	50	21	1	18	3	n/a	n/a	n/a	n/a
DQ sandwich	1	183	5	3.0	130	30	1	17	4	n/a	n/a	n/a	n/a
Peanut Buster parfait	1	710	31	18.0	340	95	3	68	17	n/a	n/a	n/a	n/a
Triple chocolate brownie dessert	1	540	25	9.0	260	74	3	57	8	n/a	n/a	n/a	n/a
Denny's													
Breakfast													
Benny w/ hash browns	1 order	730	37	12.0	2020	64	2	9	32	n/a	n/a	n/a	n/a
southwestern	1 order	950	60	20.0	2100	65	3	5	36	n/a	n/a	n/a	n/a
Chicken biscuit & gravy bowl w/ eggs	1 order	1020	61	24.0	3070	80	4	7	39	n/a	n/a	n/a	n/a
Country fried steak & eggs w/ gravy, hash browns & toast	1 order	810	43	13.0	1850	82	2	4	22	n/a	n/a	n/a	n/a
Grand Slamwich w/ hash browns	1 order	1300	79	26.0	3470	94	3	9	52	n/a	n/a	n/a	n/a
Moons Over My Hammy w/ hash browns	1 order	1040	54	18.0	2960	90	3	4	47	n/a	n/a	n/a	n/a
Sante Fe skillet w/ eggs	1 order	770	58	19.0	1890	38	4	4	27	n/a	n/a	n/a	n/a
T-bone steak & eggs w/ hash browns & toast	1 order	910	49	16.0	2190	55	1	3	59	n/a	n/a	n/a	n/a
Omelettes													
Build Your Own													
bacon	2 slices	100	8	3.0	350	1	0	1	7	n/a	n/a	n/a	n/a
caramelized onions	1 order	70	7	1.0	210	2	1	1	0	n/a	n/a	n/a	n/a
cheese													
American	1 slice	80	7	4.0	390	1	0	1	4	n/a	n/a	n/a	n/a
cheddar	1 order	80	6	3.5	120	0	0	0	5	n/a	n/a	n/a	n/a
pepper Jack queso	1 order	100	7	3.0	360	5	0	2	3	n/a	n/a	n/a	n/a
Swiss	1 slice	80	6	4.0	45	0	0	0	6	n/a	n/a	n/a	n/a
chorizo sausage	1 order	330	27	10.0	830	4	0	0	17	n/a	n/a	n/a	n/a
fire-roasted bell peppers & onions	1 order	70	6	1.0	110	4	1	2	0	n/a	n/a	n/a	n/a
fresh avocado	1 order	90	8	1.0	0	5	4	0	1	n/a	n/a	n/a	n/a
fresh spinach	1 order	5	0	0.0	10	0	0	0	0	n/a	n/a	n/a	n/a
ham	1 order	120	4	1.5	860	7	0	6	14	n/a	n/a	n/a	n/a
jalapeños	1 order	5	0	0.0	440	1	0	1	0	n/a	n/a	n/a	n/a

RESTAURANT & FAST FOOD CHAINS

Denny's

	Amount	Calories	Fat (g)	Saturated Fat (g)	Sodium (mg)	Carbohydrate (g)	Fiber (g)	Sugar (g)	Protein (g)	Vitamin D (mcg)	Calcium (mg)	Iron (mg)	Potassium (mg)
omelette, plain	1	340	26	7.0	540	2	0	0	21	n/a	n/a	n/a	n/a
egg white	1	110	2	0.0	340	1	0	1	20	n/a	n/a	n/a	n/a
pico de gallo	1 order	15	0	0.0	75	3	1	2	1	n/a	n/a	n/a	n/a
sausage	1 order	180	17	5.0	330	0	0	0	6	n/a	n/a	n/a	n/a
sautéed mushrooms	1 order	50	6	1.0	55	1	0	0	1	n/a	n/a	n/a	n/a
tomatoes	1 order	10	0	0.0	0	2	1	1	0	n/a	n/a	n/a	n/a
turkey bacon	2 slices	70	4	1.0	330	1	0	1	7	n/a	n/a	n/a	n/a
Loaded Veggie w/ hash browns & toast	1 order	920	56	16.0	1540	63	3	6	36	n/a	n/a	n/a	n/a
Mile High Denver w/ hash browns & toast	1 order	1090	67	21.0	3130	69	2	12	51	n/a	n/a	n/a	n/a
Philly Cheesesteak w/ hash browns & toast	1 order	1130	71	21.0	2010	63	2	5	54	n/a	n/a	n/a	n/a
Ultimate w/ hash browns & toast	1 order	1140	77	23.0	2110	63	3	7	44	n/a	n/a	n/a	n/a

Pancakes & Crepes

	Amount	Calories	Fat (g)	Saturated Fat (g)	Sodium (mg)	Carbohydrate (g)	Fiber (g)	Sugar (g)	Protein (g)	Vitamin D (mcg)	Calcium (mg)	Iron (mg)	Potassium (mg)
Berry vanilla crepes													
à la carte	1 order	270	12	4.5	210	30	2	22	4	n/a	n/a	n/a	n/a
breakfast	1 order	440	20	6.0	670	60	3	23	5	n/a	n/a	n/a	n/a
Choconana pancakes	2	830	25	13.0	1360	149	9	72	14	n/a	n/a	n/a	n/a
Cinnamon roll pancakes													
w/ cream cheese icing	2	1100	26	11.0	1700	207	4	146	10	n/a	n/a	n/a	n/a
w/ salted caramel	2	970	21	9.0	1750	185	4	121	11	n/a	n/a	n/a	n/a
Double berry pancakes	2	490	7	2.5	1360	97	6	32	11	n/a	n/a	n/a	n/a
Hearty 9-grain pancakes	2	410	11	4.0	880	68	5	21	10	n/a	n/a	n/a	n/a

Slams

	Amount	Calories	Fat (g)	Saturated Fat (g)	Sodium (mg)	Carbohydrate (g)	Fiber (g)	Sugar (g)	Protein (g)	Vitamin D (mcg)	Calcium (mg)	Iron (mg)	Potassium (mg)
All-American w/ hash browns & toast	1 order	1170	80	27.0	2340	57	1	3	50	n/a	n/a	n/a	n/a
FitSlam	1 order	450	12	2.5	860	59	5	22	27	n/a	n/a	n/a	n/a
French Toast	1 order	800	52	16.0	1560	52	1	12	30	n/a	n/a	n/a	n/a
Lumberjack w/ hash browns & toast	1 order	1230	56	16.0	3900	135	3	26	44	n/a	n/a	n/a	n/a

Breakfast Sides

	Amount	Calories	Fat (g)	Saturated Fat (g)	Sodium (mg)	Carbohydrate (g)	Fiber (g)	Sugar (g)	Protein (g)	Vitamin D (mcg)	Calcium (mg)	Iron (mg)	Potassium (mg)
Bacon strips	4	210	16	6.0	700	2	0	1	14	n/a	n/a	n/a	n/a
Buttermilk biscuits	2	450	26	15.0	1040	52	2	6	6	n/a	n/a	n/a	n/a
Cheddar cheese hash browns	1 order	250	14	6.0	580	24	1	1	6	n/a	n/a	n/a	n/a
Eggs													
boiled	1	60	4	1.5	60	0	0	0	6	n/a	n/a	n/a	n/a
fried/basted	1	90	8	2.0	100	0	0	0	6	n/a	n/a	n/a	n/a
scrambled	1	110	9	2.5	180	1	0	0	7	n/a	n/a	n/a	n/a
white	1	40	0	0.0	115	0	0	0	7	n/a	n/a	n/a	n/a
English muffin													
w/ margarine	1	190	6	1.0	270	29	1	1	5	n/a	n/a	n/a	n/a
w/o margarine	1	140	1	0.0	220	29	1	1	5	n/a	n/a	n/a	n/a
gluten-free													
w/ margarine	1	210	6	0.5	540	36	1	7	4	n/a	n/a	n/a	n/a
w/o margarine	1	180	2	0.0	500	36	1	7	4	n/a	n/a	n/a	n/a

RESTAURANT & FAST FOOD CHAINS

Denny's	Amount	Calories	Fat (g)	Saturated Fat (g)	Sodium (mg)	Carbohydrate (g)	Fiber (g)	Sugar (g)	Protein (g)	Vitamin D (mcg)	Calcium (mg)	Iron (mg)	Potassium (mg)
Grilled ham slice	1	120	4	1.5	860	7	0	6	14	n/a	n/a	n/a	n/a
Hash browns	1 order	180	8	1.5	460	24	1	1	1	n/a	n/a	n/a	n/a
Pancakes	2	450	11	3.5	1390	77	2	20	10	n/a	n/a	n/a	n/a
Red-skinned potatoes	1 order	250	13	2.5	800	30	3	2	4	n/a	n/a	n/a	n/a
Sausage links	4	320	30	10.0	690	0	1	1	11	n/a	n/a	n/a	n/a
Seasonal fruit	1 order	100	0	0.0	5	25	3	17	1	n/a	n/a	n/a	n/a
French toast	1 slice	320	19	8.0	470	26	1	6	9	n/a	n/a	n/a	n/a
Tortillas, flour	3	260	8	3.5	660	40	5	3	7	n/a	n/a	n/a	n/a
Turkey bacon strips	4	140	8	2.0	660	2	0	2	15	n/a	n/a	n/a	n/a
Appetizers													
Boneless chicken wings													
w/ BBQ sauce	8	740	36	5.0	2850	71	4	27	34	n/a	n/a	n/a	n/a
w/ Buffalo sauce	8	770	52	8.0	3730	42	4	0	34	n/a	n/a	n/a	n/a
w/ Nashville hot sauce	8	720	42	8.0	3280	52	5	8	35	n/a	n/a	n/a	n/a
Classic sampler													
w/ Beer-battered onion rings	5 oz	400	27	4.5	710	35	3	5	4	n/a	n/a	n/a	n/a
w/ boneless Buffalo wings	4	380	26	4.0	1860	21	2	0	17	n/a	n/a	n/a	n/a
w/ mozzarella sticks	4	350	16	6.0	840	35	0	3	16	n/a	n/a	n/a	n/a
w/ wavy-cut fries	5 oz	400	22	4.0	470	46	4	0	4	n/a	n/a	n/a	n/a
Mozzarella cheese sticks w/o sauce	1 order	690	32	13.0	1680	70	0	7	32	n/a	n/a	n/a	n/a
Premium chicken tenders w/o sauce	1 order	680	40	5.0	2520	38	3	0	45	n/a	n/a	n/a	n/a
Strawberry pancake puppies	6	620	25	11.0	760	94	2	60	5	n/a	n/a	n/a	n/a
Zesty nachos	1 order	1660	106	36.0	3370	170	11	15	44	n/a	n/a	n/a	n/a
Burgers													
Bacon avocado cheeseburger	1	1020	69	24.0	1420	54	6	11	48	n/a	n/a	n/a	n/a
Bourbon bacon burger	1	880	50	21.0	1480	62	3	21	48	n/a	n/a	n/a	n/a
Build Your Own													
avocado, fresh	1 order	90	8	1.0	0	5	4	0	1	n/a	n/a	n/a	n/a
bacon strips	2 slices	100	8	3.0	350	1	0	1	7	n/a	n/a	n/a	n/a
brioche bun	1	250	5	2.0	360	44	1	8	7	n/a	n/a	n/a	n/a
caramelized onions	1 order	70	7	1.0	210	2	1	1	0	n/a	n/a	n/a	n/a
cheese													
American	1 slice	80	7	4.0	390	1	0	1	4	n/a	n/a	n/a	n/a
cheddar	1 slice	80	7	4.0	135	0	0	0	5	n/a	n/a	n/a	n/a
Swiss	1 slice	80	6	4.0	45	0	0	0	6	n/a	n/a	n/a	n/a
chicken breast													
fried	1	410	26	5.0	1280	18	2	0	27	n/a	n/a	n/a	n/a
grilled seasoned	1	200	9	2.5	820	1	0	0	29	n/a	n/a	n/a	n/a
jalapeños	1 order	5	0	0.0	440	1	0	1	0	n/a	n/a	n/a	n/a
lettuce	1 order	5	0	0.0	5	1	0	0	0	n/a	n/a	n/a	n/a
mayonnaise	1 order	100	11	2.0	75	0	0	0	0	n/a	n/a	n/a	n/a
patties													
100% beef	1	320	24	11.0	440	0	0	0	26	n/a	n/a	n/a	n/a
Dr. Praeger's veggie	1	210	9	1.0	560	25	14	1	8	n/a	n/a	n/a	n/a

RESTAURANT & FAST FOOD CHAINS

Denny's

	Amount	Calories	Fat (g)	Saturated Fat (g)	Sodium (mg)	Carbohydrate (g)	Fiber (g)	Sugar (g)	Protein (g)	Vitamin D (mcg)	Calcium (mg)	Iron (mg)	Potassium (mg)
pickles	4 slices	0	0	0.0	10	0	0	0	0	n/a	n/a	n/a	n/a
red onions	3 rings	5	0	0.0	0	2	0	1	0	n/a	n/a	n/a	n/a
sauces													
BBQ	1 order	60	0	0.0	230	15	0	14	0	n/a	n/a	n/a	n/a
bourbon	1 order	110	0	0.0	270	26	0	24	0	n/a	n/a	n/a	n/a
diner	1 order	150	14	2.5	210	6	0	6	0	n/a	n/a	n/a	n/a
sautéed mushrooms	1 order	50	6	1.0	55	1	0	0	1	n/a	n/a	n/a	n/a
tomato	2 slices	5	0	0.0	0	2	0	1	0	n/a	n/a	n/a	n/a
Double cheeseburger	1	920	52	23.0	1260	49	2	10	61	n/a	n/a	n/a	n/a
Flamin' 5-pepper	1	1000	66	23.0	2060	53	2	13	47	n/a	n/a	n/a	n/a
Slamburger	1	840	47	20.0	1770	58	1	10	45	n/a	n/a	n/a	n/a
Dinners													
Country-fried steak	1 order	960	56	21.0	2240	78	3	4	35	n/a	n/a	n/a	n/a
Oven-baked lasagna	1 order	1130	51	23.0	2290	110	4	7	56	n/a	n/a	n/a	n/a
Plate Lickin' Chicken fried chicken	1 order	1070	62	14.0	3230	68	6	3	60	n/a	n/a	n/a	n/a
Premium chicken tenders	1 order	860	47	7.0	2860	63	3	2	51	n/a	n/a	n/a	n/a
Sirloin steak	1 order	530	25	7.0	1420	27	1	2	49	n/a	n/a	n/a	n/a
Skillets													
bourbon chicken	1 order	910	43	9.0	2070	71	6	36	65	n/a	n/a	n/a	n/a
Crazy Spicy	1 order	1040	69	23.0	3640	48	5	9	59	n/a	n/a	n/a	n/a
Mac 'n Brisket	1 order	990	60	16.0	2160	110	3	21	42	n/a	n/a	n/a	n/a
T-bone steak	1 order	680	38	14.0	1690	26	1	2	57	n/a	n/a	n/a	n/a
Wild Alaska salmon	1 order	540	31	8.0	1300	27	1	2	37	n/a	n/a	n/a	n/a
Melts & Handhelds													
Melts													
Brisk-It-All	1	1190	76	21.0	2670	75	3	12	53	n/a	n/a	n/a	n/a
Nashville hot chicken	1	1250	76	23.0	3200	95	6	12	48	n/a	n/a	n/a	n/a
slow cooker meaty	1	1060	60	18.0	2120	67	3	4	63	n/a	n/a	n/a	n/a
Sandwiches													
Cali club	1	890	55	14.0	2070	59	10	12	44	n/a	n/a	n/a	n/a
Super Bird	1	760	33	14.0	2130	69	2	6	49	n/a	n/a	n/a	n/a
Salads (w/o dressing)													
Cobb	1 order	480	34	12.0	610	23	7	6	22	n/a	n/a	n/a	n/a
House	1 order	190	9	4.5	340	19	3	6	9	n/a	n/a	n/a	n/a
Toppings													
avocado, fresh	1 order	90	8	1.0	0	5	4	0	1	n/a	n/a	n/a	n/a
grilled chicken	1 order	200	9	2.5	820	1	0	0	29	n/a	n/a	n/a	n/a
premium chicken tenders	3	410	24	3.0	1500	23	2	0	27	n/a	n/a	n/a	n/a
prime rib	1 order	140	8	2.0	430	2	0	0	14	n/a	n/a	n/a	n/a
wild Alaskan salmon	1 order	350	23	6.0	780	2	0	1	32	n/a	n/a	n/a	n/a

RESTAURANT & FAST FOOD CHAINS

Denny's

	Amount	Calories	Fat (g)	Saturated Fat (g)	Sodium (mg)	Carbohydrate (g)	Fiber (g)	Sugar (g)	Protein (g)	Vitamin D (mcg)	Calcium (mg)	Iron (mg)	Potassium (mg)
Soups													
Chicken noodle	cup	260	10	4.0	2580	28	2	4	14	n/a	n/a	n/a	n/a
	bowl	390	15	6.0	3880	43	2	5	21	n/a	n/a	n/a	n/a
Loaded baked potato	cup	340	23	11.0	1180	22	1	5	10	n/a	n/a	n/a	n/a
	bowl	440	29	15.0	1650	32	2	6	12	n/a	n/a	n/a	n/a
Vegetable beef	cup	200	11	2.0	2280	27	2	3	11	n/a	n/a	n/a	n/a
	bowl	310	16	3.0	3420	40	3	4	16	n/a	n/a	n/a	n/a
Dinner Sides													
Beer-battered onion rings	1 order	400	27	4.5	710	35	3	5	4	n/a	n/a	n/a	n/a
Fries													
seasoned	1 order	490	26	5.0	1100	57	8	1	7	n/a	n/a	n/a	n/a
wavy-cut	1 order	400	22	4.0	470	46	4	0	4	n/a	n/a	n/a	n/a
Fresh vegetable medly	1 order	70	5	1.0	110	6	2	3	2	n/a	n/a	n/a	n/a
Fruit	1 order	100	0	0.0	5	25	3	17	1	n/a	n/a	n/a	n/a
Garden salad w/o dressing	1	170	9	4.5	340	16	2	4	8	n/a	n/a	n/a	n/a
Garlic toast	2 pcs	190	7	2.0	360	25	1	2	6	n/a	n/a	n/a	n/a
Herb-glazed corn	1 order	300	18	3.5	280	30	8	13	6	n/a	n/a	n/a	n/a
Red-skinned potatoes	1 order	250	13	2.5	800	30	3	2	4	n/a	n/a	n/a	n/a
Whole grain rice	1 order	240	2.5	0.5	360	48	5	2	6	n/a	n/a	n/a	n/a
Desserts													
Caramel apple pie crisp	1 order	740	28	16.0	380	115	0	82	7	n/a	n/a	n/a	n/a
Lava cookie skillet	1 order	820	40	25.0	460	108	0	73	10	n/a	n/a	n/a	n/a
New York–style cheesecake	1 order	490	32	19.0	370	42	1	29	9	n/a	n/a	n/a	n/a
w/ strawberry topping & whipped cream	1 order	560	33	19.0	370	57	1	42	9	n/a	n/a	n/a	n/a
Domino's													
Pizza*													
Buffalo chicken	1 serving	410	19	10.0	1030	38	1	3	18	n/a	n/a	n/a	n/a
Cali chicken bacon ranch	1 serving	480	27	10.0	1060	37	1	3	19	n/a	n/a	n/a	n/a
Deluxe	1 serving	390	19	8.0	780	39	2	4	15	n/a	n/a	n/a	n/a
ExtravaganZZa	1 serving	440	22	9.0	1040	40	2	4	18	n/a	n/a	n/a	n/a
Honolulu Hawaiian	1 serving	380	17	7.0	910	40	1	5	17	n/a	n/a	n/a	n/a
MeatZZa	1 serving	420	21	9.0	1000	38	1	3	18	n/a	n/a	n/a	n/a
Memphis BBQ chicken	1 serving	410	17	8.0	800	44	1	8	18	n/a	n/a	n/a	n/a
Pacific veggie	1 serving	360	15	7.0	730	39	2	4	14	n/a	n/a	n/a	n/a
Philly cheese steak	1 serving	370	16	8.0	890	37	1	3	15	n/a	n/a	n/a	n/a
Spinach & feta	1 serving	370	17	9.0	710	37	1	2	15	n/a	n/a	n/a	n/a
Ultimate pepperoni	1 serving	420	21	9.0	960	38	1	3	17	n/a	n/a	n/a	n/a
Wisconsin 6 cheese	1 serving	390	18	9.0	790	39	1	3	17	n/a	n/a	n/a	n/a

* Based on a 12-in medium pizza with hand-tossed crust

Domino's

Build Your Own Pizza*

	Amount	Calories	Fat (g)	Saturated Fat (g)	Sodium (mg)	Carbohydrate (g)	Fiber (g)	Sugar (g)	Protein (g)	Vitamin D (mcg)	Calcium (mg)	Iron (mg)	Potassium (mg)
Cheese	1 slice	50	4	2.0	150	1	0	0	3	n/a	n/a	n/a	n/a
American	1 slice	40	3	2.0	190	1	0	0	2	n/a	n/a	n/a	n/a
cheddar blend	1 slice	25	2	1.0	55	0	0	0	1	n/a	n/a	n/a	n/a
extra	1 slice	100	7	4.5	300	2	0	0	6	n/a	n/a	n/a	n/a
feta	1 slice	15	1	1.0	65	0	0	0	1	n/a	n/a	n/a	n/a
light	1 slice	50	4	2.5	170	1	0	0	3	n/a	n/a	n/a	n/a
Parmesan Asiago, shredded	1 slice	20	2	1.0	45	0	0	0	2	n/a	n/a	n/a	n/a
provolone, shredded	1 slice	25	2	1.5	60	0	0	0	1	n/a	n/a	n/a	n/a
Crust	1 slice	110	2	0.0	115	21	1	1	4	n/a	n/a	n/a	n/a
Sauce	1 slice	10	0	0.0	65	2	0	1	0	n/a	n/a	n/a	n/a
Alfredo	1 slice	25	3	1.5	75	1	0	0	0	n/a	n/a	n/a	n/a
Garlic Parm	1 slice	60	6	1.0	90	1	0	0	0	n/a	n/a	n/a	n/a
Hearty Marinara	1 slice	10	0	0.0	105	2	0	1	0	n/a	n/a	n/a	n/a
honey BBQ	1 slice	15	0	0.0	70	4	0	4	0	n/a	n/a	n/a	n/a
ranch	1 slice	50	6	1.0	135	1	0	0	0	n/a	n/a	n/a	n/a
Toppings													
bacon	1 slice	45	4	1.5	160	0	0	0	3	n/a	n/a	n/a	n/a
beef	1 slice	40	4	1.5	90	0	0	0	2	n/a	n/a	n/a	n/a
black olives	1 slice	15	1	0.0	55	0	0	0	0	n/a	n/a	n/a	n/a
Buffalo sauce, hot	1 slice	0	0	0.0	100	0	0	0	0	n/a	n/a	n/a	n/a
chicken, premium	1 slice	20	1	0.0	70	0	0	0	2	n/a	n/a	n/a	n/a
ham	1 slice	10	1	0.0	125	0	0	0	1	n/a	n/a	n/a	n/a
Italian sausage	1 slice	50	5	1.5	80	0	0	0	2	n/a	n/a	n/a	n/a
mushrooms	1 slice	5	0	0.0	0	0	0	0	0	n/a	n/a	n/a	n/a
onions	1 slice	5	0	0.0	0	1	0	0	0	n/a	n/a	n/a	n/a
pepperoni	1 slice	30	3	1.0	125	0	0	0	1	n/a	n/a	n/a	n/a
peppers													
banana	1 slice	0	0	0.0	115	0	0	0	0	n/a	n/a	n/a	n/a
jalapeño	1 slice	0	0	0.0	120	0	0	0	0	n/a	n/a	n/a	n/a
green	1 slice	0	0	0.0	0	0	0	0	0	n/a	n/a	n/a	n/a
Philly steak	1 slice	15	1	0.0	100	0	0	0	1	n/a	n/a	n/a	n/a
pineapple	1 slice	10	0	0.0	0	2	0	2	0	n/a	n/a	n/a	n/a
salami	1 slice	30	3	1.0	130	0	0	0	1	n/a	n/a	n/a	n/a
spinach	1 slice	0	0	0.0	0	0	0	0	0	n/a	n/a	n/a	n/a
tomatoes, diced	1 slice	5	0	0.0	40	1	0	0	0	n/a	n/a	n/a	n/a

Chicken

	Amount	Calories	Fat (g)	Saturated Fat (g)	Sodium (mg)	Carbohydrate (g)	Fiber (g)	Sugar (g)	Protein (g)	Vitamin D (mcg)	Calcium (mg)	Iron (mg)	Potassium (mg)
Boneless	3 pcs	170	7	1.5	660	18	0	1	9	n/a	n/a	n/a	n/a
Specialty													
classic hot Buffalo	4 pcs	190	11	3.5	1030	14	0	1	9	n/a	n/a	n/a	n/a
crispy bacon & tomato	4 pcs	260	17	5.0	810	14	0	1	11	n/a	n/a	n/a	n/a
spicy jalapeño & pineapple	4 pcs	190	8	2.5	670	21	0	7	9	n/a	n/a	n/a	n/a
sweet BBQ bacon	4 pcs	210	10	3.5	790	20	0	7	11	n/a	n/a	n/a	n/a

* Based on a 12-in medium pizza with hand-tossed crust

RESTAURANT & FAST FOOD CHAINS

Domino's	Amount	Calories	Fat (g)	Saturated Fat (g)	Sodium (mg)	Carbohydrate (g)	Fiber (g)	Sugar (g)	Protein (g)	Vitamin D (mcg)	Calcium (mg)	Iron (mg)	Potassium (mg)
Wings	4 pcs	250	20	5.0	720	8	0	0	14	n/a	n/a	n/a	n/a
Buffalo													
hot	4 pcs	260	20	5.0	1520	9	0	0	15	n/a	n/a	n/a	n/a
mild	4 pcs	260	20	5.0	1420	10	0	0	15	n/a	n/a	n/a	n/a
garlic Parmesan	4 pcs	390	34	8.0	960	10	0	1	15	n/a	n/a	n/a	n/a
honey BBQ	4 pcs	310	20	5.0	940	22	0	13	15	n/a	n/a	n/a	n/a
sweet mango habanero	4 pcs	310	20	5.0	790	21	0	10	15	n/a	n/a	n/a	n/a
Pasta													
Chicken Alfredo	1 order	600	29	17.0	1110	60	2	5	25	n/a	n/a	n/a	n/a
Chicken carbonara	1 order	690	34	19.0	1370	63	2	6	30	n/a	n/a	n/a	n/a
Italian sausage marinara	1 order	700	36	15.0	1650	68	3	13	27	n/a	n/a	n/a	n/a
Pasta primavera	1 order	530	26	16.0	880	62	3	6	15	n/a	n/a	n/a	n/a
Sandwiches													
Buffalo chicken	½	430	21	7.0	1270	39	2	2	21	n/a	n/a	n/a	n/a
Chicken bacon ranch	½	450	22	8.0	1190	37	1	2	23	n/a	n/a	n/a	n/a
Chicken parm	½	400	15	7.0	1050	38	1	2	25	n/a	n/a	n/a	n/a
Italian	½	410	19	9.0	1440	37	0	1	21	n/a	n/a	n/a	n/a
Mediterranean veggie	½	360	15	8.0	1130	39	1	3	17	n/a	n/a	n/a	n/a
Philly cheese steak	½	380	15	8.0	1280	38	2	3	20	n/a	n/a	n/a	n/a
Sweet & spicy chicken habanero	½	390	14	7.0	1080	44	1	6	22	n/a	n/a	n/a	n/a
Bread													
Parmesan bites	4 pcs	220	10	4.5	220	27	1	1	5	n/a	n/a	n/a	n/a
Stuffed cheesy bread	1 pc	150	7	3.0	250	16	1	1	6	n/a	n/a	n/a	n/a
jalapeño bacon	1 pc	170	8	3.5	350	17	1	1	7	n/a	n/a	n/a	n/a
spinach & feta	1 pc	160	7	3.5	270	17	1	1	6	n/a	n/a	n/a	n/a
Twists													
garlic	2 pcs	220	11	4.5	220	27	1	1	5	n/a	n/a	n/a	n/a
Parmesan	2 pcs	230	11	4.5	240	27	1	1	5	n/a	n/a	n/a	n/a
Loaded Tots													
Cheddar bacon	¼ order	240	16	5.0	590	17	1	1	7	n/a	n/a	n/a	n/a
Melty 3-cheese	¼ order	210	13	6.0	510	17	1	1	6	n/a	n/a	n/a	n/a
Philly cheese steak	¼ order	200	12	5.0	530	18	1	1	6	n/a	n/a	n/a	n/a
Salads													
Chicken Caesar	1 order	220	8	3.0	490	14	2	3	19	n/a	n/a	n/a	n/a
Classic garden	1 order	80	4	2.0	125	8	1	2	3	n/a	n/a	n/a	n/a
Desserts													
Chocolate lava crunch cake	1	350	17	10.0	180	47	1	30	4	n/a	n/a	n/a	n/a
Cinnamon bread twists	2 pcs	250	12	4.5	170	31	1	6	5	n/a	n/a	n/a	n/a
Marbled cookie brownie	1	200	10	3.5	125	26	0	19	2	n/a	n/a	n/a	n/a

Dunkin'

	Amount	Calories	Fat (g)	Saturated Fat (g)	Sodium (mg)	Carbohydrate (g)	Fiber (g)	Sugar (g)	Protein (g)	Vitamin D (mcg)	Calcium (mg)	Iron (mg)	Potassium (mg)
Americano													
Hot	medium	10	0	0.0	25	2	0	0	0	0	12	0	118
Iced	medium	10	0	0.0	30	2	0	0	0	0	18	0	116
Cappuccino, Hot													
Caramel swirl													
w/ skim milk	medium	230	0	0.0	135	49	0	47	8	2	303	0	611
w/ whole milk	medium	280	6	3.5	135	48	0	47	8	2	285	0	566
French vanilla swirl													
w/ skim milk	medium	230	0	0.0	130	48	0	46	8	2	288	0	584
w/ whole milk	medium	280	6	3.5	130	48	0	45	8	2	271	0	539
Mocha swirl													
w/ skim milk	medium	220	1	0.5	105	48	2	43	7	2	233	1	614
w/ whole milk	medium	270	7	4.0	110	48	2	43	7	2	216	1	569
Regular													
w/ skim milk	medium	70	0	0.0	85	10	0	9	6	2	225	0	351
& sugar	medium	170	0	0.0	85	36	0	35	6	2	225	0	351
w/ whole milk	medium	120	6	3.5	85	10	0	9	6	2	208	0	306
& sugar	medium	220	6	3.5	85	36	0	35	6	2	208	0	306
Coffee, Cold Brew													
Nitro	small	5	0	0.0	5	0	0	0	0	0	6	0	148
w/ sweet cold foam	small	00	3	1.5	30	12	0	11	1	0	33	0	222
Regular	medium	5	0	0.0	15	0	0	0	0	0	15	0	206
w/ cream	medium	90	9	4.5	45	1	0	1	2	0	55	0	247
& sugar	medium	190	9	4.5	45	27	0	27	2	0	55	0	247
w/ sweet cold foam	medium	80	3	1.5	35	12	0	11	1	0	39	0	215
& cream	medium	170	11	6.0	65	14	0	12	2	0	79	0	255
Coffee, Hot													
Café au lait													
w/ skim milk	medium	70	0	0.0	80	9	0	9	7	2	229	0	416
w/ whole milk	medium	110	6	3.5	85	9	0	9	6	2	212	0	371
Caramel swirl													
black	medium	170	0	0.0	60	39	0	38	3	0	85	0	448
w/ cream	medium	260	9	4.5	90	40	0	40	4	0	126	0	490
French vanilla swirl													
black	medium	170	0	0.0	50	38	0	37	2	0	71	0	420
w/ cream	medium	250	9	4.5	85	40	0	38	4	0	111	0	463
Mocha swirl													
black	medium	160	1	0.0	30	38	2	34	2	0	16	1	451
w/ cream	medium	240	9	5.0	60	39	2	35	3	0	56	1	493
Regular													
black	medium	5	0	0.0	10	0	0	0	1	0	8	0	207
w/ sugar	medium	110	0	0.0	10	26	0	26	1	0	9	0	208

RESTAURANT & FAST FOOD CHAINS

Dunkin'	Amount	Calories	Fat (g)	Saturated Fat (g)	Sodium (mg)	Carbohydrate (g)	Fiber (g)	Sugar (g)	Protein (g)	Vitamin D (mcg)	Calcium (mg)	Iron (mg)	Potassium (mg)
w/ almond milk	medium	25	1	0.0	45	4	0	3	1	1	123	0	198
w/ coconut milk	medium	15	1	1.0	20	0	0	0	1	1	133	0	234
w/ cream	medium	90	9	4.5	40	1	0	1	2	0	49	0	249
& sugar	medium	190	9	4.5	40	27	0	27	2	0	49	0	250
w/ oat milk	medium	30	1	0.0	35	5	1	1	1	1	90	0	253
w/ skim milk	medium	20	0	0.0	25	2	0	2	2	1	64	0	259
& sugar	medium	120	0	0.0	25	28	0	28	2	1	64	0	260
w/ whole milk	medium	30	2	1.0	25	2	0	2	2	1	59	0	248
& sugar	medium	130	2	1.0	30	28	0	28	2	1	60	0	249
Coolattas													
Blue raspberry	medium	350	0	0.0	45	84	0	83	0	0	18	0	7
Strawberry	medium	350	0	0.0	15	86	1	83	0	0	24	0	93
Vanilla bean	medium	590	5	2.5	240	129	0	125	7	2	284	0	342
Espresso													
Café con leche	medium	250	9	5.0	125	35	0	34	9	4	312	0	427
Cortadito	1	80	1	0.5	20	16	0	16	1	0	35	0	87
Hot	1 shot	5	0	0.0	5	1	0	0	0	0	1	0	46
w/ sugar	1 shot	60	0	0.0	5	15	0	14	0	0	1	0	46
Frozen Chocolate													
Caramel swirl	medium	700	14	10.0	290	135	1	126	9	2	302	0	639
French vanilla swirl	medium	700	14	10.0	280	135	1	124	9	2	287	0	612
Regular	medium	690	15	10.0	250	134	3	121	7	2	214	2	643
Frozen Coffee													
Caramel swirl													
w/ cream	medium	860	31	17.0	220	139	0	132	8	2	267	2	1730
w/ skim milk	medium	650	5	3.0	180	142	0	135	9	2	312	2	1760
w/ whole milk	medium	680	9	6.0	180	141	0	134	8	2	299	2	1727
French vanilla swirl													
w/ cream	medium	860	31	17.0	220	138	0	130	8	2	253	2	1703
w/ skim milk	medium	640	5	3.0	180	141	0	133	9	2	297	2	1733
w/ whole milk	medium	680	9	6.0	180	141	0	132	8	2	284	2	1699
Mocha swirl													
w/ cream	medium	850	31	17.0	190	137	2	125	7	2	180	3	1734
w/ skim milk	medium	630	5	3.5	150	140	2	129	8	2	224	3	1764
w/ whole milk	medium	670	10	6.0	150	140	2	129	7	2	211	3	1730
Regular													
w/ cream	medium	590	26	14.0	150	85	0	81	5	1	153	2	1381
w/ skim milk	medium	370	0	0.0	115	88	0	84	6	2	198	2	1411
w/ whole milk	medium	410	5	2.5	115	88	0	84	5	2	185	2	1377
Hot Chocolate													
Regular	medium	330	10	9.0	320	59	2	46	3	0	50	0	220
w/ espresso shot	medium	280	9	8.0	280	51	2	39	2	0	43	0	251

	Amount	Calories	Fat (g)	Saturated Fat (g)	Sodium (mg)	Carbohydrate (g)	Fiber (g)	Sugar (g)	Protein (g)	Vitamin D (mcg)	Calcium (mg)	Iron (mg)	Potassium (mg)
Lattes, Hot													
Caramel craze signature													
w/ skim milk	medium	340	5	3.0	180	61	0	57	12	3	436	0	806
w/ whole milk	medium	410	14	8.0	190	61	0	57	11	4	410	0	739
Caramel swirl													
w/ skim milk	medium	260	0	0.0	170	53	0	52	11	3	415	0	754
w/ whole milk	medium	340	9	5.0	180	53	0	52	11	4	389	0	687
Chai													
w/ skim milk	medium	220	0	0.0	150	44	2	41	10	3	338	0	488
w/ whole milk	medium	290	9	5.0	150	43	2	40	9	4	312	0	421
Cocoa mocha signature													
w/ skim milk	medium	330	6	3.5	160	61	2	53	11	3	363	2	812
w/ whole milk	medium	400	14	9.0	160	60	2	52	10	4	337	2	744
French vanilla swirl													
w/ skim milk	medium	260	0	0.0	170	53	0	50	11	3	400	0	727
w/ whole milk	medium	330	9	5.0	170	52	0	50	11	4	374	0	659
Matcha													
w/ skim milk	medium	180	0	0.0	115	34	1	32	11	6	336	0	430
w/ whole milk	medium	250	9	5.0	120	33	1	32	10	6	362	0	310
Mocha swirl													
w/ skim milk	medium	250	1	0.5	150	52	2	48	10	3	345	1	757
w/ whole milk	medium	330	10	6.0	150	52	2	47	10	4	319	1	690
Regular													
w/ almond milk	medium	100	3	0.0	180	17	1	15	1	3	525	1	273
w/ coconut milk	medium	50	5	3.5	60	3	0	1	1	4	569	1	417
w/ oat milk	medium	130	4	0.5	135	24	3	5	2	7	377	0	502
w/ skim milk	medium	100	0	0.0	125	15	0	14	9	3	337	0	494
& sugar	medium	200	0	0.0	125	41	0	40	9	3	337	0	495
w/ whole milk	medium	170	9	5.0	125	14	0	13	9	4	311	0	427
& sugar	medium	270	9	5.0	125	40	0	39	9	4	312	0	427
Lattes, Frozen													
Chai	medium	520	9	5.0	160	99	2	96	9	4	325	0	426
Matcha													
w/ skim milk	medium	360	0	0.0	70	83	1	82	6	5	182	0	220
w/ whole milk	medium	390	5	2.5	75	83	1	81	6	5	169	0	186
Macchiatos, Hot													
Caramel swirl													
w/ skim milk	medium	240	0	0.0	140	49	0	47	8	2	303	0	657
w/ whole milk	medium	290	6	3.5	140	49	0	47	8	2	286	0	612
French vanilla													
w/ skim milk	medium	230	0	0.0	135	49	0	46	8	2	289	0	630
w/ whole milk	medium	280	6	3.5	135	49	0	45	8	2	272	0	585

RESTAURANT & FAST FOOD CHAINS

Dunkin'

	Amount	Calories	Fat (g)	Saturated Fat (g)	Sodium (mg)	Carbohydrate (g)	Fiber (g)	Sugar (g)	Protein (g)	Vitamin D (mcg)	Calcium (mg)	Iron (mg)	Potassium (mg)
Mocha swirl													
w/ skim milk	medium	230	1	0.5	110	49	2	43	7	2	234	2	660
w/ whole milk	medium	280	7	4.0	115	48	2	43	7	2	217	2	615
Regular													
w/ coconut milk	medium	40	3	2.5	50	3	0	0	0	2	380	0	345
w/ oat milk	medium	90	3	0.0	100	17	2	4	2	4	252	0	402
w/ skim milk	medium	70	0	0.0	90	11	0	9	6	2	226	0	397
& sugar	medium	170	0	0.0	90	37	0	35	6	2	226	0	397
w/ whole milk	medium	120	6	3.5	90	10	0	9	6	2	209	0	352
& sugar	medium	220	6	3.5	90	37	0	35	6	2	209	0	352
Iced Tea													
Blueberry													
sweetened	medium	110	0	0.0	20	27	0	25	0	0	6	0	149
unsweetened	medium	10	0	0.0	20	2	0	0	0	0	6	0	149
Raspberry													
sweetened	medium	110	0	0.0	20	29	0	25	0	0	6	0	149
unsweetened	medium	15	0	0.0	20	4	0	0	0	0	6	0	149
Green													
sweetened	medium	100	0	0.0	10	25	0	25	1	0	6	0	36
unsweetened	medium	5	0	0.0	10	0	0	0	1	0	6	0	36
Regular													
sweetened	medium	100	0	0.0	20	26	0	25	0	0	6	0	159
unsweetened	medium	5	0	0.0	20	1	0	0	0	0	6	0	148
Sweet tea	medium	230	0	0.0	20	60	0	58	0	0	7	0	154
blueberry	medium	250	0	0.0	20	64	0	60	0	0	7	0	167
raspberry	medium	250	0	0.0	20	65	0	60	0	0	7	0	167
Refreshers													
Peach passion fruit	medium	130	0	0.0	15	32	0	29	1	0	10	0	24
coconut	medium	180	5	3.5	65	34	0	30	1	4	579	1	356
Strawberry dragonfruit	medium	130	0	0.0	15	29	0	27	1	0	10	0	24
coconut	medium	170	5	3.5	65	31	0	28	1	4	579	1	356
Bagels													
Cinnamon raisin	1	320	1	0.0	510	67	4	13	11	0	38	3	160
Everything	1	340	3	0.5	630	67	5	8	12	0	57	4	182
Multigrain	1	380	8	1.0	550	63	8	8	15	0	52	5	297
Plain	1	300	1	0.0	620	64	4	7	11	0	20	4	126
Sesame seed	1	350	5	1.0	630	64	5	7	12	0	24	4	152
White cheddar twist	1	390	8	4.5	760	64	4	7	16	0	171	4	142
Cream Cheese													
Classic plain	1 pkt	120	12	8.0	200	3	0	3	2	0	36	0	0
Garden veggie	1 pkt	100	10	6.0	200	2	0	1	2	0	33	0	0
Strawberry	1 pkt	130	10	6.0	100	9	0	8	2	0	32	0	0

Donuts

	Amount	Calories	Fat (g)	Saturated Fat (g)	Sodium (mg)	Carbohydrate (g)	Fiber (g)	Sugar (g)	Protein (g)	Vitamin D (mcg)	Calcium (mg)	Iron (mg)	Potassium (mg)
Apple													
crumb	1	290	11	4.5	310	44	1	21	5	1	12	2	73
fritter	1	470	28	12.0	410	47	2	17	6	0	25	1	96
'n spice	1	230	10	4.0	300	31	1	10	4	1	14	2	67
stick	1	470	30	15.0	440	50	1	24	4	0	30	2	78
Bismark	1	480	22	9.0	470	63	1	34	6	2	19	3	87
Blueberry glazed	1	350	18	7.0	380	44	1	21	4	0	20	1	68
Butternut	1	430	21	10.0	320	57	1	34	4	0	25	2	79
chocolate	1	450	24	11.0	420	57	1	35	4	0	26	1	70
Chocolate													
crème	1	290	14	6.0	300	36	1	14	5	1	14	2	101
double	1	380	23	11.0	430	41	1	22	4	0	20	1	75
frosted	1	260	11	4.5	290	34	1	13	4	0	13	2	75
cake	1	360	20	9.0	340	41	1	21	4	0	25	2	85
w/ sprinkles	1	270	12	5.0	290	36	1	15	4	0	13	2	75
glazed	1	370	23	10.0	420	41	1	21	4	0	25	1	57
stick	1	410	25	10.0	480	42	2	20	4	0	31	2	126
headlight	1	310	14	6.0	310	41	1	19	5	0	15	2	105
Long John	1	320	15	6.0	400	41	1	16	5	2	17	3	101
Cinnamon	1	330	20	9.0	320	34	1	13	4	0	27	2	66
stick	1	430	30	15.0	380	39	1	16	4	0	29	2	63
Coconut	1	410	21	11.0	320	50	1	28	4	0	25	2	89
toasted	1	430	22	11.0	360	52	3	29	5	1	27	2	97
Coffee roll	1	390	19	8.0	440	48	2	17	7	0	27	3	92
Éclair	1	370	16	6.0	470	50	2	23	6	2	18	3	106
French cruller	1	230	14	7.0	135	21	0	10	3	0	12	0	17
chocolate dipped	1	280	15	7.0	150	33	0	20	3	0	13	0	37
Glazed	1	240	11	4.5	270	33	1	13	4	0	12	2	56
stick	1	470	30	15.0	380	48	1	24	4	0	27	2	64
Jelly	1	250	10	4.0	290	36	1	13	4	1	13	2	58
glazed	1	280	10	4.0	290	44	1	21	4	1	12	2	60
stick	1	540	30	15.0	430	66	1	37	4	0	29	2	67
stick	1	500	30	15.0	420	57	1	29	4	0	29	2	65
Kreme													
Bavarian	1	240	11	4.0	310	31	1	11	4	1	12	2	59
Boston	1	270	11	4.5	320	39	1	18	5	1	13	2	80
Lemon	1	230	10	4.0	310	31	1	10	4	1	12	2	59
stick	1	480	30	15.0	460	50	1	24	4	0	28	2	67
Maple													
crème	1	290	14	5.0	290	38	1	18	4	1	12	2	61
stick	1	460	22	9.0	440	59	1	34	5	2	17	2	89
vanilla	1	330	15	6.0	300	45	1	25	4	1	12	2	65
frosted	1	260	11	4.5	280	35	1	14	4	0	12	2	59
Old fashioned	1	310	19	9.0	320	30	1	10	4	0	24	2	64

Dunkin'	Amount	Calories	Fat (g)	Saturated Fat (g)	Sodium (mg)	Carbohydrate (g)	Fiber (g)	Sugar (g)	Protein (g)	Vitamin D (mcg)	Calcium (mg)	Iron (mg)	Potassium (mg)
Peanut	1	470	27	10.0	320	50	2	26	8	0	33	2	162
Plain stick	1	420	30	15.0	380	36	1	13	4	0	27	2	62
Powdered	1	330	20	9.0	320	34	1	14	4	0	24	2	64
stick	1	440	30	15.0	380	42	1	18	4	0	27	2	62
Sour cream	1	360	17	7.0	360	49	1	25	4	0	15	1	16
Strawberry														
frosted	1	260	11	4.5	280	35	1	14	4	0	12	2	59
w/ sprinkles	1	270	12	5.0	280	37	1	16	4	0	12	2	59
glazed	1	280	10	4.0	280	44	1	23	4	1	12	2	67
Sugared	1	210	11	4.5	270	24	1	5	4	0	12	2	55
stick	1	430	30	15.0	380	39	1	16	4	0	27	2	62
Taillight	1	320	15	6.0	310	41	1	21	4	0	13	2	78
Vanilla														
crème	1	300	15	6.0	290	37	1	18	4	1	12	2	61
frosted	1	330	16	6.0	310	44	1	24	5	1	13	2	81
frosted	1	260	11	4.5	280	34	1	14	4	0	12	2	58
w/ sprinkles	1	270	11	4.5	280	37	1	16	4	0	12	2	60
headlight	1	310	15	6.0	310	41	1	21	4	0	13	2	78
Long John	1	320	15	6.0	400	42	1	17	5	2	16	2	81
Munchkins														
Cinnamon	1	60	4	1.5	65	6	0	2	1	0	4	0	7
Glazed	1	60	3	1.5	60	7	0	3	1	0	2	0	11
blueberry	1	60	3	1.0	75	9	0	5	1	0	5	0	12
chocolate	1	60	4	1.5	80	8	0	4	1	0	6	0	31
old fashioned	1	70	3	1.5	65	8	0	4	1	0	3	0	7
Jelly	1	60	3	1.5	65	8	0	3	1	0	3	0	11
Old fashioned	1	50	3	1.5	65	6	0	2	1	0	3	0	6
Powdered	1	60	4	1.5	65	7	0	2	1	0	3	0	6
Muffins														
Blueberry	1	460	15	3.0	390	77	1	44	6	0	21	2	93
Chocolate chip	1	550	21	6.0	400	85	2	49	7	0	29	3	175
Coffee cake	1	590	24	8.0	370	88	2	51	7	0	36	3	101
Corn	1	460	16	3.0	670	73	1	30	7	0	17	2	85
Sandwiches														
Bacon, egg & cheese														
bagel	1	520	18	6.0	1200	67	4	8	23	1	137	5	280
croissant	1	560	36	14.0	820	41	1	6	18	4	126	3	210
English muffin	1	400	19	7.0	840	39	1	4	18	2	126	3	209
Wake-Up Wrap	1	220	13	5.0	590	15	0	1	10	1	134	1	112
Egg & cheese														
bagel	1	460	13	5.0	1010	66	4	8	19	1	135	4	222
croissant	1	500	31	13.0	640	40	1	6	15	4	125	3	153
English muffin	1	340	15	5.0	650	38	1	4	14	2	124	3	151
Wake-Up Wrap	1	180	10	4.0	470	14	0	1	7	1	132	1	74

RESTAURANT & FAST FOOD CHAINS

	Amount	Calories	Fat (g)	Saturated Fat (g)	Sodium (mg)	Carbohydrate (g)	Fiber (g)	Sugar (g)	Protein (g)	Vitamin D (mcg)	Calcium (mg)	Iron (mg)	Potassium (mg)
Dunkin'													
Sausage, egg & cheese													
bagel	1	680	34	12.0	1500	68	5	8	26	2	162	5	330
croissant	1	720	52	20.0	1120	42	2	6	21	5	152	4	261
English muffin	1	560	35	12.0	1140	40	2	4	21	2	151	3	260
Wake-Up Wrap	1	290	21	8.0	710	15	1	1	10	1	146	2	128
Turkey sausage													
English muffin	1	470	25	8.0	1080	39	1	4	23	2	130	3	249
Wake-Up Wrap	1	240	15	6.0	680	15	0	1	11	1	135	2	122
Avocado toast	1	240	11	1.5	530	34	6	1	6	0	47	2	371
bacon-topped	1	290	14	3.5	740	32	5	2	10	0	26	2	378
Grilled cheese	1	480	20	11.0	1120	54	3	1	21	0	407	4	167
Sides													
Croissant	1	340	19	8.0	250	37	1	5	6	3	10	2	57
English muffin	1	190	2	0.0	270	35	1	3	6	0	10	2	56
Hash browns	6 pcs	110	6	1.5	360	13	1	1	1	0	6	0	187
Hardee's													
Biscuits													
Bacon, egg & cheese	1	520	29	14.0	1410	44	2	4	20	n/a	n/a	n/a	n/a
Biscuit 'n' gravy	1	500	27	12.0	1460	54	2	5	10	n/a	n/a	n/a	n/a
Country-fried steak	1	550	33	14.0	1240	49	2	4	14	n/a	n/a	n/a	n/a
Country ham	1	410	21	11.0	1670	42	2	4	16	n/a	n/a	n/a	n/a
Frisco breakfast sandwich	1	450	21	8.0	1300	42	2	5	24	n/a	n/a	n/a	n/a
Hand-breaded chicken	1	610	31	11.0	2780	52	2	4	30	n/a	n/a	n/a	n/a
Loaded omelet	1	520	30	15.0	1370	46	2	4	19	n/a	n/a	n/a	n/a
Monster	1	790	52	23.0	2370	45	2	6	35	n/a	n/a	n/a	n/a
Plain	1	340	16	9.0	840	41	2	4	6	n/a	n/a	n/a	n/a
Pork chop 'n' gravy	1	600	31	12.0	1430	56	3	4	24	n/a	n/a	n/a	n/a
Sausage	1	530	34	15.0	1210	42	2	4	13	n/a	n/a	n/a	n/a
& egg	1	600	39	16.0	1290	44	2	4	19	n/a	n/a	n/a	n/a
Breakfast													
French Toast Dips	1 order	620	19	3.5	670	106	3	30	9	n/a	n/a	n/a	n/a
Hardee Breakfast Platter													
w/ bacon	1	950	54	20.0	2300	76	12	5	31	n/a	n/a	n/a	n/a
w/ chicken fillet	1	980	58	19.0	2030	63	4	6	29	n/a	n/a	n/a	n/a
w/ country ham	1	860	48	17.0	2210	75	4	6	28	n/a	n/a	n/a	n/a
w/ country steak	1	970	60	20.0	1950	62	4	6	24	n/a	n/a	n/a	n/a
w/ pork chop	1	990	56	18.0	2020	66	2	5	33	n/a	n/a	n/a	n/a
w/ sausage	1	1050	68	24.0	2310	76	12	5	30	n/a	n/a	n/a	n/a
Loaded breakfast burrito	1	580	30	12.0	1320	46	3	2	30	n/a	n/a	n/a	n/a

RESTAURANT & FAST FOOD CHAINS

Hardee's	Amount	Calories	Fat (g)	Saturated Fat (g)	Sodium (mg)	Carbohydrate (g)	Fiber (g)	Sugar (g)	Protein (g)	Vitamin D (mcg)	Calcium (mg)	Iron (mg)	Potassium (mg)
Burgers													
The Big Hardee	1	920	58	23.0	1380	55	0	12	47	n/a	n/a	n/a	n/a
Cheeseburger													
bacon	1	740	48	14.0	1410	49	0	9	36	n/a	n/a	n/a	n/a
double	1	1020	68	24.0	1930	50	0	10	58	n/a	n/a	n/a	n/a
big	1	540	24	10.0	1360	53	4	12	28	n/a	n/a	n/a	n/a
double	1	760	42	17.0	1600	53	4	13	46	n/a	n/a	n/a	n/a
double	1	530	26	11.0	1470	56	2	11	25	n/a	n/a	n/a	n/a
small	1	300	14	4.0	790	33	1	8	13	n/a	n/a	n/a	n/a
Frisco	1	850	59	19.0	1640	43	3	7	40	n/a	n/a	n/a	n/a
double	1	1130	81	28.0	2130	44	4	8	61	n/a	n/a	n/a	n/a
Hamburger, small	1	250	9	3.5	570	32	1	7	11	n/a	n/a	n/a	n/a
Monster	1	1160	79	29.0	2580	49	0	10	68	n/a	n/a	n/a	n/a
Mushroom & Swiss	1	560	29	12.0	1330	49	3	8	30	n/a	n/a	n/a	n/a
double	1	790	46	19.0	1570	49	4	8	49	n/a	n/a	n/a	n/a
Star													
Famous w/ cheese	1	670	40	13.0	1370	52	4	11	28	n/a	n/a	n/a	n/a
Super w/ cheese	1	950	62	22.0	1890	54	5	12	50	n/a	n/a	n/a	n/a
Hand-Breaded Chicken Tenders													
	3 pcs	260	13	3.0	770	13	2	0	25	n/a	n/a	n/a	n/a
	5 pcs	440	21	5.0	1290	21	3	0	41	n/a	n/a	n/a	n/a
	10 pcs	880	43	9.0	2580	43	6	1	82	n/a	n/a	n/a	n/a
Sandwiches													
Charbroiled chicken club	1	650	29	7.0	1870	53	0	5	43	n/a	n/a	n/a	n/a
Hand-breaded chicken	1	650	32	5.0	2660	59	2	7	30	n/a	n/a	n/a	n/a
BLT	1	730	38	7.0	2840	59	0	8	39	n/a	n/a	n/a	n/a
Hot Ham 'n' Cheese	1	360	9	4.0	1380	51	2	9	21	n/a	n/a	n/a	n/a
big	1	460	15	7.0	2210	50	2	8	31	n/a	n/a	n/a	n/a
Roast beef	1	390	5	2.0	1210	50	2	7	0	n/a	n/a	n/a	n/a
big	1	520	6	3.0	1860	48	2	6	29	n/a	n/a	n/a	n/a
Jumbo chili dog	1	400	26	9.0	1410	24	1	5	16	n/a	n/a	n/a	n/a
Sides													
Fries	medium	420	21	4.0	850	55	5	0	5	n/a	n/a	n/a	n/a
Crispy Curls	medium	340	17	4.0	840	43	4	0	4	n/a	n/a	n/a	n/a
Grits	1 order	100	3	0.0	320	17	0	0	2	n/a	n/a	n/a	n/a
Hash rounds	medium	320	19	4.0	400	28	3	1	3	n/a	n/a	n/a	n/a
Onion rings	1 order	670	35	6.0	750	77	0	7	10	n/a	n/a	n/a	n/a
Desserts													
Apple turnover	1	270	13	4.0	260	35	1	11	3	n/a	n/a	n/a	n/a
Cinnamon roll	1	520	16	9.0	1060	89	1	57	6	n/a	n/a	n/a	n/a

RESTAURANT & FAST FOOD CHAINS

Hardee's	Amount	Calories	Fat (g)	Saturated Fat (g)	Sodium (mg)	Carbohydrate (g)	Fiber (g)	Sugar (g)	Protein (g)	Vitamin D (mcg)	Calcium (mg)	Iron (mg)	Potassium (mg)
Ice cream shakes													
chocolate	1	710	36	24.0	270	86	1	64	13	n/a	n/a	n/a	n/a
strawberry	1	710	36	24.0	220	85	0	69	13	n/a	n/a	n/a	n/a
vanilla	1	740	36	24.0	220	87	0	76	13	n/a	n/a	n/a	n/a

IHOP

	Amount	Calories	Fat (g)	Saturated Fat (g)	Sodium (mg)	Carbohydrate (g)	Fiber (g)	Sugar (g)	Protein (g)	Vitamin D (mcg)	Calcium (mg)	Iron (mg)	Potassium (mg)
Crepes (w/o syrup)													
Breakfast	1 order	1210	83	28.0	2290	63	5	13	52	n/a	n/a	n/a	n/a
Chicken pesto	1 order	870	54	42.0	2330	41	4	13	56	n/a	n/a	n/a	n/a
Cinnamon bun	1 order	630	31	13.0	680	78	3	49	11	n/a	n/a	n/a	n/a
Fresh berry	1 order	540	22	5.0	830	71	5	24	16	n/a	n/a	n/a	n/a
Lemon ricotta blueberry	1 order	540	24	10.0	680	68	4	41	16	n/a	n/a	n/a	n/a
Eggs Benedict													
Bourbon Bacon Jam	1 order	730	48	20.0	1990	42	2	10	32	n/a	n/a	n/a	n/a
Classic	1 order	800	29	13.0	1440	33	1	3	28	n/a	n/a	n/a	n/a
Pesto veggie	1 order	670	47	16.0	1260	41	5	6	22	n/a	n/a	n/a	n/a
Spicy poblano	1 order	610	33	15.0	1530	38	3	4	39	n/a	n/a	n/a	n/a
Umelettes (w/o cheese)													
Bacon Temptation	1 (3 egg)	1190	90	35.0	2930	20	0	8	72	n/a	n/a	n/a	n/a
Big Steak	1 (3 egg)	1040	69	24.0	1750	39	5	6	66	n/a	n/a	n/a	n/a
Chicken fajita	1 (3 egg)	900	58	49.0	2040	21	4	6	74	n/a	n/a	n/a	n/a
Colorado	1 (3 egg)	1270	100	36.0	2630	18	1	6	74	n/a	n/a	n/a	n/a
Egg white	1 (3 egg)	90	3	0.0	250	0	0	0	15	n/a	n/a	n/a	n/a
pesto veggie	1 (3 egg)	480	34	6.0	610	26	7	16	21	n/a	n/a	n/a	n/a
Plain	1 (3 egg)	400	28	8.0	440	8	0	0	28	n/a	n/a	n/a	n/a
Spicy poblano	1 (3 egg)	1090	88	37.0	1990	23	6	4	55	n/a	n/a	n/a	n/a
Spinach & mushroom	1 (3 egg)	950	78	31.0	2080	20	3	5	46	n/a	n/a	n/a	n/a
Toppings													
avocado	1 order	80	7	1.0	0	4	3	0	1	n/a	n/a	n/a	n/a
bacon, diced	1 order	80	7	2.5	340	0	0	0	6	n/a	n/a	n/a	n/a
basil pesto	1 order	90	9	1.5	190	0	0	0	2	n/a	n/a	n/a	n/a
cheese													
American	1 order	100	8	5.0	480	2	0	0	5	n/a	n/a	n/a	n/a
cheddar, shredded	1 order	230	18	10.0	360	2	0	0	13	n/a	n/a	n/a	n/a
four-cheese blend, shredded	1 order	230	18	11.0	350	2	1	0	14	n/a	n/a	n/a	n/a
Jack & cheddar blend, shredded	1 order	220	17	10.0	340	2	0	0	13	n/a	n/a	n/a	n/a
cherry tomatoes, roasted	1 order	30	1	0.0	100	5	1	3	0	n/a	n/a	n/a	n/a
fire roasted poblano salsa	1 order	15	0	0.0	130	3	0	1	0	n/a	n/a	n/a	n/a
green peppers & onions, sautéed	1 order	70	7	1.5	45	2	0	0	0	n/a	n/a	n/a	n/a
ham, diced	1 order	35	1	0.0	310	1	0	0	5	n/a	n/a	n/a	n/a
hash brown	1 order	220	14	3.0	240	20	2	0	2	n/a	n/a	n/a	n/a
mushrooms, sautéed	1 order	70	7	1.5	50	2	0	1	2	n/a	n/a	n/a	n/a
pork sausage link	1 order	210	21	7.0	330	0	0	0	5	n/a	n/a	n/a	n/a
sour cream	1 order	60	6	3.5	15	1	0	0	0	n/a	n/a	n/a	n/a
spinach, sautéed	1 order	80	7	1.5	90	2	1	0	2	n/a	n/a	n/a	n/a
tomato	1 order	10	0	0.0	0	2	0	2	0	n/a	n/a	n/a	n/a

RESTAURANT & FAST FOOD CHAINS

IHOP

	Amount	Calories	Fat (g)	Saturated Fat (g)	Sodium (mg)	Carbohydrate (g)	Fiber (g)	Sugar (g)	Protein (g)	Vitamin D (mcg)	Calcium (mg)	Iron (mg)	Potassium (mg)
Pancakes (w/o syrup)													
Buttermilk	3	450	18	7.0	1560	59	3	11	13	n/a	n/a	n/a	n/a
Chocolate chip	4	750	25	10.0	2000	120	7	50	19	n/a	n/a	n/a	n/a
chocolate	4	770	25	11.0	2020	123	9	50	21	n/a	n/a	n/a	n/a
Cinn-a-Stack	4	870	29	12.0	2260	136	6	66	17	n/a	n/a	n/a	n/a
Cupcake	4	800	21	10.0	2030	136	4	67	17	n/a	n/a	n/a	n/a
Double blueberry	4	610	15	4.5	1990	101	6	32	17	n/a	n/a	n/a	n/a
Gluten friendly	4	550	23	8.0	1050	77	2	16	9	n/a	n/a	n/a	n/a
Lemon ricotta blueberry protein	4	730	23	7.0	1720	92	8	37	40	n/a	n/a	n/a	n/a
Mexican tres leches	4	690	26	11.0	2080	98	4	31	19	n/a	n/a	n/a	n/a
New York cheesecake	4	890	33	14.0	2220	126	6	48	22	n/a	n/a	n/a	n/a
Protein Power	4	660	26	9.0	1670	70	5	19	37	n/a	n/a	n/a	n/a
Strawberry banana	4	680	15	4.5	2000	119	8	41	19	n/a	n/a	n/a	n/a
protein	4	740	18	3.5	1620	109	9	44	38	n/a	n/a	n/a	n/a
Thick 'N Fluffy French Toast													
Classic	1 order	900	42	18.0	1240	108	5	28	23	n/a	n/a	n/a	n/a
Lemon ricotta	1 order	950	39	15.0	1280	125	7	42	26	n/a	n/a	n/a	n/a
Strawberry banana	1 order	960	34	13.0	1190	144	9	53	24	n/a	n/a	n/a	n/a
Waffles (w/o syrup or sauce)													
Belgian waffles	1 order	570	33	10.0	840	60	3	15	9	n/a	n/a	n/a	n/a
gluten friendly	1 order	430	19	8.0	800	58	1	12	7	n/a	n/a	n/a	n/a
Chicken & waffles	1 order	1030	54	14.0	2030	93	5	15	42	n/a	n/a	n/a	n/a
Appetizers													
Chicken quesadilla	1 order	1030	65	42.0	2750	62	4	7	51	n/a	n/a	n/a	n/a
Crispy shrimp	1 order	460	22	4.0	940	51	3	12	16	n/a	n/a	n/a	n/a
Jalapeño & cheese bites	1 order	560	35	9.0	1770	50	3	3	10	n/a	n/a	n/a	n/a
Mozza sticks w/ marinara	1 order	630	32	14.0	1730	55	4	7	31	n/a	n/a	n/a	n/a
Sampler w/ marinara	1 order	1450	74	19.0	3550	136	10	12	61	n/a	n/a	n/a	n/a
Burritos & Bowls													
The Classic													
bowl													
w/ bacon	1	850	63	22.0	1620	30	3	3	41	n/a	n/a	n/a	n/a
w/ sausage	1	900	71	25.0	1260	29	4	2	35	n/a	n/a	n/a	n/a
burrito													
w/ bacon	1	1150	71	25.0	2490	80	4	5	49	n/a	n/a	n/a	n/a
w/ sausage	1	1200	79	27.0	2130	80	5	5	42	n/a	n/a	n/a	n/a
New Mexico chicken													
bowl	1	840	46	31.0	2680	67	11	7	45	n/a	n/a	n/a	n/a
burrito	1	1160	53	33.0	3560	118	12	10	53	n/a	n/a	n/a	n/a
Southwest chicken													
bowl	1	1080	77	38.0	2490	42	8	7	56	n/a	n/a	n/a	n/a
burrito	1	1380	84	40.0	3370	92	9	10	64	n/a	n/a	n/a	n/a

RESTAURANT & FAST FOOD CHAINS

IHOP

	Amount	Calories	Fat (g)	Saturated Fat (g)	Sodium (mg)	Carbohydrate (g)	Fiber (g)	Sugar (g)	Protein (g)	Vitamin D (mcg)	Calcium (mg)	Iron (mg)	Potassium (mg)
Spicy shredded beef													
bowl	1	800	41	18.0	1960	65	10	3	44	n/a	n/a	n/a	n/a
burrito	1	1100	49	20.0	2830	115	11	6	52	n/a	n/a	n/a	n/a
Hand-Crafted Melts													
Cali roasted turkey	1	1110	71	21.0	1930	63	12	7	59	n/a	n/a	n/a	n/a
Ham & egg	1	780	44	16.0	2220	59	1	12	41	n/a	n/a	n/a	n/a
Nashville Hot Chicken Melt	1	2100	165	39.0	4030	98	8	14	62	n/a	n/a	n/a	n/a
Philly Cheese Steak Stacker	1	820	47	18.0	2140	55	3	8	47	n/a	n/a	n/a	n/a
Entrées (w/o sides)													
Buttermilk crispy chicken dinner													
w/ country gravy	1 order	630	30	6.0	1740	47	2	0	43	n/a	n/a	n/a	n/a
w/ sausage gravy	1 order	700	36	9.0	2020	49	2	0	45	n/a	n/a	n/a	n/a
Pot roast	1 order	360	20	10.0	1600	11	0	2	35	n/a	n/a	n/a	n/a
Roasted turkey breast	1 order	310	13	3.0	890	6	0	1	44	n/a	n/a	n/a	n/a
Salisbury steak	1 order	680	56	20.0	1630	11	2	4	35	n/a	n/a	n/a	n/a
Salmon	1 order	250	12	2.0	660	2	0	0	35	n/a	n/a	n/a	n/a
Sirloin steak tips	1 order	510	31	9.0	1450	21	2	16	37	n/a	n/a	n/a	n/a
T-bone steak	10 oz	290	11	4.5	580	0	0	0	49	n/a	n/a	n/a	n/a
Platters (w/ fries)													
Buttermilk crispy chicken strips	1 order	890	41	8.0	2660	83	7	0	46	n/a	n/a	n/a	n/a
w/ BBQ sauce	1 order	1140	42	8.0	4540	142	9	41	48	n/a	n/a	n/a	n/a
w/ Buffalo sauce	1 order	920	43	8.0	5280	87	7	1	47	n/a	n/a	n/a	n/a
Crispy fish	1 order	1000	61	11.0	2640	77	6	2	38	n/a	n/a	n/a	n/a
Crispy shrimp	1 order	980	58	10.0	2380	94	6	13	22	n/a	n/a	n/a	n/a
Fisherman's platter	1 order	1100	64	11.0	2920	97	6	13	34	n/a	n/a	n/a	n/a
Ultimate Steakburgers													
Big Brunch	1	920	64	21.0	2010	44	2	8	43	n/a	n/a	n/a	n/a
w/ crispy chicken	1	890	53	13.0	1940	61	2	7	42	n/a	n/a	n/a	n/a
w/ grilled chicken	1	770	43	11.0	2390	44	2	8	54	n/a	n/a	n/a	n/a
Bourbon Bacon Jam	1	1020	73	23.0	2320	49	2	13	40	n/a	n/a	n/a	n/a
w/ crispy chicken	1	980	62	15.0	2250	66	2	12	38	n/a	n/a	n/a	n/a
w/ grilled chicken	1	870	52	13.0	2700	49	2	13	51	n/a	n/a	n/a	n/a
The Classic	1	780	53	17.0	1910	45	3	9	32	n/a	n/a	n/a	n/a
w/ bacon	1	880	61	20.0	2230	46	3	10	38	n/a	n/a	n/a	n/a
& crispy chicken	1	850	50	12.0	2160	62	3	9	37	n/a	n/a	n/a	n/a
& grilled chicken	1	730	40	11.0	2610	45	3	10	49	n/a	n/a	n/a	n/a
w/ crispy chicken	1	750	42	9.0	1840	62	3	8	30	n/a	n/a	n/a	n/a
w/ grilled chicken	1	630	32	8.0	2290	45	3	9	43	n/a	n/a	n/a	n/a
Cowboy BBQ	1	1070	65	21.0	2730	80	4	21	40	n/a	n/a	n/a	n/a
w/ crispy chicken	1	1030	54	13.0	2660	97	5	20	39	n/a	n/a	n/a	n/a
w/ grilled chicken	1	920	44	11.0	3110	80	5	21	51	n/a	n/a	n/a	n/a
Jalapeño Kick	1	1260	97	33.0	2320	47	5	9	50	n/a	n/a	n/a	n/a
w/ crispy chicken	1	1220	86	25.0	2250	63	5	8	48	n/a	n/a	n/a	n/a
w/ grilled chicken	1	1110	76	23.0	2700	47	5	9	61	n/a	n/a	n/a	n/a

IHOP

	Amount	Calories	Fat (g)	Saturated Fat (g)	Sodium (mg)	Carbohydrate (g)	Fiber (g)	Sugar (g)	Protein (g)	Vitamin D (mcg)	Calcium (mg)	Iron (mg)	Potassium (mg)
Salads													
Chopped chicken													
w/ crispy chicken	1	840	57	20.0	1690	38	14	7	48	n/a	n/a	n/a	n/a
w/ grilled chicken	1	700	50	31.0	1920	23	13	8	46	n/a	n/a	n/a	n/a
Fresh berry													
w/ crispy chicken	1	470	26	4.0	640	42	14	10	22	n/a	n/a	n/a	n/a
w/ grilled chicken	1	330	19	16.0	870	26	13	11	21	n/a	n/a	n/a	n/a
w/ salmon	1	490	27	4.5	700	27	13	10	41	n/a	n/a	n/a	n/a
House	1	140	9	6.0	200	7	3	3	9	n/a	n/a	n/a	n/a
Dressings													
balsamic vinaigrette	3 fl oz	320	30	4.5	540	13	0	12	0	n/a	n/a	n/a	n/a
honey mustard	3 fl oz	340	27	4.0	660	25	0	23	1	n/a	n/a	n/a	n/a
ranch	3 fl oz	320	33	5.0	530	3	0	2	2	n/a	n/a	n/a	n/a
Sides													
Bacon	2 pcs	100	8	3.0	320	0	0	0	6	n/a	n/a	n/a	n/a
turkey	2 pcs	60	5	1.0	310	0	0	0	5	n/a	n/a	n/a	n/a
Broccoli w/ garlic butter	1 order	90	7	3.5	150	5	2	1	3	n/a	n/a	n/a	n/a
Buttered English muffin	1	180	5	3.0	290	29	1	0	5	n/a	n/a	n/a	n/a
Buttermilk biscuit	1	810	64	26.0	1360	53	1	4	6	n/a	n/a	n/a	n/a
Crispy breakfast potatoes	1 order	280	13	2.5	1120	37	5	0	5	n/a	n/a	n/a	n/a
Eggs													
fried	1	60	3	1.0	65	2	0	0	6	n/a	n/a	n/a	n/a
hardboiled	1	80	5	1.5	60	0	0	0	6	n/a	n/a	n/a	n/a
poached	1	60	4	1.5	130	0	0	0	6	n/a	n/a	n/a	n/a
scrambled	1	110	9	2.5	105	0	0	0	7	n/a	n/a	n/a	n/a
white	1	30	1	0.0	90	0	0	0	5	n/a	n/a	n/a	n/a
French fries	1 order	320	15	2.5	1170	42	4	0	5	n/a	n/a	n/a	n/a
Fresh fruit	1 order	50	0	0.0	5	14	1	11	0	n/a	n/a	n/a	n/a
Garlic bread	1 order	150	8	1.5	210	15	0	0	3	n/a	n/a	n/a	n/a
Grits	1 order	110	0	0.0	85	23	1	0	2	n/a	n/a	n/a	n/a
Ham	2 pcs	60	2	0.0	670	2	0	1	10	n/a	n/a	n/a	n/a
Hash browns	1 order	220	14	3.0	240	20	2	0	2	n/a	n/a	n/a	n/a
Macaroni & cheese	1 order	350	20	10.0	920	32	1	4	12	n/a	n/a	n/a	n/a
bacon	1 order	390	23	11.0	1090	32	1	4	15	n/a	n/a	n/a	n/a
Mashed potatoes													
loaded	1 order	410	27	9.0	1130	31	3	2	15	n/a	n/a	n/a	n/a
red skin	1 order	240	13	2.5	680	30	3	1	5	n/a	n/a	n/a	n/a
Multigrain bread	1 order	160	4	0.0	270	26	3	2	6	n/a	n/a	n/a	n/a
Oatmeal	1 order	200	3	1.0	105	41	4	20	6	n/a	n/a	n/a	n/a
Onion rings	1 order	570	31	6.0	1130	65	4	6	7	n/a	n/a	n/a	n/a
Rice & barley medley	1 order	240	2	0.0	650	49	5	0	5	n/a	n/a	n/a	n/a

IHOP	Amount	Calories	Fat (g)	Saturated Fat (g)	Sodium (mg)	Carbohydrate (g)	Fiber (g)	Sugar (g)	Protein (g)	Vitamin D (mcg)	Calcium (mg)	Iron (mg)	Potassium (mg)
Sausage													
plant-based	1 order	240	16	5.0	580	11	6	2	13	n/a	n/a	n/a	n/a
pork	2 pcs	210	21	7.0	330	0	0	0	5	n/a	n/a	n/a	n/a
turkey	2 pcs	90	7	1.5	390	0	0	0	8	n/a	n/a	n/a	n/a
Scrapple	1 order	290	18	7.0	960	16	0	0	18	n/a	n/a	n/a	n/a
Spam	4 slices	340	29	10.0	1100	3	0	1	16	n/a	n/a	n/a	n/a
Toast													
Multigrain	1 order	160	4	0.0	270	26	3	2	6	n/a	n/a	n/a	n/a
buttered w/ jam	1 order	210	6	2.0	290	35	3	10	6	n/a	n/a	n/a	n/a
Rye	1 order	200	3	0.0	450	36	4	3	6	n/a	n/a	n/a	n/a
buttered w/ jam	1 order	320	8	4.5	500	55	5	20	7	n/a	n/a	n/a	n/a
Sourdough	1 order	110	1	0.0	240	21	0	2	4	n/a	n/a	n/a	n/a
buttered w/ jam	1 order	170	5	2.5	270	30	1	10	4	n/a	n/a	n/a	n/a
Wheatberry	1 order	210	3	0.5	430	40	4	0	7	n/a	n/a	n/a	n/a
buttered w/ jam	1 order	350	11	6.0	500	58	5	17	7	n/a	n/a	n/a	n/a
White	1 order	130	2	0.0	340	25	1	3	4	n/a	n/a	n/a	n/a
buttered w/ jam	1 order	250	7	4.0	290	43	2	20	5	n/a	n/a	n/a	n/a
Whole wheat	1 order	200	3	0.5	370	34	5	3	10	n/a	n/a	n/a	n/a
buttered w/ jam	1 order	340	11	6.0	430	52	5	21	10	n/a	n/a	n/a	n/a
Tortilla													
corn	1	110	2	0.0	50	23	2	0	2	n/a	n/a	n/a	n/a
flour	1	300	8	2.5	870	50	0	3	8	n/a	n/a	n/a	n/a
Yellow & green beans w/ garlic butter	1	100	7	3.5	135	9	4	3	2	n/a	n/a	n/a	n/a
Sauces & Syrup													
Sauces													
buttermilk ranch	1 order	160	16	2.5	260	1	0	0	0	n/a	n/a	n/a	n/a
honey mustard	1 order	170	13	2.0	330	12	0	12	0	n/a	n/a	n/a	n/a
IHOP	1 order	170	10	2.5	300	5	0	5	0	n/a	n/a	n/a	n/a
Syrup													
blueberry	¼ cup	110	0	0.0	5	27	0	19	0	n/a	n/a	n/a	n/a
butter pecan	¼ cup	110	0	0.0	10	27	0	14	0	n/a	n/a	n/a	n/a
old-fashioned	¼ cup	110	0	0.0	5	28	0	16	0	n/a	n/a	n/a	n/a
strawberry	¼ cup	100	0	0.0	5	26	0	19	0	n/a	n/a	n/a	n/a
Desserts													
Cinnamon dippers	1 order	750	37	11.0	470	93	2	67	11	n/a	n/a	n/a	n/a
Ultimate chocolate cake	1 order	750	46	27.0	150	82	6	59	7	n/a	n/a	n/a	n/a
In-N-Out Burger													
Burgers													
Cheeseburger w/ onion	1	480	27	10.0	1000	39	3	10	22	n/a	n/a	n/a	257
ketchup & mustard instead of spread	1	400	18	9.0	1080	41	3	10	22	n/a	n/a	n/a	344
Protein Style	1	330	25	9.0	720	11	3	7	18	n/a	n/a	n/a	n/a

	Amount	Calories	Fat (g)	Saturated Fat (g)	Sodium (mg)	Carbohydrate (g)	Fiber (g)	Sugar (g)	Protein (g)	Vitamin D (mcg)	Calcium (mg)	Iron (mg)	Potassium (mg)
In-N-Out Burger													
Double-Double w/ onion	1	670	41	18.0	1440	39	3	10	37	n/a	n/a	n/a	297
ketchup & mustard instead of spread	1	590	32	17.0	1520	41	3	10	37	n/a	n/a	n/a	384
Protein Style	1	520	39	17.0	1160	11	3	7	33	n/a	n/a	n/a	n/a
Hamburger w/ onion	1	390	19	5.0	650	39	3	10	16	n/a	n/a	n/a	216
ketchup & mustard instead of spread	1	310	10	4.0	730	41	3	10	16	n/a	n/a	n/a	303
Protein Style	1	240	17	4.0	370	11	3	7	13	n/a	n/a	n/a	n/a
French fries	1 order	370	15	1.5	250	52	6	0	6	n/a	n/a	n/a	n/a
Shakes													
Chocolate	15 fl oz	580	28	18.0	400	84	0	65	10	n/a	n/a	n/a	n/a
Strawberry	15 fl oz	590	24	15.0	310	114	0	100	8	n/a	n/a	n/a	n/a
Vanilla	15 fl oz	570	30	19.0	360	65	0	50	10	n/a	n/a	n/a	n/a
KFC													
Chicken Sandwiches													
Chicken Littles	1	300	15	2.5	620	27	1	3	14	n/a	n/a	n/a	n/a
Classic	1	650	35	4.5	1260	49	1	6	34	n/a	n/a	n/a	n/a
Crispy Twister	1	630	34	7.0	1260	53	4	3	28	n/a	n/a	n/a	n/a
Spicy	1	620	33	4.0	2140	49	1	6	34	n/a	n/a	n/a	n/a
Extra Crispy Chicken													
Breast	1	530	35	6.0	1150	18	0	0	35	n/a	n/a	n/a	n/a
Drumstick	1	170	12	2.0	390	5	0	0	10	n/a	n/a	n/a	n/a
Thigh	1	330	23	4.5	700	9	0	0	22	n/a	n/a	n/a	n/a
Whole wing	1	170	13	2.0	340	5	0	0	10	n/a	n/a	n/a	n/a
Kentucky Grilled Chicken													
Breast	1	210	7	2.0	710	0	0	0	38	n/a	n/a	n/a	n/a
Drumstick	1	80	4	1.0	220	0	0	0	11	n/a	n/a	n/a	n/a
Thigh	1	150	9	3.0	420	0	0	0	17	n/a	n/a	n/a	n/a
Whole wing	1	70	3	1.0	180	0	0	0	9	n/a	n/a	n/a	n/a
Nashville Hot Spicy Crispy Chicken													
Breast	1	540	40	7.0	1390	14	2	1	31	n/a	n/a	n/a	n/a
Drumstick	1	190	14	2.5	510	6	1	0	9	n/a	n/a	n/a	n/a
Thigh	1	390	32	6.0	900	12	2	1	13	n/a	n/a	n/a	n/a
Whole wing	1	180	15	2.5	450	5	1	0	8	n/a	n/a	n/a	n/a
Original Recipe Chicken													
Breast	1	390	21	4.0	1190	11	2	0	39	n/a	n/a	n/a	n/a
Drumstick	1	130	8	1.5	430	4	1	0	12	n/a	n/a	n/a	n/a
Thigh	1	280	19	4.5	910	8	1	0	19	n/a	n/a	n/a	n/a
Whole wing	1	130	8	2.0	380	3	0	0	10	n/a	n/a	n/a	n/a

RESTAURANT & FAST FOOD CHAINS

	Amount	Calories	Fat (g)	Saturated Fat (g)	Sodium (mg)	Carbohydrate (g)	Fiber (g)	Sugar (g)	Protein (g)	Vitamin D (mcg)	Calcium (mg)	Iron (mg)	Potassium (mg)
Spicy Crispy Chicken													
Breast	1	350	20	3.5	1100	11	1	0	30	n/a	n/a	n/a	n/a
Drumstick	1	130	8	1.5	420	5	1	0	9	n/a	n/a	n/a	n/a
Thigh	1	270	20	3.5	720	10	1	0	13	n/a	n/a	n/a	n/a
Whole wing	1	120	8	1.5	350	5	0	0	7	n/a	n/a	n/a	n/a
Other Chicken													
Extra crispy tenders	1	140	7	1.0	320	8	0	0	10	n/a	n/a	n/a	n/a
Kentucky Fried Nuggets	1	35	2	0.0	140	1	0	0	3	n/a	n/a	n/a	n/a
KFC Famous Bowl	1	590	23	5.0	2160	67	4	2	31	n/a	n/a	n/a	n/a
Pot pie	1	720	41	25.0	1750	60	7	5	26	n/a	n/a	n/a	n/a
Sides													
BBQ baked beans	1 order	190	1	0.0	650	34	7	15	11	n/a	n/a	n/a	n/a
Biscuit	1	180	8	4.5	520	22	1	1	4	n/a	n/a	n/a	n/a
Coleslaw	1 order	170	12	2.0	180	14	4	10	1	n/a	n/a	n/a	n/a
Corn on the cob	1	70	1	0.0	0	17	2	3	2	n/a	n/a	n/a	n/a
Green beans	1 order	25	0	0.0	300	5	3	1	1	n/a	n/a	n/a	n/a
KFC Cornbread muffin	1	210	9	1.5	240	28	0	11	3	n/a	n/a	n/a	n/a
Macaroni & cheese	1 order	140	6	1.5	600	17	1	2	6	n/a	n/a	n/a	n/a
Macaroni salad	1 order	140	8	1.0	290	14	0	9	1	n/a	n/a	n/a	n/a
Mashed potatoes	1 order	110	4	0.5	330	17	1	0	2	n/a	n/a	n/a	n/a
w/ gravy	1 order	130	5	1.0	520	20	1	0	3	n/a	n/a	n/a	n/a
Potato salad	1	340	28	4.5	290	19	2	3	2	n/a	n/a	n/a	n/a
Secret recipe fries	1 order	320	15	2.0	1100	41	3	0	5	n/a	n/a	n/a	n/a
Sweet kernel corn	1 order	70	1	0.0	0	16	2	2	2	n/a	n/a	n/a	n/a
Salads													
Side Salads													
Caesar	1	40	2	1.0	90	2	1	1	3	n/a	n/a	n/a	n/a
House	1	15	0	0.0	10	3	2	2	1	n/a	n/a	n/a	n/a
Parmesan garlic croutons	1 order	60	3	0.0	135	8	0	0	2	n/a	n/a	n/a	n/a
Dressings													
Heinz buttermilk	1 pkt	160	17	2.0	220	1	0	1	0	n/a	n/a	n/a	n/a
Hidden Valley fat-free ranch	1 pkt	35	0	0.0	410	8	0	2	1	n/a	n/a	n/a	n/a
KFC creamy Parmesan Caesar	1 pkt	260	26	5.0	540	4	0	2	2	n/a	n/a	n/a	n/a
Marzetti light Italian	1 pkt	15	1	0.0	510	2	0	1	0	n/a	n/a	n/a	n/a
Desserts													
Apple turnover	1	230	10	2.5	140	32	0	12	2	n/a	n/a	n/a	n/a
Café Valley chocolate chip cake	1 slice	300	15	3.0	260	39	1	27	4	n/a	n/a	n/a	n/a
mini	1	300	12	2.5	190	49	1	35	3	n/a	n/a	n/a	n/a
Café Valley lemon cake	1 slice	220	10	2.0	170	30	0	20	2	n/a	n/a	n/a	n/a
mini	1	300	13	2.5	230	43	0	31	3	n/a	n/a	n/a	n/a

Pizza*

	Amount	Calories	Fat (g)	Saturated Fat (g)	Sodium (mg)	Carbohydrate (g)	Fiber (g)	Sugar (g)	Protein (g)	Vitamin D (mcg)	Calcium (mg)	Iron (mg)	Potassium (mg)
Detroit-style deep dish													
3 Meat Treat	1 slice	435	22	9.0	898	40	2	2	20	n/a	n/a	n/a	n/a
5 Meat Feast	1 slice	438	22	9.0	1011	40	2	2	21	n/a	n/a	n/a	n/a
cheese	1 slice	313	11	5.0	521	40	2	2	15	n/a	n/a	n/a	n/a
Hula Hawaiian	1 slice	336	11	5.0	694	43	2	4	17	n/a	n/a	n/a	n/a
Italian sausage	1 slice	353	14	6.0	634	40	2	2	17	n/a	n/a	n/a	n/a
pepperoni	1 slice	346	14	6.0	652	40	2	2	16	n/a	n/a	n/a	n/a
seasoned beef	1 slice	343	13	6.0	626	40	2	2	16	n/a	n/a	n/a	n/a
Ultimate Supreme	1 slice	381	16	7.0	778	42	3	3	18	n/a	n/a	n/a	n/a
veggie	1 slice	341	12	5.5	713	42	3	3	15	n/a	n/a	n/a	n/a
Large classic													
cheese	1 slice	244	11	4.0	460	31	2	2	12	n/a	n/a	n/a	n/a
Italian sausage	1 slice	284	11	5.0	560	32	2	2	14	n/a	n/a	n/a	n/a
pepperoni	1 slice	288	12	5.5	624	31	2	2	14	n/a	n/a	n/a	n/a
seasoned beef	1 slice	274	11	5.0	551	32	2	1	14	n/a	n/a	n/a	n/a
Large ExtraMostBestest													
cheese	1 slice	278	11	5.5	546	32	2	2	15	n/a	n/a	n/a	n/a
Italian sausage	1 slice	333	16	6.5	703	32	2	2	16	n/a	n/a	n/a	n/a
pepperoni	1 slice	313	14	6.5	698	32	2	2	15	n/a	n/a	n/a	n/a
seasoned beef	1 slice	319	15	6.5	703	31	2	2	16	n/a	n/a	n/a	n/a
Large specialty													
3 Meat Treat	1 slice	359	19	7.5	820	32	2	2	17	n/a	n/a	n/a	n/a
5 Meat Feast	1 slice	354	18	7.5	886	32	2	2	18	n/a	n/a	n/a	n/a
Hula Hawaiian	1 slice	273	9	4.0	689	34	2	4	15	n/a	n/a	n/a	n/a
Slices-N-Stix	1 slice	288	12	5.0	644	25	2	2	20	n/a	n/a	n/a	n/a
Stuffed crust pepperoni	1 slice	373	19	9.0	873	32	2	2	18	n/a	n/a	n/a	n/a
Ultimate Supreme	1 slice	314	14	6.0	719	32	2	2	15	n/a	n/a	n/a	n/a
veggie	1 slice	280	11	5.0	671	33	3	3	13	n/a	n/a	n/a	n/a
Thin crust													
cheese	1 slice	248	14	6.0	424	19	1	1	12	n/a	n/a	n/a	n/a
pepperoni	1 slice	266	16	6.5	534	19	1	0	12	n/a	n/a	n/a	n/a
Add stuffed crust													
Detroit-style deep dish	1 slice	66	5	3.0	214	1	0	0	4	n/a	n/a	n/a	n/a
round pizza	1 slice	70	6	3.0	201	1	0	0	4	n/a	n/a	n/a	n/a
Toppings, Detroit-Style Deep Dish													
Base pizza	1 slice	346	11	5.0	521	40	2	14	15	n/a	n/a	n/a	n/a
Bacon	1 slice	48	4	1.5	133	0	0	0	2	n/a	n/a	n/a	n/a
Black olives	1 slice	26	2	1.0	101	0	0	0	0	n/a	n/a	n/a	n/a
Extra cheese	1 slice	34	10	1.5	86	1	0	0	7	n/a	n/a	n/a	n/a
Green peppers	1 slice	2	0	0.0	0	1	0	0	0	n/a	n/a	n/a	n/a
Italian sausage	1 slice	41	6	1.5	113	0	0	0	2	n/a	n/a	n/a	n/a
Jalapeño peppers	1 slice	8	1	0.0	183	0	0	0	0	n/a	n/a	n/a	n/a

* Based on a 14-in large pizza (8 slices).

RESTAURANT & FAST FOOD CHAINS

Little Caesars	Amount	Calories	Fat (g)	Saturated Fat (g)	Sodium (mg)	Carbohydrate (g)	Fiber (g)	Sugar (g)	Protein (g)	Vitamin D (mcg)	Calcium (mg)	Iron (mg)	Potassium (mg)
Mild banana peppers	1 slice	4	0	0.0	365	1	0	1	0	n/a	n/a	n/a	n/a
Mozzarella	1 slice	25	2	1.5	45	0	0	0	2	n/a	n/a	n/a	n/a
Mushrooms													
canned	1 slice	5	0	0.0	70	1	0	0	0	n/a	n/a	n/a	n/a
fresh	1 slice	4	0	0.0	1	1	0	0	1	n/a	n/a	n/a	n/a
Onions	1 slice	3	0	0.0	0	1	0	0	0	n/a	n/a	n/a	n/a
Pepperoni	1 slice	35	3	1.0	131	0	0	0	1	n/a	n/a	n/a	n/a
Pineapple	1 slice	11	0	0.0	0	3	0	2	0	n/a	n/a	n/a	n/a
Seasoned beef	1 slice	31	3	1.0	104	0	0	0	2	n/a	n/a	n/a	n/a
Smoky ham	1 slice	14	0	0.0	173	0	0	0	1	n/a	n/a	n/a	n/a
Toppings, Round Pizza													
Base pizza	1 slice	244	8	4.0	460	31	2	2	12	n/a	n/a	n/a	n/a
Bacon	1 slice	48	4	1.5	133	0	0	0	2	n/a	n/a	n/a	n/a
Black olives	1 slice	35	3	1.0	135	1	1	0	0	n/a	n/a	n/a	n/a
Extra cheese	1 slice	34	2	1.5	86	1	0	0	3	n/a	n/a	n/a	n/a
Green peppers	1 slice	3	0	0.0	0	1	0	0	0	n/a	n/a	n/a	n/a
Italian sausage	1 slice	54	5	1.5	148	0	0	0	2	n/a	n/a	n/a	n/a
Jalapeño peppers	1 slice	10	1	0.0	250	1	1	0	0	n/a	n/a	n/a	n/a
Mild banana peppers	1 slice	6	0	0.0	355	1	0	1	0	n/a	n/a	n/a	n/a
Mozzarella	1 slice	25	2	1.0	45	0	0	0	2	n/a	n/a	n/a	n/a
Mushrooms													
canned	1 slice	5	0	0.0	70	1	0	0	0	n/a	n/a	n/a	n/a
fresh	1 slice	4	0	0.0	1	1	0	0	1	n/a	n/a	n/a	n/a
Onions	1 slice	4	0	0.0	0	1	0	1	0	n/a	n/a	n/a	n/a
Pepperoni	1 slice	53	4	1.5	164	0	0	0	2	n/a	n/a	n/a	n/a
Pineapple	1 slice	11	0	0.0	0	3	0	2	0	n/a	n/a	n/a	n/a
Seasoned beef	1 slice	38	4	1.5	135	0	0	0	2	n/a	n/a	n/a	n/a
Smoky ham	1 slice	18	1	0.0	229	0	0	0	3	n/a	n/a	n/a	n/a
Wings													
BBQ	1 order	620	35	9.0	2300	32	0	24	48	n/a	n/a	n/a	n/a
Buffalo	1 order	510	35	9.0	3600	3	0	0	47	n/a	n/a	n/a	n/a
Garlic parmesan	1 order	670	51	13.0	2510	5	0	0	49	n/a	n/a	n/a	n/a
Oven roasted	1 order	510	35	9.0	1740	3	0	0	47	n/a	n/a	n/a	n/a
Sides													
Cheese bread													
Italian	1 pc	134	5	2.0	225	14	1	1	6	n/a	n/a	n/a	n/a
pepperoni	1 pc	152	7	2.5	284	16	1	1	6	n/a	n/a	n/a	n/a
zesty	1 pc	149	7	2.5	249	16	1	1	6	n/a	n/a	n/a	n/a
Cookie dough brownie													
w/ M&M's minis	1	210	11	5.0	75	24	1	17	3	n/a	n/a	n/a	n/a
w/ Twix	1	200	11	4.0	150	30	1	20	2	n/a	n/a	n/a	n/a
Crazy Bread	1 pc	100	3	0.5	161	16	1	1	3	n/a	n/a	n/a	n/a
stuffed w/ Crazy Sauce	1 pc	327	13	4.5	653	42	1	2	12	n/a	n/a	n/a	n/a

RESTAURANT & FAST FOOD CHAINS

Little Caesars	Amount	Calories	Fat (g)	Saturated Fat (g)	Sodium (mg)	Carbohydrate (g)	Fiber (g)	Sugar (g)	Protein (g)	Vitamin D (mcg)	Calcium (mg)	Iron (mg)	Potassium (mg)
Sauces													
Buffalo ranch	1 order	230	23	3.5	580	4	0	3	1	n/a	n/a	n/a	n/a
Butter garlic flavor	1 order	370	42	8.0	330	0	0	0	0	n/a	n/a	n/a	n/a
Cheddar cheese	1 order	110	8	2.5	770	7	0	2	4	n/a	n/a	n/a	n/a
Cheezy jalapeño	1 order	210	21	3.5	460	3	0	2	1	n/a	n/a	n/a	n/a
Ranch	1 order	230	23	3.5	480	4	0	3	2	n/a	n/a	n/a	n/a
McDonald's													
Breakfast													
Big Breakfast	1 order	760	48	18.0	1530	57	3	3	26	2	140	5	560
w/ hotcakes	1 order	1340	63	24.0	2070	158	5	48	36	2	280	8	980
Biscuits													
bacon	1	340	18	9.0	1030	36	1	3	9	0	70	2	150
w/ cheese	1	390	22	12.0	1240	38	2	3	11	0	150	2	170
egg & cheese	1	460	26	13.0	1330	39	2	3	17	0	180	3	240
egg	1	340	17	9.0	910	37	1	2	11	0	100	3	170
w/ cheese	1	390	21	11.0	1110	39	2	3	13	0	180	3	190
sausage	1	460	30	13.0	1090	37	2	2	11	0	70	3	200
w/ egg	1	530	35	15.0	1190	38	2	3	17	0	110	4	260
Fruit & maple oatmeal	1 order	320	5	1.5	150	64	4	31	6	0	80	2	330
Hash browns	1 order	140	8	1.0	310	18	2	0	2	0	8	1	240
Hotcakes	1 order	580	15	6.0	530	101	3	45	9	0	130	3	430
w/ sausage	1 order	770	33	12.0	810	102	2	46	15	0	140	3	520
McGriddles													
bacon, egg & cheese	1	430	21	9.0	1230	44	2	15	17	0	190	3	220
sausage	1	430	24	9.0	990	41	2	14	11	0	80	3	180
w/ egg & cheese	1	550	33	13.0	1290	44	2	15	19	0	190	3	270
McMuffins													
egg	1	310	13	6.0	770	30	2	3	17	2	170	3	200
sausage	1	400	26	10.0	760	29	2	2	14	0	140	3	190
w/ egg	1	480	31	12.0	830	30	2	2	20	4	170	3	260
Sausage burrito	1	310	17	7.0	800	25	1	2	13	0	140	3	170
Burgers													
Big Mac	1	590	34	11.0	1050	46	3	9	25	0	120	5	390
Cheeseburger	1	300	13	6.0	720	32	2	7	15	0	100	3	220
double	1	450	24	11.0	1120	34	2	7	25	0	180	4	350
Hamburger	1	250	9	3.5	510	31	1	6	12	0	20	3	200
McDouble	1	400	20	9.0	920	33	2	7	22	0	100	4	330
Quarter Pounder	1	420	18	8.0	730	40	2	9	25	0	35	4	370
cheesy jalapeño bacon w/ cheese	1	650	38	17	1410	40	2	8	36	0	210	5	450
double	1	870	54	24	1630	41	2	8	55	0	220	6	690
w/ cheese	1	520	26	12	1140	42	2	10	30	0	190	4	420
deluxe	1	630	37	14.0	1210	44	3	11	30	0	200	5	500
double	1	740	42	20.0	1360	43	2	10	48	0	200	6	660
w/ bacon	1	630	35	15.0	1470	43	3	10	36	0	190	5	490

RESTAURANT & FAST FOOD CHAINS

McDonald's

	Amount	Calories	Fat (g)	Saturated Fat (g)	Sodium (mg)	Carbohydrate (g)	Fiber (g)	Sugar (g)	Protein (g)	Vitamin D (mcg)	Calcium (mg)	Iron (mg)	Potassium (mg)
Chicken McNuggets													
	4 pcs	170	10	1.5	330	10	0	0	9	0	6	1	140
	6 pcs	250	15	2.5	500	15	1	0	14	0	10	1	220
	10 pcs	410	24	4.0	850	26	1	0	23	0	15	1	360
Chicken & Fish Sandwiches													
Filet-O-Fish	1	390	19	4.0	580	39	2	5	16	0	60	2	290
McChicken	1	400	21	3.5	560	39	1	5	14	0	20	3	320
McCrispy	1	470	20	5.0	1140	46	1	9	26	0	30	2	420
deluxe	1	530	26	4.0	1050	48	2	10	27	0	30	3	490
spicy	1	530	26	4.0	1320	48	2	9	27	0	30	3	440
deluxe	1	530	26	4.0	1200	49	2	10	27	0	30	3	510
Sides													
Apple slices	1 order	15	0	0.0	0	4	0	3	0	0	10	0	35
French fries	medium	320	15	2.0	260	43	4	0	5	0	15	1	670
McCafé Coffee													
Americano	medium	0	0	0.0	15	1	0	0	0	0	15	0	100
Cappuccino	medium	160	7	4.5	100	14	0	11	9	2	290	0	470
caramel	medium	200	6	3.5	370	44	0	39	8	0	200	0	400
French vanilla	medium	260	6	3.5	80	47	0	34	7	0	220	0	400
Caramel macchiato	medium	320	8	5.0	400	51	0	44	11	2	380	0	600
iced	medium	240	6	3.5	320	41	0	35	8	0	270	0	450
Iced coffee	medium	190	6	4.0	50	32	0	25	2	0	50	0	230
caramel	medium	190	7	4.5	300	31	0	26	4	0	100	0	290
French vanilla	medium	200	6	4.0	50	33	0	22	2	0	50	0	230
Frappés													
caramel	medium	490	20	13.0	90	70	1	62	8	0	240	0	420
mocha	medium	490	20	13.0	140	72	0	60	8	0	250	1	510
Iced mocha	medium	320	11	7.0	125	48	2	43	8	2	250	1	390
Premium roast coffee	medium	10	0	0.0	10	0	0	0	1	0	8	0	210
Latte	medium	190	10	6.0	135	15	0	15	10	4	350	0	490
caramel	medium	320	8	5.0	410	50	0	43	11	2	390	0	630
iced	medium	220	5	3.0	300	36	0	32	7	0	250	0	420
French vanilla	medium	310	8	5.0	115	50	0	37	10	2	330	0	540
iced	medium	220	5	3.0	75	38	0	28	6	0	200	0	340
iced	medium	120	6	3.5	90	10	0	9	6	0	220	0	250
mocha	medium	380	12	7.0	150	57	2	52	10	4	320	1	490
Desserts													
Apple fritter	1	510	29	9.0	360	56	2	25	5	0	90	2	100
Baked apple pie	1	230	11	6.0	100	33	1	14	2	0	6	1	70
Blueberry muffin	1	440	20	3.0	330	60	2	34	5	0	40	2	150
Chocolate chip cookie	1	170	8	4.0	95	22	1	15	2	0	10	2	60
Cinnamon roll w/ cream cheese icing	1	540	16	7.0	450	90	4	43	10	0	50	4	210

RESTAURANT & FAST FOOD CHAINS

McDonald's	Amount	Calories	Fat (g)	Saturated Fat (g)	Sodium (mg)	Carbohydrate (g)	Fiber (g)	Sugar (g)	Protein (g)	Vitamin D (mcg)	Calcium (mg)	Iron (mg)	Potassium (mg)
McFlurrys													
M&M's	regular	640	21	14.0	200	96	2	83	13	0	440	1	670
Oreo	regular	510	16	8.0	260	80	1	60	12	0	380	2	540
Shakes													
chocolate	medium	650	17	11.0	310	107	1	85	15	0	500	1	800
strawberry	medium	600	16	10.0	210	99	0	74	13	0	460	0	650
vanilla	medium	570	15	9.0	260	97	0	62	12	0	410	0	560
Sundaes													
hot caramel	1	330	7	4.5	150	58	0	41	7	0	240	0	320
hot fudge	1	330	10	7.0	170	51	2	44	8	0	260	1	420
Vanilla cone	1	200	5	3.0	80	33	0	23	5	0	180	1	240
Olive Garden													
Appetizers													
Calamari	1 order	670	42	3.5	1600	48	2	3	24	n/a	n/a	n/a	n/a
w/ marinara sauce	1 order	705	44	3.5	1920	52	2	5	24	n/a	n/a	n/a	n/a
w/ spicy ranch	1 order	910	68	8.0	2340	50	2	3	25	n/a	n/a	n/a	n/a
Fried mozzarella	1 order	800	49	17.0	1990	57	4	3	33	n/a	n/a	n/a	n/a
w/ marinara	1 order	835	51	17.0	2310	61	4	5	33	n/a	n/a	n/a	n/a
Lasagna Fritta	1 order	1130	76	31.0	1800	75	5	6	39	n/a	n/a	n/a	n/a
Meatballs Parmigiana	1 order	1040	83	40.0	2800	27	6	5	51	n/a	n/a	n/a	n/a
Shrimp Fritto misto	1 order	1280	79	5.0	5010	101	9	9	41	n/a	n/a	n/a	n/a
w/ marinara sauce	1 order	1315	81	5.0	5330	105	9	11	41	n/a	n/a	n/a	n/a
w/ spicy ranch	1 order	1520	105	9.5	5750	103	9	9	42	n/a	n/a	n/a	n/a
Spinach-artichoke dip w/ flatbread crisps	1 order	1160	81	21.0	2440	75	7	8	33	n/a	n/a	n/a	n/a
Stuffed Ziti Fritta	1 order	500	26	11.0	1040	40	3	0	27	n/a	n/a	n/a	n/a
w/ Alfredo sauce	1 order	720	48	25.0	1340	43	3	0	31	n/a	n/a	n/a	n/a
w/ marinara sauce	1 order	535	28	11.0	1360	44	3	2	27	n/a	n/a	n/a	n/a
Toasted ravioli	1 order	650	31	10.0	1330	69	4	5	25	n/a	n/a	n/a	n/a
w/ marinara sauce	1 order	685	33	10.0	1650	73	4	7	25	n/a	n/a	n/a	n/a
Entrées													
Cheese ravioli													
w/ marinara sauce	lunch	440	22	11.0	1330	38	3	4	25	n/a	n/a	n/a	n/a
	dinner	750	38	19.0	2370	63	5	8	41	n/a	n/a	n/a	n/a
w/ meat sauce	lunch	500	26	14.0	1240	39	2	6	29	n/a	n/a	n/a	n/a
	dinner	860	46	24.0	2190	65	4	11	50	n/a	n/a	n/a	n/a
Chicken Alfredo													
w/ crispy chicken fritta	dinner	1790	114	57.0	2670	123	6	7	70	n/a	n/a	n/a	n/a
w/ grilled chicken	dinner	1570	95	56.0	2290	96	5	6	81	n/a	n/a	n/a	n/a
Chicken & shrimp carbonara	dinner	1370	91	47.0	2050	75	3	10	64	n/a	n/a	n/a	n/a
Chicken Marsala fettuccine	dinner	1400	77	36.0	2580	112	4	12	55	n/a	n/a	n/a	n/a

Olive Garden

	Amount	Calories	Fat (g)	Saturated Fat (g)	Sodium (mg)	Carbohydrate (g)	Fiber (g)	Sugar (g)	Protein (g)	Vitamin D (mcg)	Calcium (mg)	Iron (mg)	Potassium (mg)
Chicken Parmigiana													
	lunch	630	29	7.0	1970	61	5	10	36	n/a	n/a	n/a	n/a
	dinner	1020	51	14.0	3300	80	7	13	64	n/a	n/a	n/a	n/a
Chicken scampi	dinner	1050	45	16.0	2470	106	5	8	49	n/a	n/a	n/a	n/a
Chicken tortellini Alfredo	dinner	1980	131	76.0	3720	95	5	9	112	n/a	n/a	n/a	n/a
Eggplant Parmigiana													
	lunch	660	32	7.0	1540	75	7	13	21	n/a	n/a	n/a	n/a
	dinner	1070	58	14.0	2440	108	11	20	35	n/a	n/a	n/a	n/a
Fettuccine Alfredo													
	lunch	650	45	27.0	610	47	2	3	15	n/a	n/a	n/a	n/a
	dinner	1310	90	55.0	1210	95	4	5	30	n/a	n/a	n/a	n/a
Five cheese ziti al forno													
	lunch	630	35	18.0	1220	57	4	9	24	n/a	n/a	n/a	n/a
	dinner	1170	69	36.0	2440	98	6	16	46	n/a	n/a	n/a	n/a
Grilled chicken Margherita	dinner	690	39	11.0	2120	15	5	5	63	n/a	n/a	n/a	n/a
Herb-grilled salmon	dinner	610	45	11.0	1360	9	4	3	45	n/a	n/a	n/a	n/a
Lasagna classico													
	lunch	500	30	16.0	1290	33	3	7	29	n/a	n/a	n/a	n/a
	dinner	940	55	30.0	2260	61	6	11	54	n/a	n/a	n/a	n/a
Ravioli carbonara	dinner	1390	104	63.0	2660	63	3	6	53	n/a	n/a	n/a	n/a
Seafood Alfredo	dinner	1450	93	55.0	1690	97	4	5	56	n/a	n/a	n/a	n/a
Shrimp Alfredo	dinner	1470	93	55.0	1620	96	4	6	63	n/a	n/a	n/a	n/a
Shrimp scampi													
	lunch	460	18	7.0	1020	52	4	5	20	n/a	n/a	n/a	n/a
	dinner	490	18	7.0	1120	52	4	5	29	n/a	n/a	n/a	n/a
Sirloin steak	dinner	980	62	36.0	1840	49	2	3	57	n/a	n/a	n/a	n/a
Spaghetti													
w/ marinara sauce	lunch	290	6	0.0	650	50	4	7	9	n/a	n/a	n/a	n/a
	dinner	490	12	1.0	1290	83	6	13	15	n/a	n/a	n/a	n/a
w/ meat sauce	lunch	360	12	3.5	530	51	3	9	14	n/a	n/a	n/a	n/a
	dinner	640	22	7.0	1050	85	4	17	26	n/a	n/a	n/a	n/a
w/ meat sauce & meatballs	lunch	680	38	17.0	1230	56	4	9	30	n/a	n/a	n/a	n/a
	dinner	1120	62	27.0	2110	92	7	17	49	n/a	n/a	n/a	n/a
w/ meat sauce & sausage	dinner	1110	62	21.0	2190	87	5	19	52	n/a	n/a	n/a	n/a
Tour of Italy	dinner	1550	97	50.0	3220	99	7	12	72	n/a	n/a	n/a	n/a
Gluten-Sensitive													
Grilled chicken parmigiana w/ rotini & marinara sauce	1 order	810	33	13.0	3040	59	7	10	75	n/a	n/a	n/a	n/a
Herb-grilled salmon	1 order	610	45	11.0	1360	9	4	3	45	n/a	n/a	n/a	n/a
Rotini pasta													
w/ marinara sauce	1 order	530	12	0.5	1530	94	8	10	13	n/a	n/a	n/a	n/a
w/ meat sauce	1 order	680	22	7.0	1300	96	6	13	23	n/a	n/a	n/a	n/a
Tuscan sirloin	6 oz	480	30	10.0	1680	9	4	2	46	n/a	n/a	n/a	n/a

RESTAURANT & FAST FOOD CHAINS

Olive Garden	Amount	Calories	Fat (g)	Saturated Fat (g)	Sodium (mg)	Carbohydrate (g)	Fiber (g)	Sugar (g)	Protein (g)	Vitamin D (mcg)	Calcium (mg)	Iron (mg)	Potassium (mg)
Breadsticks													
Breadstick	1	140	3	0.5	460	25	0	1	4	n/a	n/a	n/a	n/a
Sauces													
Alfredo	regular	440	43	27.0	600	5	0	1	8	n/a	n/a	n/a	n/a
marinara	regular	70	5	0.0	640	8	2	5	2	n/a	n/a	n/a	n/a
five cheese	regular	200	17	9.0	650	9	1	5	5	n/a	n/a	n/a	n/a
Salads													
w/o dressing	1	70	2	0.0	250	11	2	2	2	n/a	n/a	n/a	n/a
w/ low-fat Italian dressing	1	30	2	0.0	410	2	0	2	0	n/a	n/a	n/a	n/a
w/ signature Italian dressing	1	150	10	1.5	770	13	2	4	3	n/a	n/a	n/a	n/a
Soups													
Chicken & gnocchi	1 cup	230	12	4.5	1290	22	1	4	11	n/a	n/a	n/a	n/a
Minestrone	1 cup	110	1	0.0	810	17	4	4	5	n/a	n/a	n/a	n/a
Pasta fagioli	1 cup	150	5	2.0	710	16	3	4	8	n/a	n/a	n/a	n/a
Zuppa Toscana	1 cup	220	15	7.0	790	15	2	2	7	n/a	n/a	n/a	n/a
Desserts													
Black Tie Mousse Cake	1 order	750	50	30.0	290	76	4	59	9	n/a	n/a	n/a	n/a
Chocolate brownie lasagna	1 order	910	52	27.0	580	144	6	103	13	n/a	n/a	n/a	n/a
Sicilian cheesecake w/ strawberry topping	1 order	730	42	26.0	450	78	2	63	12	n/a	n/a	n/a	n/a
Smoothies													
peach	1	190	0	0.0	10	49	0	47	0	n/a	n/a	n/a	n/a
strawberry	1	220	0	0.0	0	60	0	55	0	n/a	n/a	n/a	n/a
Strawberry cream cake	1 order	540	26	17.0	370	69	2	47	9	n/a	n/a	n/a	n/a
Tiramisu	1 order	470	27	17.0	125	54	0	35	6	n/a	n/a	n/a	n/a
Warm Italian donuts	1 order	810	28	3.5	510	119	6	25	20	n/a	n/a	n/a	n/a
w/ chocolate sauce	1 order	1030	31	5.5	620	167	6	67	22	n/a	n/a	n/a	n/a
w/ raspberry sauce	1 order	1020	28	3.5	520	170	6	60	20	n/a	n/a	n/a	n/a
P.F. Chang's													
Appetizers													
Chang's lettuce wraps													
chicken	1 order	660	26	6.0	1840	66	8	28	38	n/a	n/a	n/a	n/a
vegetarian	1 order	520	28	3.0	1880	46	8	16	16	n/a	n/a	n/a	n/a
Crispy green beans	1 serving	1000	78	12.0	1500	70	8	12	8	n/a	n/a	n/a	n/a
Dynamite shrimp	1 order	580	42	7.0	1020	40	4	6	14	n/a	n/a	n/a	n/a
Edamame	1 order	400	16	3.0	1960	24	12	0	36	n/a	n/a	n/a	n/a
Kung pao brussel sprouts	1 order	740	42	6.0	1100	86	12	54	16	n/a	n/a	n/a	n/a
Spare ribs													
BBQ pork	1 order	860	28	14.0	1120	34	2	30	38	n/a	n/a	n/a	n/a
Northern style	1 order	760	28	14.0	900	10	2	8	38	n/a	n/a	n/a	n/a

RESTAURANT & FAST FOOD CHAINS

	Amount	Calories	Fat (g)	Saturated Fat (g)	Sodium (mg)	Carbohydrate (g)	Fiber (g)	Sugar (g)	Protein (g)	Vitamin D (mcg)	Calcium (mg)	Iron (mg)	Potassium (mg)
Dim Sum													
Crab wontons	1	100	5	2.0	290	11	0	5	2	n/a	n/a	n/a	n/a
Dumplings													
pork													
pan fried	1	90	5	1.5	230	7	0	2	3	n/a	n/a	n/a	n/a
steamed	1	80	4	1.0	230	7	0	2	3	n/a	n/a	n/a	n/a
shrimp													
pan fried	1	60	3	0.0	270	6	0	2	4	n/a	n/a	n/a	n/a
steamed	1	50	1	0.0	270	6	0	2	4	n/a	n/a	n/a	n/a
Egg rolls, pork	1	350	19	3.5	460	34	3	7	9	n/a	n/a	n/a	n/a
Spring rolls, vegetable	1	350	16	2.5	450	48	2	20	4	n/a	n/a	n/a	n/a
Entrées													
Beef w/ broccoli	1 order	600	30	9.0	2000	40	4	32	52	n/a	n/a	n/a	n/a
Buddha's feast	1 order	300	8	0.0	1620	36	12	14	22	n/a	n/a	n/a	n/a
steamed	1 order	240	5	0.0	380	32	12	10	22	n/a	n/a	n/a	n/a
Cantonese style lobster	1 order	1220	60	20.0	3780	112	6	22	58	n/a	n/a	n/a	n/a
Chang's spicy chicken	1 order	1140	58	10.0	1900	98	4	62	78	n/a	n/a	n/a	n/a
steamed	1 order	600	14	3.0	1420	64	0	62	58	n/a	n/a	n/a	n/a
Crispy honey chicken	1 order	1140	62	10.0	780	88	2	38	46	n/a	n/a	n/a	n/a
Crispy honey shrimp	1 order	1020	56	8.0	1180	80	0	38	46	n/a	n/a	n/a	n/a
Fire braised short ribs	1 order	1540	100	46.0	2300	102	2	34	52	n/a	n/a	n/a	n/a
Ginger chicken w/ broccoli	1 order	500	14	3.0	1600	36	6	26	60	n/a	n/a	n/a	n/a
Kung pao chicken	1 order	1040	68	12.0	1920	30	6	20	54	n/a	n/a	n/a	n/a
steamed	1 order	600	28	4.0	1900	26	4	18	64	n/a	n/a	n/a	n/a
Kung pao shrimp	1 order	1020	70	12.0	3260	54	8	20	48	n/a	n/a	n/a	n/a
steamed	1 order	420	20	3.0	2700	26	4	20	34	n/a	n/a	n/a	n/a
Ma po tofu	1 order	980	62	9.0	2780	66	16	30	58	n/a	n/a	n/a	n/a
Miso glazed salmon	1 order	640	36	6.0	1340	28	4	18	50	n/a	n/a	n/a	n/a
Mongolian beef	1 order	760	38	12.0	2480	42	2	30	62	n/a	n/a	n/a	n/a
Oolong Chilean sea bass	1 order	560	36	6.0	2320	30	4	16	34	n/a	n/a	n/a	n/a
Orange chicken	1 order	1160	58	9.0	1820	88	4	56	66	n/a	n/a	n/a	n/a
Pepper steak	1 order	600	30	9.0	2320	30	4	16	48	n/a	n/a	n/a	n/a
steamed	1 order	520	28	7.0	1900	28	4	16	38	n/a	n/a	n/a	n/a
Salt & pepper prawns	1 order	920	68	22.0	2980	44	6	12	36	n/a	n/a	n/a	n/a
Sesame chicken	1 order	980	48	9.0	2060	60	4	48	48	n/a	n/a	n/a	n/a
steamed	1 order	660	18	3.0	2020	60	4	48	66	n/a	n/a	n/a	n/a
Shrimp w/ lobster sauce	1 order	420	22	4.0	3080	12	2	4	36	n/a	n/a	n/a	n/a
steamed	1 order	380	20	3.0	2780	14	2	4	32	n/a	n/a	n/a	n/a
Stir-fried eggplant	1 order	560	36	5.0	2220	58	8	36	4	n/a	n/a	n/a	n/a
Sweet & sour chicken	1 order	880	42	7.0	560	88	4	46	36	n/a	n/a	n/a	n/a
Wagyu steak	1 order	460	32	12.0	1060	20	2	12	26	n/a	n/a	n/a	n/a

P.F. Chang's

	Amount	Calories	Fat (g)	Saturated Fat (g)	Sodium (mg)	Carbohydrate (g)	Fiber (g)	Sugar (g)	Protein (g)	Vitamin D (mcg)	Calcium (mg)	Iron (mg)	Potassium (mg)
Lunch Rice Bowls (w/o rice)													
Beef & broccoli	1 order	390	17	5.0	1600	34	3	24	26	n/a	n/a	n/a	n/a
Chang's spicy chicken	1 order	810	44	8.0	1210	58	3	32	59	n/a	n/a	n/a	n/a
Crispy honey chicken	1 order	840	42	7.0	680	71	1	38	35	n/a	n/a	n/a	n/a
Crispy honey shrimp	1 order	700	40	6.0	780	56	1	38	23	n/a	n/a	n/a	n/a
Ginger chicken w/ broccoli	1 order	350	10	2.0	1450	31	3	24	34	n/a	n/a	n/a	n/a
Kung pao chicken	1 order	590	39	7.0	1290	19	3	13	29	n/a	n/a	n/a	n/a
Kung pao shrimp	1 order	450	31	5.0	1660	27	4	13	19	n/a	n/a	n/a	n/a
Mongolian beef	1 order	460	24	7.0	1460	26	1	19	35	n/a	n/a	n/a	n/a
Orange chicken	1 order	670	34	5.0	1010	55	3	31	34	n/a	n/a	n/a	n/a
Sesame chicken	1 order	590	29	5.0	1320	44	5	34	26	n/a	n/a	n/a	n/a
Sweet & sour chicken	1 order	630	30	5.0	420	64	2	35	24	n/a	n/a	n/a	n/a
Noodles & Rice													
Fried rice													
beef	1 order	1180	30	8.0	1900	156	4	18	46	n/a	n/a	n/a	n/a
chicken	1 order	840	20	4.0	1760	152	4	18	50	n/a	n/a	n/a	n/a
combo	1 order	1060	28	7.0	2220	154	4	18	60	n/a	n/a	n/a	n/a
pork	1 order	1100	30	8.0	1740	152	4	18	50	n/a	n/a	n/a	n/a
short rib	1 order	1680	86	26.0	2960	174	8	32	48	n/a	n/a	n/a	n/a
shrimp	1 order	920	16	3.0	2220	152	4	18	36	n/a	n/a	n/a	n/a
vegetable	1 order	900	16	3.0	1540	162	8	22	24	n/a	n/a	n/a	n/a
Korean glass noodles	1 order	740	24	4.0	1840	120	6	36	10	n/a	n/a	n/a	n/a
beef	1 order	980	40	9.0	2240	120	6	36	36	n/a	n/a	n/a	n/a
chicken	1 order	920	32	6.0	2100	120	6	36	40	n/a	n/a	n/a	n/a
combo	1 order	1000	38	8.0	2580	120	6	38	48	n/a	n/a	n/a	n/a
shrimp	1 order	840	30	5.0	2640	120	6	38	28	n/a	n/a	n/a	n/a
Lo mein													
beef	1 order	900	28	7.0	3440	118	6	24	44	n/a	n/a	n/a	n/a
chicken	1 order	660	18	3.0	3280	114	6	24	48	n/a	n/a	n/a	n/a
combo	1 order	840	24	6.0	3820	116	6	24	54	n/a	n/a	n/a	n/a
pork	1 order	880	26	6.0	3260	114	6	24	44	n/a	n/a	n/a	n/a
shrimp	1 order	760	18	3.0	3960	116	6	24	34	n/a	n/a	n/a	n/a
vegetable	1 order	720	14	2.0	3100	126	10	28	22	n/a	n/a	n/a	n/a
Pad thai													
chicken	1 order	1340	36	6.0	2900	190	8	52	68	n/a	n/a	n/a	n/a
combo	1 order	1300	38	7.0	3100	186	8	50	56	n/a	n/a	n/a	n/a
shrimp	1 order	1260	36	6.0	3380	186	8	50	48	n/a	n/a	n/a	n/a
Singapore street noodles	1 order	1220	14	3.0	2920	224	6	22	52	n/a	n/a	n/a	n/a
Sushi Rolls													
California	1 pc	50	2	0.0	170	7	0	2	1	n/a	n/a	n/a	n/a
Dynamite shrimp	1 pc	100	6	1.0	340	9	1	3	2	n/a	n/a	n/a	n/a
Kung pao dragon	1 pc	60	3	0.0	190	7	0	2	3	n/a	n/a	n/a	n/a
Shrimp tempura	1 pc	70	3	0.0	230	9	0	2	3	n/a	n/a	n/a	n/a
Spicy tuna	1 pc	45	2	0.0	140	6	0	2	2	n/a	n/a	n/a	n/a

RESTAURANT & FAST FOOD CHAINS

P.F. Chang's

	Amount	Calories	Fat (g)	Saturated Fat (g)	Sodium (mg)	Carbohydrate (g)	Fiber (g)	Sugar (g)	Protein (g)	Vitamin D (mcg)	Calcium (mg)	Iron (mg)	Potassium (mg)
Gluten-Free Appetizers & Soups													
Chicken lettuce wraps	1 order	480	20	3.0	1700	46	4	22	30	n/a	n/a	n/a	n/a
Egg drop soup	cup	40	1	0.0	560	6	0	2	1	n/a	n/a	n/a	n/a
	bowl	270	7	2.0	3760	42	1	14	7	n/a	n/a	n/a	n/a
Gluten-Free Entrées													
Beef w/ broccoli	1 order	680	32	9.0	2000	42	6	32	56	n/a	n/a	n/a	n/a
Chang's spicy chicken	1 order	1160	60	12.0	1900	96	4	62	78	n/a	n/a	n/a	n/a
Ginger chicken w/ broccoli	1 order	500	14	3.0	1760	40	6	28	58	n/a	n/a	n/a	n/a
Mongolian beef	1 order	740	40	12.0	1960	28	2	24	66	n/a	n/a	n/a	n/a
Shrimp w/ lobster sauce	1 order	420	22	4.0	3080	12	2	4	36	n/a	n/a	n/a	n/a
Gluten-Free Lunch Bowls (w/o rice)													
Beef w/ broccoli	1 order	500	19	4.0	1040	31	3	24	22	n/a	n/a	n/a	n/a
Chang's spicy chicken	1 order	810	44	8.0	1210	50	3	32	59	n/a	n/a	n/a	n/a
Ginger chicken w/ broccoli	1 order	500	14	3.0	1750	39	5	28	58	n/a	n/a	n/a	n/a
Mongolian beef	1 order	500	28	6.0	1500	22	1	18	39	n/a	n/a	n/a	n/a
Gluten-Free Noodles & Rice													
Fried rice													
beef	1 order	1100	30	8.0	1680	154	4	20	46	n/a	n/a	n/a	n/a
chicken	1 order	1080	22	5.0	1560	164	8	22	54	n/a	n/a	n/a	n/a
combo	1 order	1200	34	8.0	2000	158	4	20	60	n/a	n/a	n/a	n/a
pork	1 order	1140	34	8.0	1580	160	4	20	42	n/a	n/a	n/a	n/a
shrimp	1 order	960	18	3.0	1980	153	4	20	36	n/a	n/a	n/a	n/a
vegetable	1 order	900	16	3.0	1300	164	10	22	26	n/a	n/a	n/a	n/a
side	1 order	510	15	3.0	670	77	2	10	13	n/a	n/a	n/a	n/a
Pad thai													
chicken	1 order	1260	34	6.0	2740	184	8	50	56	n/a	n/a	n/a	n/a
combo	1 order	1220	32	6.0	3020	184	8	50	50	n/a	n/a	n/a	n/a
shrimp	1 order	1180	30	5.0	3300	184	8	50	44	n/a	n/a	n/a	n/a
Singapore street noodles	1 order	1220	14	3.0	2920	224	6	22	52	n/a	n/a	n/a	n/a
Salads													
Asian Caesar	1 order	420	30	7.0	880	22	4	2	16	n/a	n/a	n/a	n/a
Mandarin Crunch	1 order	740	46	6.0	1500	76	8	42	14	n/a	n/a	n/a	n/a
Toppings													
chicken	1 order	280	14	2.0	200	2	0	2	30	n/a	n/a	n/a	n/a
salmon	1 order	320	26	4.0	60	0	0	0	22	n/a	n/a	n/a	n/a
Soups													
Chicken noodle	cup	170	2	0.0	1310	30	1	6	9	n/a	n/a	n/a	n/a
Egg drop	cup	40	1	0.0	560	6	0	2	1	n/a	n/a	n/a	n/a
Hot & sour	cup	70	2	0.0	580	9	0	1	4	n/a	n/a	n/a	n/a
Wonton	cup	130	4	1.0	770	14	1	2	9	n/a	n/a	n/a	n/a

RESTAURANT & FAST FOOD CHAINS

P.F. Chang's	Amount	Calories	Fat (g)	Saturated Fat (g)	Sodium (mg)	Carbohydrate (g)	Fiber (g)	Sugar (g)	Protein (g)	Vitamin D (mcg)	Calcium (mg)	Iron (mg)	Potassium (mg)
Sides													
Brown rice	1 order	190	0	0.0	0	40	3	0	4	n/a	n/a	n/a	n/a
Fried rice	1 order	500	15	3.0	800	76	2	9	13	n/a	n/a	n/a	n/a
White rice	1 order	220	0	0.0	0	49	1	1	4	n/a	n/a	n/a	n/a
Desserts													
Banana spring rolls	1 order	940	34	14.0	480	150	2	46	14	n/a	n/a	n/a	n/a
Chang's apple crunch	1 order	920	42	18.0	460	124	4	64	12	n/a	n/a	n/a	n/a
Chocolate souffle	1 order	800	50	32.0	100	84	6	72	12	n/a	n/a	n/a	n/a
The Great Wall of Chocolate	1 order	1940	80	30.0	1580	308	16	230	20	n/a	n/a	n/a	n/a
New York–style cheesecake	1 order	960	62	36.0	660	84	6	70	16	n/a	n/a	n/a	n/a
Sticky toffee pudding	1 order	860	48	30.0	580	102	2	78	12	n/a	n/a	n/a	n/a
Panda Express													
Appetizers													
Chicken egg roll	1	200	10	2.0	340	20	2	2	6	n/a	n/a	n/a	n/a
Chicken pot stickers	3	160	6	1.5	250	20	1	2	6	n/a	n/a	n/a	n/a
Cream cheese rangoons	3	190	8	5.0	180	24	2	1	5	n/a	n/a	n/a	n/a
Vegetable spring rolls	2	240	14	2.0	560	24	2	0	4	n/a	n/a	n/a	n/a
Entrées													
Beef													
Beijing	1 order	480	27	5.0	600	46	2	21	14	n/a	n/a	n/a	n/a
broccoli	1 order	150	7	1.5	520	13	2	7	9	n/a	n/a	n/a	n/a
Black pepper Angus steak	1 order	210	10	2.5	560	13	1	7	19	n/a	n/a	n/a	n/a
Chicken													
Asian	1 order	340	13	3.5	630	14	3	10	41	n/a	n/a	n/a	n/a
grilled	1 order	275	10	3.0	470	14	0	9	33	n/a	n/a	n/a	n/a
black pepper	1 order	280	19	3.5	1130	15	1	7	13	n/a	n/a	n/a	n/a
kung pao	1 order	290	19	3.5	970	14	2	6	16	n/a	n/a	n/a	n/a
mushroom	1 order	220	14	2.5	840	10	1	5	13	n/a	n/a	n/a	n/a
orange	1 order	490	23	5.0	820	51	2	19	25	n/a	n/a	n/a	n/a
Beyond	1 order	440	22	5.0	810	47	5	15	13	n/a	n/a	n/a	n/a
potato	1 order	190	10	2.0	680	18	2	4	8	n/a	n/a	n/a	n/a
teriyaki	1 order	340	13	3.5	630	14	3	10	41	n/a	n/a	n/a	n/a
grilled	1 order	275	10	3.0	470	14	0	9	33	n/a	n/a	n/a	n/a
Chicken breast													
honey sesame	1 order	340	15	2.5	540	35	1	16	16	n/a	n/a	n/a	n/a
string bean	1 order	210	12	2.0	560	13	5	5	12	n/a	n/a	n/a	n/a
sweet & sour	1 order	300	12	3.0	260	40	1	24	10	n/a	n/a	n/a	n/a
sweetfire	1 order	360	15	3.0	370	40	2	19	15	n/a	n/a	n/a	n/a

RESTAURANT & FAST FOOD CHAINS

Panda Express	Amount	Calories	Fat (g)	Saturated Fat (g)	Sodium (mg)	Carbohydrate (g)	Fiber (g)	Sugar (g)	Protein (g)	Vitamin D (mcg)	Calcium (mg)	Iron (mg)	Potassium (mg)
Shrimp													
golden treasure	1 order	360	18	3.0	440	35	2	14	14	n/a	n/a	n/a	n/a
honey walnut	1 order	360	24	3.5	590	27	1	8	11	n/a	n/a	n/a	n/a
wok-fired	1 order	190	5	1.0	1140	19	1	15	17	n/a	n/a	n/a	n/a
Steamed ginger fish	1 order	200	12	2.5	1990	8	0	6	15	n/a	n/a	n/a	n/a
Sides													
Chow fun	1 order	410	9	1.0	1110	73	1	6	9	n/a	n/a	n/a	n/a
Chow mein	1 order	510	20	3.5	860	80	6	9	13	n/a	n/a	n/a	n/a
Eggplant tofu	1 order	340	24	3.5	520	23	3	17	7	n/a	n/a	n/a	n/a
Fried rice	1 order	520	16	3.0	850	85	1	3	11	n/a	n/a	n/a	n/a
Hot & sour soup	cup	120	5	0.5	880	14	1	4	7	n/a	n/a	n/a	n/a
	bowl	170	6	1.0	1260	20	1	6	10	n/a	n/a	n/a	n/a
Steamed rice													
brown	1 order	420	4	1.0	15	86	4	1	9	n/a	n/a	n/a	n/a
white	1 order	380	0	0.0	0	87	0	0	7	n/a	n/a	n/a	n/a
Super greens	1 order	90	3	0.0	260	10	5	4	6	n/a	n/a	n/a	n/a
Sauces													
Chili	1 order	10	0	0.0	125	2	0	2	0	n/a	n/a	n/a	n/a
Hot mustard	1 order	10	1	0.0	115	0	0	0	0	n/a	n/a	n/a	n/a
Plum	1 order	15	0	0.0	55	3	0	3	0	n/a	n/a	n/a	n/a
Potsticker	1 order	10	0	0.0	290	3	0	2	0	n/a	n/a	n/a	n/a
Soy	1 order	5	0	0.0	375	0	0	0	0	n/a	n/a	n/a	n/a
Sweet & sour	1 order	70	0	0.0	115	21	0	20	0	n/a	n/a	n/a	n/a
Teriyaki	1 order	70	0	0.0	380	16	0	14	0	n/a	n/a	n/a	n/a
Desserts													
Chocolate chunk cookie	1	160	7	3.0	125	25	1	14	2	n/a	n/a	n/a	n/a
Fortune cookie	1	20	0	0.0	0	5	0	2	0	n/a	n/a	n/a	n/a
Panera Bread													
Breakfast													
Artisan ciabatta, breakfast portion	¼ loaf	200	2	0.0	360	38	2	1	7	n/a	n/a	n/a	n/a
Avocado, egg white, spinach & cheese on sprouted grain bagel flat	1	350	14	5.0	680	39	5	5	19	n/a	n/a	n/a	n/a
Bacon, scrambled egg & cheese													
artisan ciabatta	1	440	21	9.0	900	40	2	2	24	n/a	n/a	n/a	n/a
brioche	1	450	26	13.0	840	33	2	6	24	n/a	n/a	n/a	n/a
Chipotle chicken, scrambled egg & avocado on artisan ciabatta	1	550	31	12.0	910	44	4	2	27	n/a	n/a	n/a	n/a
scrambled egg	1	550	31	12.0	910	44	4	2	27	n/a	n/a	n/a	n/a

RESTAURANT & FAST FOOD CHAINS

Panera Bread

	Amount	Calories	Fat (g)	Saturated Fat (g)	Sodium (mg)	Carbohydrate (g)	Fiber (g)	Sugar (g)	Protein (g)	Vitamin D (mcg)	Calcium (mg)	Iron (mg)	Potassium (mg)
Sausage, scrambled egg & cheese													
artisan ciabatta	1	590	35	15.0	880	40	2	1	27	n/a	n/a	n/a	n/a
Asiago bagel	1	820	51	20.0	1300	58	2	5	33	n/a	n/a	n/a	n/a
brioche	1	590	40	19.0	820	33	2	6	28	n/a	n/a	n/a	n/a
Scrambled egg & cheese													
artisan ciabatta	1	380	16	7.0	610	40	2	1	20	n/a	n/a	n/a	n/a
brioche	1	390	20	11.0	560	32	2	6	21	n/a	n/a	n/a	n/a
Sandwich options													
aioli sauce													
chipotle	1 order	45	5	1.0	55	0	0	0	0	n/a	n/a	n/a	n/a
garlic	1 order	50	5	1.0	30	0	0	0	0	n/a	n/a	n/a	n/a
egg													
scrambled	1	90	7	3.0	90	1	0	0	8	n/a	n/a	n/a	n/a
whites	1 order	30	0	0.0	100	1	0	0	6	n/a	n/a	n/a	n/a
Steel cut oatmeal w/ strawberries, pecans & cinnamon crunch topping	1 bowl	370	15	2.0	150	52	9	17	8	n/a	n/a	n/a	n/a
w/o pecans	1 bowl	260	4	1.0	150	50	8	16	7	n/a	n/a	n/a	n/a
Souffles													
Four cheese	1	470	30	16.0	830	36	1	8	14	n/a	n/a	n/a	n/a
Spinach & artichoke	1	530	35	19.0	930	37	3	8	18	n/a	n/a	n/a	n/a
Spinach & bacon	1	550	37	19.0	970	36	1	8	19	n/a	n/a	n/a	n/a
Baked Goods													
Bear claw	1	500	23	10.0	350	65	3	30	10	n/a	n/a	n/a	n/a
mini	1	160	8	3.5	115	20	1	8	3	n/a	n/a	n/a	n/a
Brownie	1	470	18	6.0	95	69	4	50	7	n/a	n/a	n/a	n/a
mini	1	120	5	1.5	25	17	1	12	2	n/a	n/a	n/a	n/a
Cookies													
candy	1	480	22	13.0	310	68	1	37	4	n/a	n/a	n/a	n/a
mini	1	130	6	3.5	75	18	0	10	1	n/a	n/a	n/a	n/a
Chocolate Chipper	1	390	19	11.0	290	52	2	31	4	n/a	n/a	n/a	n/a
mini	1	100	5	3.0	75	13	0	8	1	n/a	n/a	n/a	n/a
kitchen sink	1	820	44	29.0	760	99	2	56	8	n/a	n/a	n/a	n/a
lemon drop	1	440	20	13.0	260	60	1	34	5	n/a	n/a	n/a	n/a
mini	1	110	5	3.5	65	15	0	9	1	n/a	n/a	n/a	n/a
oatmeal raisin w/ berries	1	350	13	7.0	170	55	2	33	4	n/a	n/a	n/a	n/a
mini	1	90	3	2.0	45	14	1	8	1	n/a	n/a	n/a	n/a
shortbread													
pumpkin-shaped	1	450	21	13.0	210	62	1	37	4	n/a	n/a	n/a	n/a
Croissant	1	270	15	11.0	240	28	1	4	5	n/a	n/a	n/a	n/a
chocolate	1	410	21	13.0	300	49	2	16	7	n/a	n/a	n/a	n/a

RESTAURANT & FAST FOOD CHAINS

	Amount	Calories	Fat (g)	Saturated Fat (g)	Sodium (mg)	Carbohydrate (g)	Fiber (g)	Sugar (g)	Protein (g)	Vitamin D (mcg)	Calcium (mg)	Iron (mg)	Potassium (mg)
Muffins													
blueberry	1	510	18	3.5	390	79	8	35	7	n/a	n/a	n/a	n/a
chocolate chip	1	670	26	9.0	390	101	6	44	9	n/a	n/a	n/a	n/a
muffie	1	340	13	4.5	200	51	3	22	5	n/a	n/a	n/a	n/a
cranberry orange	1	530	20	3.5	340	82	4	42	7	n/a	n/a	n/a	n/a
mini	1	80	3	0.5	55	13	1	7	1	n/a	n/a	n/a	n/a
pumpkin	1	570	24	4.5	430	78	5	40	8	n/a	n/a	n/a	n/a
Pecan braid	1	450	25	9.0	160	52	3	25	6	n/a	n/a	n/a	n/a
Scones													
blueberry	1	460	19	12.0	900	65	2	26	8	n/a	n/a	n/a	n/a
mini	1	150	6	4.0	300	21	1	9	3	n/a	n/a	n/a	n/a
orange	1	550	20	13.0	810	80	2	38	9	n/a	n/a	n/a	n/a
mini	1	180	7	4.5	270	27	1	13	3	n/a	n/a	n/a	n/a
Vanilla cinnamon roll	1	620	18	8.0	490	106	1	71	9	n/a	n/a	n/a	n/a
mini	1	310	9	4.0	240	53	1	35	4	n/a	n/a	n/a	n/a
Bagels													
Asiago cheese	1	320	6	3.5	560	56	2	5	14	n/a	n/a	n/a	n/a
Blueberry	1	300	1	0.0	430	66	3	11	10	n/a	n/a	n/a	n/a
Chocolate chip	1	330	6	3.0	400	64	2	14	10	n/a	n/a	n/a	n/a
Cinnamon crunch	1	420	7	5.0	400	84	2	34	9	n/a	n/a	n/a	n/a
Cinnamon swirl & raisin	1	310	2	1.0	430	68	3	13	10	n/a	n/a	n/a	n/a
Everything	1	300	2	0.0	610	63	3	5	11	n/a	n/a	n/a	n/a
Jalapeño cheddar	1	300	3	1.5	750	56	2	4	13	n/a	n/a	n/a	n/a
Plain	1	280	1	0.0	460	62	2	5	10	n/a	n/a	n/a	n/a
Poppyseed	1	300	2	0.0	460	63	3	5	11	n/a	n/a	n/a	n/a
Salt	1	280	1	0.0	2020	62	2	5	10	n/a	n/a	n/a	n/a
Sesame	1	300	3	0.5	460	63	3	5	11	n/a	n/a	n/a	n/a
Sprouted grain bagel flat	1	180	2	0.0	410	34	3	4	7	n/a	n/a	n/a	n/a
Bread													
Artisan ciabatta	1 slice	150	2	0.0	280	30	1	0	6	n/a	n/a	n/a	n/a
Asiago cheese focaccia	1 slice	150	3	1.0	320	24	1	0	6	n/a	n/a	n/a	n/a
Black pepper focaccia	1 slice	140	2	0.0	370	26	1	0	5	n/a	n/a	n/a	n/a
Brioche roll	1	220	7	4.0	270	31	2	5	8	n/a	n/a	n/a	n/a
Classic sourdough	1 slice	150	0	0.0	320	31	1	0	6	n/a	n/a	n/a	n/a
Classic white miche	1 slice	160	4	2.0	260	27	1	4	6	n/a	n/a	n/a	n/a
Country rustic sourdough	1 slice	130	0	0.0	240	28	1	0	5	n/a	n/a	n/a	n/a
French baguette	1 slice	150	5	0.0	370	30	1	1	5	n/a	n/a	n/a	n/a
New England roll	1	250	5	1.5	440	44	1	5	9	n/a	n/a	n/a	n/a
Sourdough bread bowl	1	670	5	0.0	1160	130	4	2	27	n/a	n/a	n/a	n/a
Tomato basil miche	1 slice	130	0	0.0	330	27	1	1	5	n/a	n/a	n/a	n/a
White whole grain	1 slice	130	1	0.0	290	25	2	3	6	n/a	n/a	n/a	n/a
Whole grain lahvash	1	170	4	0.5	310	25	9	3	12	n/a	n/a	n/a	n/a

Panera Bread

	Amount	Calories	Fat (g)	Saturated Fat (g)	Sodium (mg)	Carbohydrate (g)	Fiber (g)	Sugar (g)	Protein (g)	Vitamin D (mcg)	Calcium (mg)	Iron (mg)	Potassium (mg)
Entrées													
Bowls													
Baja	1	630	34	6.0	1280	70	13	12	17	n/a	n/a	n/a	n/a
w/ chicken	1	690	35	7.0	1440	71	13	12	28	n/a	n/a	n/a	n/a
Mediterranean	1	510	28	6.0	1100	52	7	7	15	n/a	n/a	n/a	n/a
w/ chicken	1	570	29	6.0	1260	53	7	8	26	n/a	n/a	n/a	n/a
Teriyaki chicken & broccoli	1	610	17	4.0	1630	69	5	27	46	n/a	n/a	n/a	n/a
Flatbread pizza													
cheese	1	920	41	19.0	2100	95	3	8	40	n/a	n/a	n/a	n/a
chipotle chicken & bacon	1	1030	51	19.0	2400	97	3	10	44	n/a	n/a	n/a	n/a
Margherita	1	870	35	16.0	1840	98	4	10	35	n/a	n/a	n/a	n/a
pepperoni	1	1070	55	24.0	2580	95	3	8	43	n/a	n/a	n/a	n/a
Mac & cheese													
broccoli cheddar													
large		740	48	23.0	1930	53	5	10	25	n/a	n/a	n/a	n/a
bread bowl		1040	28	12.0	2120	157	7	7	39	n/a	n/a	n/a	n/a
regular													
large		960	64	35.0	2300	67	0	15	32	n/a	n/a	n/a	n/a
bread bowl		1150	36	18.0	2310	164	4	9	43	n/a	n/a	n/a	n/a
Sandwiches													
Avocado	1	210	5	0.5	330	37	4	2	7	n/a	n/a	n/a	n/a
Bacon Turkey Bravo	1	1000	41	19.0	2660	104	4	11	54	n/a	n/a	n/a	n/a
Classic grilled cheese	1	880	51	29.0	2370	68	2	9	37	n/a	n/a	n/a	n/a
Deli turkey	1	590	17	3.0	1690	76	4	8	35	n/a	n/a	n/a	n/a
Green Goddess caprese melt	1	970	40	13.0	1900	118	5	8	36	n/a	n/a	n/a	n/a
Mediterranean veggie	1	640	14	4.0	1660	106	7	11	23	n/a	n/a	n/a	n/a
Napa almond chicken salad	1	640	25	4.5	920	78	4	12	27	n/a	n/a	n/a	n/a
Pepperoni mozzarella melt	1	1010	39	20.0	2600	115	4	6	48	n/a	n/a	n/a	n/a
Smoky Buffalo chicken melt	1	830	19	9.0	3010	115	4	4	50	n/a	n/a	n/a	n/a
The Chef's Chicken Sandwich													
The Signature Take	1	560	29	10.0	1140	41	2	7	36	n/a	n/a	n/a	n/a
The Spicy Take	1	570	29	8.0	1410	45	2	8	33	n/a	n/a	n/a	n/a
Toasted Frontega Chicken	1	810	36	10.0	1890	79	4	6	43	n/a	n/a	n/a	n/a
Toasted smokehouse BBQ chicken	1	760	29	14.0	1640	81	3	18	45	n/a	n/a	n/a	n/a
Toasted steak & white cheddar	1	950	47	15.0	1550	87	4	7	44	n/a	n/a	n/a	n/a
Tuna salad	1	720	33	5.0	1670	78	6	6	29	n/a	n/a	n/a	n/a
Salads													
Asian sesame w/ chicken	1	410	22	3.0	690	26	6	7	29	n/a	n/a	n/a	n/a
Caesar	1	350	25	6.0	640	18	4	4	10	n/a	n/a	n/a	n/a
w/ chicken	1	450	27	7.0	960	20	4	4	32	n/a	n/a	n/a	n/a

Panera Bread	Amount	Calories	Fat (g)	Saturated Fat (g)	Sodium (mg)	Carbohydrate (g)	Fiber (g)	Sugar (g)	Protein (g)	Vitamin D (mcg)	Calcium (mg)	Iron (mg)	Potassium (mg)
Citrus Asian crunch	1	430	25	3.0	850	44	8	25	10	n/a	n/a	n/a	n/a
w/ chicken	1	620	33	5.0	1320	46	8	26	36	n/a	n/a	n/a	n/a
Fuji apple w/ chicken	1	560	34	7.0	740	37	6	22	29	n/a	n/a	n/a	n/a
w/o pecans	1	460	23	6.0	740	35	4	22	28	n/a	n/a	n/a	n/a
Greek	1	410	35	9.0	1080	16	5	7	8	n/a	n/a	n/a	n/a
Green Goddess Cobb w/ chicken	1	500	28	6.0	930	26	8	14	38	n/a	n/a	n/a	n/a
Southwest Caesar	1	530	46	9.0	650	20	8	5	10	n/a	n/a	n/a	n/a
w/ chicken	1	640	48	10.0	980	21	8	5	32	n/a	n/a	n/a	n/a
Strawberry poppyseed	1	240	12	1.0	140	34	8	25	5	n/a	n/a	n/a	n/a
w/ chicken	1	350	14	2.0	470	36	8	26	26	n/a	n/a	n/a	n/a
Soups													
Bistro French onion													
bowl		310	12	5.0	1990	39	3	16	12	n/a	n/a	n/a	n/a
bread bowl		860	12	4.0	2450	153	6	12	34	n/a	n/a	n/a	n/a
Broccoli cheddar													
bowl		380	25	17.0	1680	25	2	9	13	n/a	n/a	n/a	n/a
bread bowl		910	20	11.0	2220	130	6	8	35	n/a	n/a	n/a	n/a
Chicken tikka masala													
bowl		380	18	10.0	1000	37	5	8	16	n/a	n/a	n/a	n/a
bread bowl		900	16	7.0	1820	154	8	8	37	n/a	n/a	n/a	n/a
Cream of chicken & wild rice													
bowl		260	16	7.0	1390	27	5	4	10	n/a	n/a	n/a	n/a
bread bowl		840	15	5.0	2090	148	8	5	33	n/a	n/a	n/a	n/a
Homestyle chicken noodle													
bowl		100	1	0.0	1280	13	0	4	9	n/a	n/a	n/a	n/a
bread bowl		730	5	0.5	2020	139	4	5	33	n/a	n/a	n/a	n/a
Ten vegetable													
bowl		100	2	0.0	1090	15	4	6	5	n/a	n/a	n/a	n/a
bread bowl		730	6	0.5	1890	140	7	6	30	n/a	n/a	n/a	n/a
Vegetarian creamy tomato													
bowl		350	21	11.0	1100	34	1	17	5	n/a	n/a	n/a	n/a
bread bowl		910	19	8.0	1910	154	5	13	31	n/a	n/a	n/a	n/a
Sides													
Apple	1	80	0	0.0	0	22	5	16	0	n/a	n/a	n/a	n/a
Banana	1	90	0	0.0	0	23	3	12	1	n/a	n/a	n/a	n/a
French baguette	1 slice	180	1	0.0	450	36	1	1	7	n/a	n/a	n/a	n/a
Greek yogurt w/ mixed berries	1 order	240	8	4.5	80	27	2	17	15	n/a	n/a	n/a	n/a
Kettle-cooked potato chips	1 pkg	150	9	1.0	75	17	1	0	2	n/a	n/a	n/a	n/a
Pickle spear	1	5	0	0.0	240	1	0	0	0	n/a	n/a	n/a	n/a
Seasonal fruit cup	1	60	0	0.0	15	17	1	12	1	n/a	n/a	n/a	n/a

RESTAURANT & FAST FOOD CHAINS

Dressings, Sauces & Spreads

	Amount	Calories	Fat (g)	Saturated Fat (g)	Sodium (mg)	Carbohydrate (g)	Fiber (g)	Sugar (g)	Protein (g)	Vitamin D (mcg)	Calcium (mg)	Iron (mg)	Potassium (mg)
Dressings													
Asian sesame vinaigrette	1 order	90	8	1.0	200	4	0	4	0	n/a	n/a	n/a	n/a
Caesar	1 order	180	18	3.0	290	2	0	2	1	n/a	n/a	n/a	n/a
Greek	1 order	230	25	3.5	290	1	0	0	0	n/a	n/a	n/a	n/a
Green Goddess	1 order	80	7	1.0	160	4	0	3	2	n/a	n/a	n/a	n/a
lemon tahini	1 order	70	7	1.0	210	2	1	0	1	n/a	n/a	n/a	n/a
poppyseed	1 order	30	0	0.0	125	7	1	6	0	n/a	n/a	n/a	n/a
tangerine soy ginger	1 order	160	14	2.0	500	9	0	8	1	n/a	n/a	n/a	n/a
white balsamic vinaigrette flavored w/ apple	1 order	160	13	2.0	170	11	0	10	0	n/a	n/a	n/a	n/a
Sauces													
apple cider vinegar BBQ	1 order	20	0	0.0	90	5	0	4	0	n/a	n/a	n/a	n/a
Buffalo	1 order	10	1	0.0	320	1	0	1	0	n/a	n/a	n/a	n/a
chipotle	1 order	100	10	1.5	105	2	0	1	0	n/a	n/a	n/a	n/a
garlic aoli	1 order	110	12	2.0	65	0	0	0	0	n/a	n/a	n/a	n/a
horseradish	1 order	100	11	2.0	85	1	0	0	0	n/a	n/a	n/a	n/a
hummus	1 order	60	5	0.5	150	4	1	1	2	n/a	n/a	n/a	n/a
mayonnaise	1 order	130	14	2.0	115	0	0	0	0	n/a	n/a	n/a	n/a
salsa verde	1 order	90	10	1.0	170	1	0	0	0	n/a	n/a	n/a	n/a
signature	1 order	90	8	1.0	90	4	0	2	0	n/a	n/a	n/a	n/a
spicy brown mustard	1 order	10	0	0.0	80	1	0	0	0	n/a	n/a	n/a	n/a
teriyaki	1 order	120	1	0.0	680	26	0	22	2	n/a	n/a	n/a	n/a
Cream cheese													
plain	2 tbsp	110	10	7.0	85	3	0	1	1	n/a	n/a	n/a	n/a
chive & onion, reduced fat	2 tbsp	80	6	4.0	115	1	0	1	3	n/a	n/a	n/a	n/a
honey walnut, reduced fat	2 tbsp	80	6	3.5	105	5	0	5	2	n/a	n/a	n/a	n/a
Smoothies													
Green Passion	16 fl oz	250	2	0.0	50	59	0	50	2	n/a	n/a	n/a	n/a
Mango w/ Greek yogurt	16 fl oz	300	5	3.0	65	51	0	42	13	n/a	n/a	n/a	n/a
Peach & blueberry w/ almond milk	16 fl oz	220	2	0.0	50	49	1	41	2	n/a	n/a	n/a	n/a
Strawberry w/ Greek yogurt	16 fl oz	270	5	2.5	65	44	2	39	13	n/a	n/a	n/a	n/a
Strawberry banana w/ Greek yogurt	16 fl oz	250	3	1.5	35	52	4	38	8	n/a	n/a	n/a	n/a
Drinks													
Iced tea													
honey ginseng green, bottled passion papaya	16 fl oz	0	0	0.0	0	0	0	0	0	n/a	n/a	n/a	n/a
	20 fl oz	140	0	0.0	20	35	0	35	0	n/a	n/a	n/a	n/a
	30 fl oz	210	0	0.0	30	52	0	52	0	n/a	n/a	n/a	n/a
sweet													
	20 fl oz	110	0	0.0	10	27	0	27	1	n/a	n/a	n/a	n/a
	30 fl oz	150	0	0.0	10	36	0	36	2	n/a	n/a	n/a	n/a

RESTAURANT & FAST FOOD CHAINS

Panera Bread

	Amount	Calories	Fat (g)	Saturated Fat (g)	Sodium (mg)	Carbohydrate (g)	Fiber (g)	Sugar (g)	Protein (g)	Vitamin D (mcg)	Calcium (mg)	Iron (mg)	Potassium (mg)
unsweetened													
	20 fl oz	10	0	0.0	10	0	0	0	2	n/a	n/a	n/a	n/a
	30 fl oz	20	0	0.0	20	0	0	0	4	n/a	n/a	n/a	n/a
Lemonade													
agave													
	20 fl oz	200	0	0.0	10	48	0	45	0	n/a	n/a	n/a	n/a
	30 fl oz	300	0	0.0	15	73	0	67	0	n/a	n/a	n/a	n/a
strawberry, frozen w/ fresh strawberries	16 fl oz	140	0	0.0	10	35	1	31	1	n/a	n/a	n/a	n/a
Lemonade, charged													
mango yuzu citrus													
	20 fl oz	350	0	0.0	10	86	0	82	0	n/a	n/a	n/a	n/a
	30 fl oz	530	1	0.0	15	130	0	124	1	n/a	n/a	n/a	n/a
strawberry lemon mint													
	20 fl oz	280	0	0.0	10	70	0	65	0	n/a	n/a	n/a	n/a
	30 fl oz	430	1	0.0	15	105	0	98	1	n/a	n/a	n/a	n/a

Pizza Hut

Slices

	Amount	Calories	Fat (g)	Saturated Fat (g)	Sodium (mg)	Carbohydrate (g)	Fiber (g)	Sugar (g)	Protein (g)	Vitamin D (mcg)	Calcium (mg)	Iron (mg)	Potassium (mg)
Hand-tossed													
Backyard BBQ Chicken	1 slice	230	7	3.0	390	31	2	6	10	n/a	n/a	n/a	n/a
Buffalo chicken	1 slice	200	6	2.5	560	28	2	1	10	n/a	n/a	n/a	n/a
cheese	1 slice	210	7	4.0	390	26	2	2	10	n/a	n/a	n/a	n/a
cheesesteak	1 slice	220	9	5.0	410	25	2	1	11	n/a	n/a	n/a	n/a
Hawaiian chicken	1 slice	200	6	3.0	420	27	2	3	9	n/a	n/a	n/a	n/a
Meat Lover's	1 slice	280	15	6.0	590	26	2	2	13	n/a	n/a	n/a	n/a
popperoni	1 slice	220	9	4.0	420	25	2	2	10	n/a	n/a	n/a	n/a
Pepperoni Lover's	1 slice	260	12	6.0	530	26	2	2	12	n/a	n/a	n/a	n/a
Supreme	1 slice	230	10	4.0	440	26	2	2	10	n/a	n/a	n/a	n/a
Veggie Lover's	1 slice	190	6	2.5	370	27	2	2	9	n/a	n/a	n/a	n/a
Original pan													
Backyard BBQ Chicken	1 slice	260	9	3.5	440	33	2	6	11	n/a	n/a	n/a	n/a
Buffalo chicken	1 slice	240	8	3.0	610	31	2	1	10	n/a	n/a	n/a	n/a
cheese	1 slice	240	10	4.0	440	28	2	2	10	n/a	n/a	n/a	n/a
cheesesteak	1 slice	260	12	5.0	450	27	2	1	11	n/a	n/a	n/a	n/a
Hawaiian chicken	1 slice	240	9	3.0	460	29	2	3	11	n/a	n/a	n/a	n/a
Meat Lover's	1 slice	310	17	6.0	630	28	2	2	13	n/a	n/a	n/a	n/a
pepperoni	1 slice	250	11	4.0	460	28	2	2	10	n/a	n/a	n/a	n/a
Pepperoni Lover's	1 slice	290	15	6.0	570	28	2	2	13	n/a	n/a	n/a	n/a
Supreme	1 slice	260	12	4.5	490	28	2	2	11	n/a	n/a	n/a	n/a
Veggie Lover's	1 slice	230	9	3.0	410	29	2	2	9	n/a	n/a	n/a	n/a

RESTAURANT & FAST FOOD CHAINS

Pizza Hut	Amount	Calories	Fat (g)	Saturated Fat (g)	Sodium (mg)	Carbohydrate (g)	Fiber (g)	Sugar (g)	Protein (g)	Vitamin D (mcg)	Calcium (mg)	Iron (mg)	Potassium (mg)
Personal pan													
Backyard BBQ Chicken	1 slice	180	6	2.0	350	25	1	8	7	n/a	n/a	n/a	n/a
Buffalo chicken	1 slice	160	5	2.0	550	22	1	2	6	n/a	n/a	n/a	n/a
cheese	1 slice	150	6	2.5	310	17	1	2	7	n/a	n/a	n/a	n/a
Hawaiian chicken	1 slice	150	5	2.0	310	18	1	3	7	n/a	n/a	n/a	n/a
Meat Lover's	1 slice	190	9	3.5	400	17	1	2	8	n/a	n/a	n/a	n/a
pepperoni	1 slice	150	7	2.5	320	17	1	2	6	n/a	n/a	n/a	n/a
Pepperoni Lover's	1 slice	180	9	3.5	370	18	1	2	8	n/a	n/a	n/a	n/a
Supreme	1 slice	160	7	2.5	330	18	1	2	7	n/a	n/a	n/a	n/a
Veggie Lover's	1 slice	140	5	2.0	290	18	1	3	6	n/a	n/a	n/a	n/a
Thin 'N Crispy													
Backyard BBQ Chicken	1 slice	210	7	3.0	440	27	1	7	10	n/a	n/a	n/a	n/a
Buffalo chicken	1 slice	180	5	2.5	620	25	1	3	9	n/a	n/a	n/a	n/a
cheese	1 slice	180	7	3.5	420	22	2	3	9	n/a	n/a	n/a	n/a
cheesesteak	1 slice	210	9	5.0	460	21	1	2	11	n/a	n/a	n/a	n/a
Hawaiian chicken	1 slice	190	6	3.0	470	24	2	5	11	n/a	n/a	n/a	n/a
Meat Lover's	1 slice	280	16	6.0	680	22	2	3	13	n/a	n/a	n/a	n/a
pepperoni	1 slice	200	9	4.0	470	22	1	3	9	n/a	n/a	n/a	n/a
Pepperoni Lover's	1 slice	250	13	6.0	580	22	2	3	12	n/a	n/a	n/a	n/a
Supreme	1 slice	220	10	4.5	490	23	2	4	10	n/a	n/a	n/a	n/a
Veggie Lover's	1 slice	170	5	2.5	410	24	2	4	8	n/a	n/a	n/a	n/a
Rectangle													
Backyard BBQ Chicken	1 slice	260	9	3.5	480	34	2	6	11	n/a	n/a	n/a	n/a
Buffalo chicken	1 slice	240	8	3.0	650	32	2	2	10	n/a	n/a	n/a	n/a
cheese	1 slice	240	9	4.0	470	29	2	2	11	n/a	n/a	n/a	n/a
Hawaiian chicken	1 slice	240	8	3.0	500	30	2	3	11	n/a	n/a	n/a	n/a
Meat Lover's	1 slice	320	17	6.0	680	29	2	2	13	n/a	n/a	n/a	n/a
pepperoni	1 slice	250	11	4.0	500	29	2	2	10	n/a	n/a	n/a	n/a
Pepperoni Lover's	1 slice	300	15	6.0	600	29	2	2	13	n/a	n/a	n/a	n/a
Supreme	1 slice	270	12	4.5	520	30	2	2	11	n/a	n/a	n/a	n/a
Veggie Lover's	1 slice	230	8	3.0	450	30	3	2	9	n/a	n/a	n/a	n/a
P'Zones (w/ marinara sauce)													
Meaty	1	1150	50	21.0	2270	124	9	9	50	n/a	n/a	n/a	n/a
Pepperoni	1	970	34	16.0	1780	123	9	8	42	n/a	n/a	n/a	n/a
Supremo	1	980	35	16.0	1760	125	9	9	42	n/a	n/a	n/a	n/a
Pasta													
Oven-baked													
cheesy Alfredo	1 order	880	48	31.0	1180	84	5	5	30	n/a	n/a	n/a	n/a
chicken Alfredo	1 order	930	49	32.0	1340	85	5	5	37	n/a	n/a	n/a	n/a
Italian meats	1 order	860	37	15.0	1640	97	8	17	36	n/a	n/a	n/a	n/a
veggie	1 order	640	16	8.0	1170	99	9	18	27	n/a	n/a	n/a	n/a
Penne													
w/ marinara	1 order	810	23	13.0	2050	112	12	31	38	n/a	n/a	n/a	n/a
& meatballs	1 order	1120	46	21.0	2750	121	12	33	57	n/a	n/a	n/a	n/a
& mushrooms	1 order	820	24	13.0	2050	114	13	32	39	n/a	n/a	n/a	n/a

RESTAURANT & FAST FOOD CHAINS

Pizza Hut	Amount	Calories	Fat (g)	Saturated Fat (g)	Sodium (mg)	Carbohydrate (g)	Fiber (g)	Sugar (g)	Protein (g)	Vitamin D (mcg)	Calcium (mg)	Iron (mg)	Potassium (mg)
Wings													
Breaded boneless													
Buffalo													
Burnin' Hot	1 pc	90	4	1.0	340	9	0	1	5	n/a	n/a	n/a	n/a
medium	1 pc	90	4	1.0	330	9	0	1	5	n/a	n/a	n/a	n/a
mild	1 pc	90	4	1.0	340	10	0	1	5	n/a	n/a	n/a	n/a
Cajun style dry rub	1 pc	80	4	1.0	210	6	0	0	5	n/a	n/a	n/a	n/a
garlic Parmesan	1 pc	130	9	1.5	270	6	0	0	5	n/a	n/a	n/a	n/a
honey BBQ	1 pc	100	4	1.0	220	11	0	4	5	n/a	n/a	n/a	n/a
lemon pepper dry rub	1 pc	80	4	1.0	200	6	0	0	5	n/a	n/a	n/a	n/a
naked	1 pc	80	4	0.5	160	6	0	0	5	n/a	n/a	n/a	n/a
spicy garlic	1 pc	110	6	1.0	290	8	0	0	5	n/a	n/a	n/a	n/a
sweet chili	1 pc	100	5	1.0	230	10	0	4	5	n/a	n/a	n/a	n/a
Traditional													
Buffalo													
Burnin' Hot	1 pc	100	5	1.0	390	5	0	1	9	n/a	n/a	n/a	n/a
medium	1 pc	100	5	1.0	370	5	0	1	9	n/a	n/a	n/a	n/a
mild	1 pc	100	5	1.0	380	5	0	1	9	n/a	n/a	n/a	n/a
Cajun style dry rub	1 pc	80	5	1.0	220	1	0	0	9	n/a	n/a	n/a	n/a
garlic Parmesan	1 pc	140	11	2.5	300	1	0	0	10	n/a	n/a	n/a	n/a
honey BBQ	1 pc	110	5	1.0	230	7	0	5	9	n/a	n/a	n/a	n/a
lemon pepper dry rub	1 pc	80	5	1.0	200	1	0	0	9	n/a	n/a	n/a	n/a
naked	1 pc	80	5	1.0	160	0	0	0	9	n/a	n/a	n/a	n/a
spicy garlic	1 pc	120	8	2.0	330	3	0	1	9	n/a	n/a	n/a	n/a
sweet chili	1 pc	100	5	1.5	220	4	0	4	9	n/a	n/a	n/a	n/a
Sides													
Breadsticks	1 pc	140	5	1.0	260	19	1	1	4	n/a	n/a	n/a	n/a
Cheese sticks	1 pc	150	5	2.5	330	20	1	1	7	n/a	n/a	n/a	n/a
Fries w/ ketchup	1 order	500	24	4.5	1230	67	3	7	4	n/a	n/a	n/a	n/a
Mozzarella sticks	1 pc	80	5	2.0	200	7	0	1	2	n/a	n/a	n/a	n/a
Desserts													
Apple pies	1 pc	170	9	2.5	100	22	1	12	1	n/a	n/a	n/a	n/a
Cinnabon mini rolls	1 pc	80	3	1.5	15	12	0	6	2	n/a	n/a	n/a	n/a
Cinnamon sticks	1 pc	80	3	0.0	100	13	0	4	2	n/a	n/a	n/a	n/a
Triple chocolate brownie	1	230	10	3.5	80	34	2	25	3	n/a	n/a	n/a	n/a
Ultimate chocolate chip cookie	1	190	9	4.5	110	26	1	17	2	n/a	n/a	n/a	n/a
Popeyes													
Breakfast													
Biscuit													
bacon	1	400	25	12.0	780	37	3	2	8	n/a	n/a	n/a	n/a
chicken	1	490	26	14.0	1280	47	1	2	17	n/a	n/a	n/a	n/a
egg	1	510	29	15.0	1160	41	1	2	13	n/a	n/a	n/a	n/a
& sausage	1	690	45	22.0	1520	43	1	2	20	n/a	n/a	n/a	n/a
sausage & gravy	1	510	33	14.0	1090	42	3	3	10	n/a	n/a	n/a	n/a

RESTAURANT & FAST FOOD CHAINS

Popeyes

	Amount	Calories	Fat (g)	Saturated Fat (g)	Sodium (mg)	Carbohydrate (g)	Fiber (g)	Sugar (g)	Protein (g)	Vitamin D (mcg)	Calcium (mg)	Iron (mg)	Potassium (mg)
Grits	1 order	370	5	0.5	30	80	7	0	5	n/a	n/a	n/a	n/a
Hash rounds	1 order	360	20	9.0	450	41	4	0	3	n/a	n/a	n/a	n/a
Chicken													
Breast	1 pc	380	20	8.0	1230	16	2	0	35	n/a	n/a	n/a	n/a
Leg	1 pc	160	9	4.0	460	5	1	0	14	n/a	n/a	n/a	n/a
Nuggets	12 pc	570	36	16.0	1320	28	2	1	34	n/a	n/a	n/a	n/a
Tenders													
blackened	5 pcs	280	3	0.0	920	3	0	0	43	n/a	n/a	n/a	n/a
classic or spicy	5 pcs	740	34	14.0	3040	48	3	0	63	n/a	n/a	n/a	n/a
Thigh	1 pc	280	21	8.0	640	7	1	0	14	n/a	n/a	n/a	n/a
Wing	1 pc	210	14	4.0	610	8	1	0	13	n/a	n/a	n/a	n/a
Seafood													
Popcorn shrimp	¼ lb	390	25	8.0	1390	28	3	0	14	n/a	n/a	n/a	n/a
Chicken Sandwiches													
Classic	1	700	42	14.0	1440	50	2	8	28	n/a	n/a	n/a	n/a
Spicy	1	700	42	14.0	1470	50	2	8	28	n/a	n/a	n/a	n/a
Sides													
Biscuit	1	210	13	6.0	440	20	1	1	3	n/a	n/a	n/a	n/a
Cajun fries	large	800	42	15.0	1760	97	9	1	10	n/a	n/a	n/a	n/a
Cinnamon apple pie	1	240	16	6.0	260	35	1	12	3	n/a	n/a	n/a	n/a
Coleslaw	large	420	30	5.0	570	36	3	27	3	n/a	n/a	n/a	n/a
Homestyle mac & cheese	large	850	63	36.0	1540	48	1	9	33	n/a	n/a	n/a	n/a
Mashed potatoes w/ Cajun gravy	large	330	12	6.0	1770	54	3	3	9	n/a	n/a	n/a	n/a
Red beans & rice	large	610	40	13.0	1490	51	15	0	19	n/a	n/a	n/a	n/a
Sauces													
Bayou Buffalo	1 oz	60	6	1.0	450	2	0	0	0	n/a	n/a	n/a	n/a
BoldBQ	1 oz	70	0	0.0	440	16	0	13	0	n/a	n/a	n/a	n/a
Creole Cocktail	1 oz	40	0	0.0	400	9	0	7	0	n/a	n/a	n/a	n/a
Mardi Gras Mustard	1 oz	100	8	1.0	240	5	1	4	1	n/a	n/a	n/a	n/a
Ranch													
blackened	1 oz	120	12	2.0	250	2	0	1	0	n/a	n/a	n/a	n/a
buttermilk	1 oz	140	15	3.0	230	2	0	1	0	n/a	n/a	n/a	n/a
Sweet Heat	1 oz	70	0	0.0	290	19	0	16	0	n/a	n/a	n/a	n/a
Tartar	1 oz	140	15	3.0	230	1	0	1	0	n/a	n/a	n/a	n/a

Shake Shack

	Amount	Calories	Fat (g)	Saturated Fat (g)	Sodium (mg)	Carbohydrate (g)	Fiber (g)	Sugar (g)	Protein (g)	Vitamin D (mcg)	Calcium (mg)	Iron (mg)	Potassium (mg)
Breakfast													
Sandwiches													
bacon	1	400	23	10.0	890	25	0	5	23	n/a	n/a	n/a	n/a
double egg	1	490	30	12.0	990	26	0	6	29	n/a	n/a	n/a	n/a
egg and cheese	1	340	19	9.0	610	25	0	5	17	n/a	n/a	n/a	n/a
double egg	1	430	25	11.0	700	25	0	5	23	n/a	n/a	n/a	n/a

RESTAURANT & FAST FOOD CHAINS

Shake Shack	Amount	Calories	Fat (g)	Saturated Fat (g)	Sodium (mg)	Carbohydrate (g)	Fiber (g)	Sugar (g)	Protein (g)	Vitamin D (mcg)	Calcium (mg)	Iron (mg)	Potassium (mg)
egg white light	1	320	18	8.0	440	26	0	6	15	n/a	n/a	n/a	n/a
double egg	1	340	18	8.0	500	26	0	6	19	n/a	n/a	n/a	n/a
sausage	1	530	32	14.0	1220	28	0	8	30	n/a	n/a	n/a	n/a
double egg	1	620	39	16.0	1310	28	0	8	36	n/a	n/a	n/a	n/a
Wake Up Shack	1	510	30	11.0	1110	34	1	7	24	n/a	n/a	n/a	n/a
double egg	1	600	37	13.0	1210	34	1	7	30	n/a	n/a	n/a	n/a
Tots	1 order	270	13	3.5	550	32	3	2	3	n/a	n/a	n/a	n/a
Add-ons													
egg	1	90	7	2.0	95	0	0	0	6	n/a	n/a	n/a	n/a
white	1	15	0	0.0	55	0	0	0	4	n/a	n/a	n/a	n/a
sausage patty	1	190	14	5.0	610	3	0	2	13	n/a	n/a	n/a	n/a
Burgers													
Avocado bacon	1	610	39	14.0	1540	28	2	5	36	n/a	n/a	n/a	n/a
double	1	870	57	22.0	2560	29	2	6	58	n/a	n/a	n/a	n/a
Bacon cheeseburger	1	500	29	13.0	1480	25	0	5	35	n/a	n/a	n/a	n/a
double	1	760	47	21.0	2510	25	0	6	58	n/a	n/a	n/a	n/a
Brat burger	1	860	61	20.0	1850	34	0	6	44	n/a	n/a	n/a	n/a
double	1	1050	73	25.0	2530	34	0	6	62	n/a	n/a	n/a	n/a
Cheeseburger	1	440	24	11.0	1200	25	0	5	29	n/a	n/a	n/a	n/a
double	1	700	42	20.0	2220	25	0	5	51	n/a	n/a	n/a	n/a
Golden State	1	560	37	13.0	1310	26	0	5	31	n/a	n/a	n/a	n/a
double	1	840	56	22.0	2130	27	0	5	54	n/a	n/a	n/a	n/a
Green Chile CheddarShack	1	470	26	12.0	1380	28	1	6	30	n/a	n/a	n/a	n/a
double	1	750	46	22.0	2190	28	1	6	53	n/a	n/a	n/a	n/a
Grilled cheese	1	320	18	10.0	850	25	0	5	14	n/a	n/a	n/a	n/a
Hamburger	1	370	18	8.0	850	24	0	5	25	n/a	n/a	n/a	n/a
double	1	560	30	12.0	1540	24	0	5	44	n/a	n/a	n/a	n/a
Link	1	680	46	18.0	2010	27	0	6	39	n/a	n/a	n/a	n/a
double	1	930	64	26.0	3040	28	0	6	61	n/a	n/a	n/a	n/a
triple	1	1190	82	34.0	4070	28	0	7	83	n/a	n/a	n/a	n/a
Lockhart	1	780	56	21.0	2050	27	0	5	39	n/a	n/a	n/a	n/a
double	1	1040	74	29.0	3080	28	0	5	61	n/a	n/a	n/a	n/a
triple	1	1300	92	38.0	4110	29	0	6	83	n/a	n/a	n/a	n/a
Montlake	1	670	45	19.0	1560	36	0	5	29	n/a	n/a	n/a	n/a
double	1	980	68	31.0	2470	36	0	5	54	n/a	n/a	n/a	n/a
Mound City Double	1	780	48	20.0	2380	26	0	6	56	n/a	n/a	n/a	n/a
Roadside Double	1	770	46	20.0	2300	32	0	7	53	n/a	n/a	n/a	n/a
ShackBurger	1	500	30	12.0	1250	26	0	6	29	n/a	n/a	n/a	n/a
double	1	760	48	20.0	2280	27	0	6	51	n/a	n/a	n/a	n/a
Shack Stack	1	770	45	18.0	1700	50	0	7	40	n/a	n/a	n/a	n/a
Shroom Burger	1	510	27	10.0	670	49	0	7	18	n/a	n/a	n/a	n/a
SilverLake Shack	1	530	33	13.0	1520	28	0	6	30	n/a	n/a	n/a	n/a
double	1	790	51	22.0	2540	28	0	7	52	n/a	n/a	n/a	n/a

Shake Shack	Amount	Calories	Fat (g)	Saturated Fat (g)	Sodium (mg)	Carbohydrate (g)	Fiber (g)	Sugar (g)	Protein (g)	Vitamin D (mcg)	Calcium (mg)	Iron (mg)	Potassium (mg)
Slap Shot	1	490	27	10.0	1150	33	0	6	28	n/a	n/a	n/a	n/a
double	1	680	40	15.0	1840	33	0	6	47	n/a	n/a	n/a	n/a
Smokeshack	1	570	35	13.0	2010	28	0	7	36	n/a	n/a	n/a	n/a
double	1	830	53	22.0	3030	28	0	7	58	n/a	n/a	n/a	n/a
Veggie Shack	1	630	31	16.0	1630	53	2	8	20	n/a	n/a	n/a	n/a
double	1	910	41	27.0	2730	73	3	10	31	n/a	n/a	n/a	n/a
Add-ons													
American cheese	1 order	70	6	3.5	340	1	0	0	4	n/a	n/a	n/a	n/a
avocado	1 order	60	5	0.5	0	3	2	0	1	n/a	n/a	n/a	n/a
bacon	2 slices	70	5	1.5	290	0	0	0	6	n/a	n/a	n/a	n/a
cherry peppers	1 order	10	0	0.0	470	2	0	2	0	n/a	n/a	n/a	n/a
gluten-free bun	1	160	3	0.0	350	31	2	5	3	n/a	n/a	n/a	n/a
lettuce	1 order	1	0	0.0	0	0	0	0	0	n/a	n/a	n/a	n/a
wrap	1	5	0	0.0	15	1	1	0	1	n/a	n/a	n/a	n/a
Martin's potato roll	1	180	6	3.0	170	24	0	5	7	n/a	n/a	n/a	n/a
onions	1 order	5	0	0.0	0	1	0	0	0	n/a	n/a	n/a	n/a
patties													
burger	1	190	12	4.5	690	0	0	0	19	n/a	n/a	n/a	n/a
veggie	1	210	4	7.0	760	20	2	2	8	n/a	n/a	n/a	n/a
crispy onions	1 order	110	8	1.5	95	7	0	0	1	n/a	n/a	n/a	n/a
pickles	1 order	1	0	0.0	140	0	0	0	0	n/a	n/a	n/a	n/a
ShakeSauce	1 order	60	6	1.0	60	0	0	0	0	n/a	n/a	n/a	n/a
tomatoes	1 order	5	0	0.0	0	1	0	0	0	n/a	n/a	n/a	n/a
Chicken													
Avocado bacon	1	680	42	9.0	1480	37	2	6	40	n/a	n/a	n/a	n/a
Chicken bites	6 pcs	300	19	3.5	780	15	0	1	17	n/a	n/a	n/a	n/a
	10 pcs	510	32	6.0	1300	26	0	2	29	n/a	n/a	n/a	n/a
Chicken Shack	1	550	31	7.0	1170	34	0	6	33	n/a	n/a	n/a	n/a
Summer citrus BBQ sandwich	1	590	30	7.0	1430	54	1	23	34	n/a	n/a	n/a	n/a
Add-ons													
BBQ sauce	1 order	70	0	0.0	380	16	0	14	1	n/a	n/a	n/a	n/a
herb mayonnaise	1 order	90	10	0.5	140	0	0	0	0	n/a	n/a	n/a	n/a
honey mustard	1 order	180	19	2.5	230	4	0	4	1	n/a	n/a	n/a	n/a
ranch	1 order	140	14	1.5	250	1	0	1	1	n/a	n/a	n/a	n/a
Flat-Top Dogs													
Garden Dog	1	180	3	0.0	1060	27	1	7	8	n/a	n/a	n/a	n/a
Hot dog	1	350	22	10.0	800	25	0	6	16	n/a	n/a	n/a	n/a
Sausage link	1	240	20	7.0	682	2	0	0	16	n/a	n/a	n/a	n/a
Shack-Cago Dog	1	390	22	10.0	1490	32	0	12	17	n/a	n/a	n/a	n/a
Shackmeister Cheddar Brat	1	690	51	21.0	1210	33	0	6	27	n/a	n/a	n/a	n/a
Add cheese	1 order	80	7	5.0	95	1	0	0	2	n/a	n/a	n/a	n/a

RESTAURANT & FAST FOOD CHAINS

	Amount	Calories	Fat (g)	Saturated Fat (g)	Sodium (mg)	Carbohydrate (g)	Fiber (g)	Sugar (g)	Protein (g)	Vitamin D (mcg)	Calcium (mg)	Iron (mg)	Potassium (mg)
Fries													
Cheese	1 order	710	44	19.0	1020	64	7	1	12	n/a	n/a	n/a	n/a
bacon	1 order	840	52	21.0	1570	65	7	1	24	n/a	n/a	n/a	n/a
Double Down	1 order	1910	117	49.0	4020	164	16	5	41	n/a	n/a	n/a	n/a
Hot	1 order	630	38	6.0	1030	66	0	2	7	n/a	n/a	n/a	n/a
cheese	1 order	870	60	20.0	1310	68	0	2	13	n/a	n/a	n/a	n/a
add extra spice	1 order	10	0	0.0	75	2	0	1	0	n/a	n/a	n/a	n/a
Regular	1 order	470	22	4.5	740	63	7	1	6	n/a	n/a	n/a	n/a
Summer BBQ	1 order	540	23	4.5	1610	79	1	12	6	n/a	n/a	n/a	n/a
cheese	1 order	780	45	19.0	1890	80	1	13	12	n/a	n/a	n/a	n/a
Floats													
Creamsicle	1	440	15	9.0	240	75	0	74	7	n/a	n/a	n/a	n/a
Root beer	1	430	15	9.0	220	70	0	69	7	n/a	n/a	n/a	n/a
Shakes													
Black & white	regular	770	42	26.0	460	80	0	76	19	n/a	n/a	n/a	n/a
	mini	390	21	13.0	240	30	0	38	9	n/a	n/a	n/a	n/a
Bourbon salted honey	regular	890	44	27.0	700	89	0	87	18	n/a	n/a	n/a	n/a
Chocolate shake	regular	750	45	27.0	310	76	0	69	16	n/a	n/a	n/a	n/a
	mini	380	23	14.0	160	38	2	35	8	n/a	n/a	n/a	n/a
non-dairy	regular	850	47	39.0	470	99	5	73	11	n/a	n/a	n/a	n/a
	mini	420	24	20.0	240	49	3	37	6	n/a	n/a	n/a	n/a
Cookies & cream	regular	850	44	24.0	580	98	0	86	19	n/a	n/a	n/a	n/a
	mini	430	22	12.0	290	49	1	43	10	n/a	n/a	n/a	n/a
Oreo funnel cake	regular	1080	55	29.0	980	129	2	100	19	n/a	n/a	n/a	n/a
	mini	540	27	15.0	490	65	1	50	10	n/a	n/a	n/a	n/a
Salted caramel	regular	840	42	26.0	950	99	0	96	17	n/a	n/a	n/a	n/a
Strawberry	regular	690	35	21.0	430	77	0	75	17	n/a	n/a	n/a	n/a
	mini	350	18	11.0	210	38	0	37	9	n/a	n/a	n/a	n/a
Triple chocolate brownie	regular	950	58	34.0	940	101	5	88	19	n/a	n/a	n/a	n/a
	mini	480	29	17.0	470	51	2	44	10	n/a	n/a	n/a	n/a
Vanilla	regular	680	36	22.0	430	72	0	71	18	n/a	n/a	n/a	n/a
	mini	340	18	11.0	220	36	0	36	9	n/a	n/a	n/a	n/a
Sundaes & Cups													
Chocolate cup	1	310	19	11.0	120	32	0	29	6	n/a	n/a	n/a	n/a
double	1	490	30	18.0	190	51	0	47	9	n/a	n/a	n/a	n/a
Non-dairy chocolate custard cup	1	400	22	19.0	190	48	2	36	5	n/a	n/a	n/a	n/a
double	1	800	44	39.0	380	96	4	72	10	n/a	n/a	n/a	n/a
Shack Attack Sundae	1	800	45	24.0	780	93	4	70	13	n/a	n/a	n/a	n/a
Strawberry shortcake sundae	1	560	26	14.0	400	73	1	58	10	n/a	n/a	n/a	n/a
Vanilla cup	1	280	15	9.0	180	30	0	30	7	n/a	n/a	n/a	n/a
double	1	450	24	14.0	280	49	0	48	11	n/a	n/a	n/a	n/a
Vanilla & choclate cup	1	290	17	10.0	150	31	0	29	6	n/a	n/a	n/a	n/a
double	1	470	27	16.0	230	50	0	47	10	n/a	n/a	n/a	n/a

RESTAURANT & FAST FOOD CHAINS

Shake Shack	Amount	Calories	Fat (g)	Saturated Fat (g)	Sodium (mg)	Carbohydrate (g)	Fiber (g)	Sugar (g)	Protein (g)	Vitamin D (mcg)	Calcium (mg)	Iron (mg)	Potassium (mg)
Add-ons													
brownie pieces	1 order	60	3	1.5	70	9	1	5	1	n/a	n/a	n/a	n/a
fudge sauce	1 order	100	7	4.5	40	9	0	7	1	n/a	n/a	n/a	n/a
maraschino cherry	1 order	10	0	0.0	0	2	0	2	0	n/a	n/a	n/a	n/a
Oreo cookie crumbs	1 order	110	5	1.5	90	16	1	9	1	n/a	n/a	n/a	n/a
rainbow sprinkles	1 order	35	2	0.0	0	6	0	4	0	n/a	n/a	n/a	n/a
Shark Attack Crunch	1 order	70	4	2.0	300	11	1	7	1	n/a	n/a	n/a	n/a
strawberry sauce	1 order	25	0	0.0	5	6	0	5	0	n/a	n/a	n/a	n/a
whipped cream	1 order	35	3	1.5	10	2	0	2	1	n/a	n/a	n/a	n/a
Sonic													
Breakfast													
Burrito													
bacon	1	470	25	11.0	1540	35	1	1	25	n/a	n/a	n/a	n/a
sausage	1	500	30	13.0	1430	35	1	1	23	n/a	n/a	n/a	n/a
SuperSONIC	1	610	35	14.0	1800	49	3	3	24	n/a	n/a	n/a	n/a
Ultimate Meat & Cheese	1	840	58	19.0	2220	47	2	1	30	n/a	n/a	n/a	n/a
Breakfast Toaster													
bacon	1	520	29	12.0	1430	43	3	4	23	n/a	n/a	n/a	n/a
sausage	1	670	45	18.0	1500	43	3	4	25	n/a	n/a	n/a	n/a
Cinnabon Cinnasnacks w/o frosting	5 pcs	630	37	11.0	350	63	4	21	10	n/a	n/a	n/a	n/a
French toast sticks w/o syrup	4 pcs	480	25	4.5	460	54	3	12	8	n/a	n/a	n/a	n/a
Burgers													
Cheeseburger	1	720	42	11.0	1400	52	2	12	31	n/a	n/a	n/a	n/a
double	1	1070	71	21.0	2020	54	2	12	53	n/a	n/a	n/a	n/a
bacon	1	1140	77	23.0	2020	52	5	10	58	n/a	n/a	n/a	n/a
quarter pound	1	560	35	12.0	1290	34	1	6	26	n/a	n/a	n/a	n/a
Add-ons													
American cheese	1 order	70	6	3.0	330	1	0	0	4	n/a	n/a	n/a	n/a
crispy bacon	1 order	80	7	2.5	290	1	0	0	6	n/a	n/a	n/a	n/a
grilled onions	1 order	5	0	0.0	5	1	0	0	0	n/a	n/a	n/a	n/a
hot chili	1 order	60	4	1.5	170	3	1	1	3	n/a	n/a	n/a	n/a
spicy jalapeños	1 order	5	0	0.0	140	1	0	1	0	n/a	n/a	n/a	n/a
Chicken													
Chicken Slinger	1	350	16	3.5	680	35	3	6	14	n/a	n/a	n/a	n/a
Crispy tenders	5 pcs	430	20	2.0	1210	27	3	0	35	n/a	n/a	n/a	n/a
Jumbo popcorn chicken	medium	490	28	5.0	1640	36	4	1	23	n/a	n/a	n/a	n/a
Buffalo	medium	620	41	7.0	3260	38	5	2	24	n/a	n/a	n/a	n/a
honey BBQ	medium	640	28	5.0	2780	73	5	36	24	n/a	n/a	n/a	n/a
Hot Dogs & Sandwiches													
All-American dog	1	410	21	8.0	1120	41	2	12	13	n/a	n/a	n/a	n/a
All beef regular hot dog	1	360	21	8.0	800	31	2	4	12	n/a	n/a	n/a	n/a

RESTAURANT & FAST FOOD CHAINS

Sonic	Amount	Calories	Fat (g)	Saturated Fat (g)	Sodium (mg)	Carbohydrate (g)	Fiber (g)	Sugar (g)	Protein (g)	Vitamin D (mcg)	Calcium (mg)	Iron (mg)	Potassium (mg)
Chili cheese coney	1	470	29	12.0	1260	34	2	5	18	n/a	n/a	n/a	n/a
Crispy chicken sandwich	1	550	30	6.0	870	48	4	10	21	n/a	n/a	n/a	n/a
Footlong quarter pound coney	1	790	49	19.0	2300	55	3	9	31	n/a	n/a	n/a	n/a
Grilled cheese sandwich	1	430	19	7.0	1090	51	2	7	14	n/a	n/a	n/a	n/a
Sides													
Chd 'R' Peppers	6 pcs	490	48	12.0	2130	56	3	4	13	n/a	n/a	n/a	n/a
Corn dog	1	230	13	4.0	480	23	1	5	6	n/a	n/a	n/a	n/a
Fries	medium	290	13	2.5	300	38	3	0	3	n/a	n/a	n/a	n/a
chili cheese	medium	450	26	10.0	940	42	4	2	12	n/a	n/a	n/a	n/a
Mozzarella sticks	6 pcs	560	29	11.0	1490	61	3	8	23	n/a	n/a	n/a	n/a
Onion rings	medium	635	34	7.0	990	75	3	12	7	n/a	n/a	n/a	n/a
Soft pretzel twist	1	250	7	1.0	440	39	2	6	7	n/a	n/a	n/a	n/a
Tots	medium	360	19	3.5	890	43	4	0	3	n/a	n/a	n/a	n/a
chili cheese	medium	530	32	10.0	1540	47	5	2	12	n/a	n/a	n/a	n/a
Limeade													
Cherry	medium	250	0	0.0	50	66	0	65	0	n/a	n/a	n/a	n/a
diet	medium	20	0	0.0	20	3	0	2	0	n/a	n/a	n/a	n/a
Diet lime	medium	10	0	0.0	15	1	0	0	0	n/a	n/a	n/a	n/a
Minute Maid cranberry	medium	240	0	0.0	45	64	0	62	0	n/a	n/a	n/a	n/a
Regular	medium	180	0	0.0	40	47	0	46	0	n/a	n/a	n/a	n/a
Strawberry	medium	220	0	0.0	50	59	1	57	0	n/a	n/a	n/a	n/a
Shakes													
Butterfinger	medium	980	48	28.0	550	118	2	75	18	n/a	n/a	n/a	n/a
Caramel	medium	830	41	28.0	520	97	0	67	12	n/a	n/a	n/a	n/a
Cheesecake	medium	840	43	28.0	680	101	1	68	12	n/a	n/a	n/a	n/a
Chocolate	medium	810	43	29.0	540	95	1	67	12	n/a	n/a	n/a	n/a
Chocolate chip cookie dough	medium	920	45	25.0	450	118	1	73	13	n/a	n/a	n/a	n/a
Fresh banana	medium	850	41	27.0	390	108	3	70	13	n/a	n/a	n/a	n/a
Hot fudge	medium	940	48	33.0	480	113	2	80	13	n/a	n/a	n/a	n/a
M&M's minis	medium	1060	54	34.0	430	127	2	98	15	n/a	n/a	n/a	n/a
Oreo	medium	860	44	24.0	620	103	2	66	13	n/a	n/a	n/a	n/a
cheesecake	medium	1030	51	30.0	900	131	2	84	13	n/a	n/a	n/a	n/a
chocolate	medium	1000	51	32.0	760	125	3	84	13	n/a	n/a	n/a	n/a
Reese's peanut butter	medium	1130	67	33.0	740	116	3	75	18	n/a	n/a	n/a	n/a
Reese's peanut butter	medium	940	59	30.0	520	87	2	58	17	n/a	n/a	n/a	n/a
cups	medium	990	55	29.0	610	110	2	82	18	n/a	n/a	n/a	n/a
Snickers	medium	890	46	26.0	490	103	1	73	15	n/a	n/a	n/a	n/a
Strawberry	medium	790	41	27.0	400	92	1	66	11	n/a	n/a	n/a	n/a
Strawberry cheesecake	medium	890	43	28.0	680	112	2	78	12	n/a	n/a	n/a	n/a
Vanilla	medium	820	45	30.0	430	89	0	61	13	n/a	n/a	n/a	n/a

RESTAURANT & FAST FOOD CHAINS

Sonic

	Amount	Calories	Fat (g)	Saturated Fat (g)	Sodium (mg)	Carbohydrate (g)	Fiber (g)	Sugar (g)	Protein (g)	Vitamin D (mcg)	Calcium (mg)	Iron (mg)	Potassium (mg)
Slushes													
Blue coconut	medium	270	0	0.0	45	72	0	72	0	n/a	n/a	n/a	n/a
Blue raspberry	medium	270	0	0.0	45	71	0	71	0	n/a	n/a	n/a	n/a
Cherry	medium	280	0	0.0	45	74	0	74	0	n/a	n/a	n/a	n/a
Grape	medium	290	0	0.0	45	77	1	76	0	n/a	n/a	n/a	n/a
Lemonade	medium	280	0	0.0	40	74	0	72	0	n/a	n/a	n/a	n/a
Limeade	medium	280	0	0.0	40	74	0	72	0	n/a	n/a	n/a	n/a
Strawberry	medium	290	0	0.0	50	78	1	77	0	n/a	n/a	n/a	n/a
Other Drinks													
Lemonade	medium	270	0	0.0	0	69	0	64	0	n/a	n/a	n/a	n/a
Iced tea													
sweet	medium	170	0	0.0	15	45	0	45	0	n/a	n/a	n/a	n/a
unsweet	medium	0	0	0.0	15	0	0	0	0	n/a	n/a	n/a	n/a
Ocean Water	medium	200	0	0.0	45	52	0	52	0	n/a	n/a	n/a	n/a
Sundaes & Cones													
Caramel	1	490	22	15.0	350	61	0	43	7	n/a	n/a	n/a	n/a
Chocolate	1	430	22	15.0	280	51	1	36	7	n/a	n/a	n/a	n/a
Hot fudge	1	520	26	18.0	270	65	1	46	7	n/a	n/a	n/a	n/a
Strawberry	1	440	21	14.0	220	55	1	40	7	n/a	n/a	n/a	n/a
Vanilla cone	1	250	12	8.0	140	30	0	17	4	n/a	n/a	n/a	n/a
Toppings													
peanuts	1 order	40	4	0.5	0	2	1	0	2	n/a	n/a	n/a	n/a
whipped topping	1 order	70	5	5.0	0	5	0	5	0	n/a	n/a	n/a	n/a

Starbucks

	Amount	Calories	Fat (g)	Saturated Fat (g)	Sodium (mg)	Carbohydrate (g)	Fiber (g)	Sugar (g)	Protein (g)	Vitamin D (mcg)	Calcium (mg)	Iron (mg)	Potassium (mg)
Cold Coffee													
Cold brew	grande (16 fl oz)	5	0	0.0	15	0	0	0	0	n/a	n/a	n/a	n/a
w/ milk	grande (16 fl oz)	35	2	1.0	40	3	0	3	2	n/a	n/a	n/a	n/a
chocolate cream	grande (16 fl oz)	250	14	9.0	35	29	0	28	2	n/a	n/a	n/a	n/a
cinnamon caramel cream	grande (16 fl oz)	250	12	8.0	125	33	0	32	2	n/a	n/a	n/a	n/a
nitro	grande (16 fl oz)	5	0	0.0	10	0	0	0	0	n/a	n/a	n/a	n/a
cinnamon caramel cream	grande (16 fl oz)	260	13	8.0	125	34	0	33	2	n/a	n/a	n/a	n/a
vanilla sweet cream	grande (16 fl oz)	70	5	3.5	20	4	0	4	1	n/a	n/a	n/a	n/a
vanilla sweet cream	grande (16 fl oz)	110	5	3.5	20	14	0	14	1	n/a	n/a	n/a	n/a
white chocolate macadamia cream	grande (16 fl oz)	240	11	7.0	140	31	0	30	2	n/a	n/a	n/a	n/a
Iced caffè Americano	grande (16 fl oz)	15	0	0.0	15	2	0	0	1	n/a	n/a	n/a	n/a
Iced caramel macchiato	grande (16 fl oz)	250	7	4.5	150	37	0	34	10	n/a	n/a	n/a	n/a
Iced coffee	grande (16 fl oz)	80	0	0.0	10	20	0	20	0	n/a	n/a	n/a	n/a
w/ milk	grande (16 fl oz)	110	2	1.0	40	23	0	23	2	n/a	n/a	n/a	n/a

RESTAURANT & FAST FOOD CHAINS

Starbucks

	Amount	Calories	Fat (g)	Saturated Fat (g)	Sodium (mg)	Carbohydrate (g)	Fiber (g)	Sugar (g)	Protein (g)	Vitamin D (mcg)	Calcium (mg)	Iron (mg)	Potassium (mg)
Iced espresso	grande (16 fl oz)	10	0	0.0	0	2	0	0	1	n/a	n/a	n/a	n/a
shaken	grande (16 fl oz)	100	2	1.0	50	17	0	14	4	n/a	n/a	n/a	n/a
brown sugar oatmilk	grande (16 fl oz)	120	3	0.0	115	22	1	12	2	n/a	n/a	n/a	n/a
chocolate almondmilk	grande (16 fl oz)	110	3	0.0	80	20	1	16	2	n/a	n/a	n/a	n/a
toasted vanilla oatmilk	grande (16 fl oz)	140	5	0.0	60	23	1	11	2	n/a	n/a	n/a	n/a
Iced flat white	grande (16 fl oz)	150	8	4.5	110	13	0	11	8	n/a	n/a	n/a	n/a
honey almondmilk	grande (16 fl oz)	100	3	0.0	70	20	1	17	1	n/a	n/a	n/a	n/a
Iced latte													
caffè	grande (16 fl oz)	130	5	2.5	115	13	0	11	8	n/a	n/a	n/a	n/a
cinnamon dolce	grande (16 fl oz)	300	13	8.0	115	38	0	35	8	n/a	n/a	n/a	n/a
Starbucks Blonde vanilla	grande (16 fl oz)	190	4	2.0	100	30	0	28	7	n/a	n/a	n/a	n/a
Iced mocha													
caffè	grande (16 fl oz)	350	17	11.0	100	38	4	30	10	n/a	n/a	n/a	n/a
white chocolate	grande (16 fl oz)	420	20	14.0	200	49	0	48	11	n/a	n/a	n/a	n/a
Cold Drinks													
BAYA Energy													
mango guava	12 fl oz	90	0	0.0	10	23	0	23	0	n/a	n/a	n/a	n/a
raspberry lime	12 fl oz	90	0	0.0	0	23	0	22	0	n/a	n/a	n/a	n/a
Milk	grande (16 fl oz)	260	10	6.0	250	25	0	25	17	n/a	n/a	n/a	n/a
Lemonade	grande (16 fl oz)	120	0	0.0	10	28	0	27	0	n/a	n/a	n/a	n/a
blended strawberry	grande (16 fl oz)	190	0	0.0	200	46	0	45	0	n/a	n/a	n/a	n/a
Refresher													
dragon drink	grande (16 fl oz)	130	3	2.5	65	26	1	23	1	n/a	n/a	n/a	n/a
mango dragonfruit	grande (16 fl oz)	90	0	0.0	15	22	0	19	0	n/a	n/a	n/a	n/a
lemonade	grande (16 fl oz)	140	0	0.0	15	34	1	31	0	n/a	n/a	n/a	n/a
paradise drink	grande (16 fl oz)	140	3	2.5	65	27	1	23	1	n/a	n/a	n/a	n/a
pineapple passionfruit	grande (16 fl oz)	100	0	0.0	15	23	0	19	0	n/a	n/a	n/a	n/a
lemonade	grande (16 fl oz)	140	0	0.0	15	35	0	30	0	n/a	n/a	n/a	n/a
pink drink	grande (16 fl oz)	140	3	2.5	65	28	1	25	1	n/a	n/a	n/a	n/a
strawberry açaí	grande (16 fl oz)	100	0	0.0	15	23	1	21	0	n/a	n/a	n/a	n/a
lemonade	grande (16 fl oz)	140	0	0.0	15	35	1	32	0	n/a	n/a	n/a	n/a
Frappucino Blended Beverages													
Caffè vanilla	grande (16 fl oz)	410	15	9.0	230	64	0	63	4	n/a	n/a	n/a	n/a
Caramel	grande (16 fl oz)	380	16	10.0	230	55	0	54	4	n/a	n/a	n/a	n/a
crème	grande (16 fl oz)	420	22	14.0	280	50	0	46	5	n/a	n/a	n/a	n/a
ribbon crunch	grande (16 fl oz)	470	22	14.0	280	65	0	60	5	n/a	n/a	n/a	n/a
Chai crème	grande (16 fl oz)	340	16	10.0	230	46	0	45	5	n/a	n/a	n/a	n/a
Chocolate cookie crumble crème	grande (16 fl oz)	460	25	16.0	290	52	2	46	7	n/a	n/a	n/a	n/a
Chocolate java mint	grande (16 fl oz)	490	20	13.0	300	73	2	69	6	n/a	n/a	n/a	n/a
Chocolate mint crème	grande (16 fl oz)	450	21	14.0	310	60	2	57	7	n/a	n/a	n/a	n/a
Coffee	grande (16 fl oz)	230	3	2.0	230	46	0	45	3	n/a	n/a	n/a	n/a

Starbucks	Amount	Calories	Fat (g)	Saturated Fat (g)	Sodium (mg)	Carbohydrate (g)	Fiber (g)	Sugar (g)	Protein (g)	Vitamin D (mcg)	Calcium (mg)	Iron (mg)	Potassium (mg)
Double chocolaty chip crème	grande (16 fl oz)	410	20	13.0	270	51	2	47	7	n/a	n/a	n/a	n/a
Espresso	grande (16 fl oz)	210	3	1.5	210	43	0	42	3	n/a	n/a	n/a	n/a
Java chip	grande (16 fl oz)	440	19	12.0	260	64	2	59	6	n/a	n/a	n/a	n/a
Matcha crème	grande (16 fl oz)	420	16	10.0	240	62	1	61	6	n/a	n/a	n/a	n/a
Mocha	grande (16 fl oz)	370	15	10.0	220	54	1	51	5	n/a	n/a	n/a	n/a
cookie crumble	grande (16 fl oz)	480	24	15.0	270	62	2	55	6	n/a	n/a	n/a	n/a
Strawberry crème	grande (16 fl oz)	370	16	10.0	240	51	0	51	5	n/a	n/a	n/a	n/a
Vanilla bean crème	grande (16 fl oz)	380	16	10.0	250	53	0	52	5	n/a	n/a	n/a	n/a
White chocolate crème	grande (16 fl oz)	380	18	12.0	280	49	0	49	6	n/a	n/a	n/a	n/a
White chocolate mocha	grande (16 fl oz)	420	17	11.0	260	61	0	61	5	n/a	n/a	n/a	n/a
Hot Coffee													
Caffè americano	grande (16 fl oz)	15	0	0.0	10	2	0	0	1	n/a	n/a	n/a	n/a
Caffè misto	grande (16 fl oz)	110	4	2.0	100	10	0	10	7	n/a	n/a	n/a	n/a
Cappuccino	grande (16 fl oz)	140	5	3.0	120	14	0	12	9	n/a	n/a	n/a	n/a
Decaf Pike Place roast	grande (16 fl oz)	5	0	0.0	10	0	0	0	1	n/a	n/a	n/a	n/a
Espresso shot	1.5 fl oz	10	0	0.0	0	2	0	0	1	n/a	n/a	n/a	n/a
con panna	1.5 fl oz	35	3	1.5	0	2	0	0	1	n/a	n/a	n/a	n/a
Featured roasts	grande (16 fl oz)	5	0	0.0	10	0	0	0	1	n/a	n/a	n/a	n/a
Flat white	grande (16 fl oz)	220	11	7.0	150	18	0	17	12	n/a	n/a	n/a	n/a
honey almondmilk	grande (16 fl oz)	170	5	0.0	135	30	1	24	3	n/a	n/a	n/a	n/a
Green Apron Blend	grande (16 fl oz)	10	0	0.0	10	0	0	0	1	n/a	n/a	n/a	n/a
Lattes													
caffè	grande (16 fl oz)	190	7	4.5	170	19	0	18	13	n/a	n/a	n/a	n/a
cinnamon dolce	grande (16 fl oz)	340	14	9.0	160	43	0	40	12	n/a	n/a	n/a	n/a
Starbucks Blonde vanilla	grande (16 fl oz)	250	6	3.5	150	37	0	35	12	n/a	n/a	n/a	n/a
Macchiato													
caramel	grande (16 fl oz)	250	7	4.5	150	35	0	33	10	n/a	n/a	n/a	n/a
espresso	1.6 fl oz	15	0	0.0	0	2	0	0	1	n/a	n/a	n/a	n/a
Mocha													
caffè	grande (16 fl oz)	370	15	10.0	150	43	4	35	14	n/a	n/a	n/a	n/a
white chocolate	grande (16 fl oz)	430	18	12.0	240	54	0	53	15	n/a	n/a	n/a	n/a
Hot Drinks													
Hot chocolate	grande (16 fl oz)	370	16	10.0	160	43	4	37	14	n/a	n/a	n/a	n/a
white	grande (16 fl oz)	440	19	13.0	260	55	0	55	15	n/a	n/a	n/a	n/a
Juice													
caramel apple spice	grande (16 fl oz)	380	8	5.0	35	77	0	70	1	n/a	n/a	n/a	n/a
steamed apple	grande (16 fl oz)	220	0	0.0	20	55	0	50	0	n/a	n/a	n/a	n/a
Steamed milk	grande (16 fl oz)	200	8	4.0	190	19	0	19	13	n/a	n/a	n/a	n/a
Vanilla crème	grande (16 fl oz)	350	14	9.0	180	44	0	43	13	n/a	n/a	n/a	n/a

RESTAURANT & FAST FOOD CHAINS

	Amount	Calories	Fat (g)	Saturated Fat (g)	Sodium (mg)	Carbohydrate (g)	Fiber (g)	Sugar (g)	Protein (g)	Vitamin D (mcg)	Calcium (mg)	Iron (mg)	Potassium (mg)
Hot Tea													
All tea	grande (16 fl oz)	0	0	0.0	0	0	0	0	0	n/a	n/a	n/a	n/a
Lattes													
chai	grande (16 fl oz)	240	5	2.0	115	45	0	42	8	n/a	n/a	n/a	n/a
Teavana London fog	grande (16 fl oz)	180	4	2.5	105	29	0	29	7	n/a	n/a	n/a	n/a
matcha	grande (16 fl oz)	240	7	4.5	160	34	1	32	12	n/a	n/a	n/a	n/a
royal English breakfast	grande (16 fl oz)	150	4	2.5	105	21	0	21	7	n/a	n/a	n/a	n/a
Iced Tea													
Black	grande (16 fl oz)	0	0	0.0	10	0	0	0	0	n/a	n/a	n/a	n/a
lemonade	grande (16 fl oz)	50	0	0.0	10	12	0	11	0	n/a	n/a	n/a	n/a
Green	grande (16 fl oz)	0	0	0.0	10	0	0	0	0	n/a	n/a	n/a	n/a
lemonade	grande (16 fl oz)	50	0	0.0	10	12	0	11	0	n/a	n/a	n/a	n/a
Lattes													
chai	grande (16 fl oz)	240	4	2.0	110	44	0	42	7	n/a	n/a	n/a	n/a
London fog	grande (16 fl oz)	140	3	1.5	70	25	0	25	4	n/a	n/a	n/a	n/a
matcha	grande (16 fl oz)	200	5	3.0	120	29	1	28	9	n/a	n/a	n/a	n/a
royal English breakfast	grande (16 fl oz)	140	3	1.5	70	25	0	25	4	n/a	n/a	n/a	n/a
Matcha lemonade	grande (16 fl oz)	120	0	0.0	10	29	1	27	1	n/a	n/a	n/a	n/a
Passion Tango	grande (16 fl oz)	0	0	0.0	10	0	0	0	0	n/a	n/a	n/a	n/a
lemonade	grande (16 fl oz)	50	0	0.0	10	12	0	11	0	n/a	n/a	n/a	n/a
Peach green	grande (16 fl oz)	60	0	0.0	20	15	0	12	0	n/a	n/a	n/a	n/a
lemonade	grande (16 fl oz)	80	0	0.0	20	21	0	18	0	n/a	n/a	n/a	n/a
Teavana mango black	14.5 fl oz	100	0	0.0	10	24	0	22	0	n/a	n/a	n/a	n/a
Breakfast													
Avocado spread	1 order	90	8	1.0	210	5	4	0	1	n/a	n/a	n/a	n/a
Berry trio parfait	1	240	3	0.0	125	39	2	25	14	n/a	n/a	n/a	n/a
Rolled & steel-cut oatmeal	1 order	410	12	1.5	140	67	7	34	8	n/a	n/a	n/a	n/a
Sandwiches													
bacon, Gouda & egg	1	360	18	7.0	720	35	1	2	19	n/a	n/a	n/a	n/a
double-smoked bacon, cheddar & egg	1	500	27	13.0	960	43	2	8	21	n/a	n/a	n/a	n/a
Impossible breakfast	1	420	22	8.0	800	36	2	4	21	n/a	n/a	n/a	n/a
sausage, cheddar & egg	1	480	29	10.0	890	34	1	2	18	n/a	n/a	n/a	n/a
turkey bacon, cheddar & egg white	1	230	5	2.5	560	28	3	2	17	n/a	n/a	n/a	n/a
Sous vide egg bites													
bacon & Gruyère	2	300	20	12.0	680	9	0	2	19	n/a	n/a	n/a	n/a
egg white & roasted red pepper	2	170	8	5.0	470	11	0	3	12	n/a	n/a	n/a	n/a
kale & mushroom	2	230	14	9.0	340	11	2	1	15	n/a	n/a	n/a	n/a
Strawberry overnight grains	1 order	300	16	11.0	15	35	4	20	5	n/a	n/a	n/a	n/a
Wraps													
bacon, sausage & egg	1	640	33	13.0	1090	58	3	2	28	n/a	n/a	n/a	n/a
spinach, feta & egg white	1	290	8	3.5	840	34	3	5	20	n/a	n/a	n/a	n/a

Starbucks

	Amount	Calories	Fat (g)	Saturated Fat (g)	Sodium (mg)	Carbohydrate (g)	Fiber (g)	Sugar (g)	Protein (g)	Vitamin D (mcg)	Calcium (mg)	Iron (mg)	Potassium (mg)
Baked Goods													
Bagels													
everything	1	290	3	0.5	530	57	3	5	10	n/a	n/a	n/a	n/a
plain	1	290	1	0.0	570	60	2	6	10	n/a	n/a	n/a	n/a
Blueberry muffin	1	330	14	2.5	250	47	1	29	5	n/a	n/a	n/a	n/a
Cake pops													
birthday	1	160	8	4.5	95	21	0	16	2	n/a	n/a	n/a	n/a
chocolate	1	150	8	5.0	60	21	1	16	2	n/a	n/a	n/a	n/a
cookies & cream	1	140	7	4.0	70	20	0	15	1	n/a	n/a	n/a	n/a
Cheese danish	1	290	14	9.0	400	33	1	11	7	n/a	n/a	n/a	n/a
Chocolate chip cookie	1	370	19	11.0	230	47	2	31	5	n/a	n/a	n/a	n/a
Cinnamon coffee cake	1	380	15	8.0	270	57	1	35	4	n/a	n/a	n/a	n/a
Croissants													
butter	1	250	14	8.0	300	26	1	4	5	n/a	n/a	n/a	n/a
chocolate	1	300	18	10.0	300	34	2	11	5	n/a	n/a	n/a	n/a
ham & Swiss	1	320	17	9.0	490	28	1	5	14	n/a	n/a	n/a	n/a
Double chocolate brownie	1	480	28	9.0	220	55	3	37	6	n/a	n/a	n/a	n/a
Glazed doughnut	1	440	19	9.0	430	60	2	34	5	n/a	n/a	n/a	n/a
Loaves													
banana walnut & pecan	1	410	20	3.0	320	50	2	28	6	n/a	n/a	n/a	n/a
iced lemon	1	450	19	9.0	300	64	1	39	6	n/a	n/a	n/a	n/a
pumpkin & pepita	1	390	14	2.5	470	59	2	38	6	n/a	n/a	n/a	n/a
Marshmallow dream bar	1	230	5	3.5	220	44	0	24	1	n/a	n/a	n/a	n/a
Scones													
blueberry	1	410	18	11.0	380	56	2	22	7	n/a	n/a	n/a	n/a
petite vanilla bean	1	130	6	3.0	110	19	0	9	2	n/a	n/a	n/a	n/a
Lunches													
Crispy grilled cheese on sourdough	1	520	27	16.0	1040	47	4	1	21	n/a	n/a	n/a	n/a
Paninis													
ham & Swiss on baguette	1	500	24	10.0	1250	43	2	1	25	n/a	n/a	n/a	n/a
tomato & mozzarella on foccacia	1	360	12	4.5	590	47	1	2	15	n/a	n/a	n/a	n/a
turkey, provolone & pesto on ciabatta	1	520	19	6.0	1190	53	3	3	32	n/a	n/a	n/a	n/a
Protein Boxes													
Cheese & fruit	1	470	28	16.0	770	37	3	17	20	n/a	n/a	n/a	n/a
Eggs & cheddar	1	460	24	7.0	450	40	5	21	22	n/a	n/a	n/a	n/a
PB&J	1	520	28	8.0	650	51	6	30	20	n/a	n/a	n/a	n/a
Snacks & Sweets													
Butter popcorn	1 pkg	150	7	1.0	240	18	3	1	2	n/a	n/a	n/a	n/a
Chocolate covered espresso beans	1 pkg	260	15	8.0	10	29	3	22	3	n/a	n/a	n/a	n/a

RESTAURANT & FAST FOOD CHAINS

	Amount	Calories	Fat (g)	Saturated Fat (g)	Sodium (mg)	Carbohydrate (g)	Fiber (g)	Sugar (g)	Protein (g)	Vitamin D (mcg)	Calcium (mg)	Iron (mg)	Potassium (mg)
Starbucks													
Madeleines	3	220	11	7.0	105	26	0	17	3	n/a	n/a	n/a	n/a
Potato chips													
perfectly salted	1 pkg	280	14	1.5	240	34	2	0	5	n/a	n/a	n/a	n/a
salt & vinegar kettle	1 pkg	270	13	1.5	640	34	2	0	5	n/a	n/a	n/a	n/a
Salted almond chocolate bites	1 pkg	300	22	7.0	200	24	4	19	7	n/a	n/a	n/a	n/a
String cheese	1	80	6	3.5	200	1	0	0	7	n/a	n/a	n/a	n/a
Vanilla biscotti w/ almonds	1	200	9	2.5	135	25	2	10	5	n/a	n/a	n/a	n/a
Subway													
Breakfast													
Black forest ham, egg & cheese													
artisan flatbread	6 in	480	23	6.0	1040	44	2	3	23	n/a	104	4	n/a
artisan Italian	6 in	450	21	6.0	1050	41	2	5	24	n/a	104	4	n/a
plain wrap	6 in	770	42	10.0	1720	57	2	4	40	n/a	195	5	n/a
Black forest ham, egg white & cheese													
artisan flatbread	6 in	390	12	4.0	1110	45	2	4	23	n/a	78	3	n/a
artisan Italian	6 in	360	10	4.0	1120	41	2	5	23	n/a	78	2	n/a
plain wrap	6 in	580	21	5.0	1860	59	2	5	39	n/a	130	4	n/a
Egg & cheese													
artisan flatbread	6 in	450	22	6.0	790	43	2	3	19	n/a	104	4	n/a
artisan Italian	6 in	420	20	6.0	800	40	2	4	19	n/a	104	3	n/a
plain wrap	6 in	700	40	10.0	1230	55	2	3	30	n/a	195	5	n/a
Egg white & cheese													
artisan flatbread	6 in	350	11	4.0	870	44	2	3	18	n/a	78	3	n/a
artisan Italian	6 in	330	9	4.0	870	40	2	4	19	n/a	78	2	n/a
plain wrap	6 in	510	19	4.0	1370	56	2	3	29	n/a	130	3	n/a
Bacon, egg & cheese													
artisan flatbread	6 in	530	28	8.0	970	44	2	3	24	n/a	104	4	n/a
artisan Italian	6 in	500	26	8.0	970	40	2	5	24	n/a	104	4	n/a
plain wrap	6 in	860	53	14.0	1570	56	2	4	40	n/a	195	5	n/a
Bacon, egg white & cheese													
artisan flatbread	6 in	430	17	6.0	1040	44	2	4	23	n/a	78	3	n/a
artisan Italian	6 in	410	16	6.0	1040	41	2	5	24	n/a	78	2	n/a
plain wrap	6 in	670	32	9.0	1720	57	2	5	39	n/a	195	4	n/a
Steak, egg & cheese													
artisan flatbread	6 in	520	25	7.0	1070	44	2	3	29	n/a	104	5	n/a
artisan Italian	6 in	490	23	7.0	1070	41	2	4	29	n/a	104	4	n/a
plain wrap	6 in	820	45	12.0	1680	56	2	4	47	n/a	195	6	n/a
Steak, egg white & cheese													
artisan flatbread	6 in	420	14	5.0	1140	45	2	3	28	n/a	78	4	n/a
artisan Italian	6 in	400	12	5.0	1140	41	2	5	29	n/a	78	3	n/a
plain wrap	6 in	630	24	6.0	1830	58	2	4	46	n/a	130	5	n/a

	Amount	Calories	Fat (g)	Saturated Fat (g)	Sodium (mg)	Carbohydrate (g)	Fiber (g)	Sugar (g)	Protein (g)	Vitamin D (mcg)	Calcium (mg)	Iron (mg)	Potassium (mg)
Build Your Own Sandwiches													
Black Forest ham	6 in	280	4	1.0	860	42	5	7	20	n/a	26	3	n/a
wrap	1	440	11	2.0	1570	58	3	6	28	n/a	104	5	n/a
Buffalo chicken	6 in	380	12	3.0	1380	42	3	6	25	n/a	26	3	n/a
wrap	1	560	19	4.0	1800	56	3	5	42	n/a	104	5	n/a
Cold Cut Combo	6 in	320	10	3.0	1000	41	3	6	17	n/a	78	3	n/a
wrap	1	530	23	5.0	1820	55	3	5	27	n/a	195	5	n/a
Grilled chicken	6 in	290	4	1.0	580	40	5	6	27	n/a	52	3	n/a
wrap	1	470	11	2.0	1010	54	3	5	42	n/a	104	5	n/a
Italian B.M.T.	6 in	400	16	6.0	1180	43	3	6	19	n/a	52	3	n/a
wrap	1	680	36	11.0	2180	58	3	5	32	n/a	130	5	n/a
Meatball marinara	6 in	440	18	7.0	1100	50	4	8	20	n/a	78	4	n/a
wrap	1	780	38	14.0	2010	76	7	11	34	n/a	195	6	n/a
Oven roasted turkey	6 in	270	4	1.0	840	40	5	6	22	n/a	26	5	n/a
wrap	1	430	10	2.0	1540	54	3	4	32	n/a	104	6	n/a
Roast beef	6 in	310	5	2.0	790	42	5	8	25	n/a	52	5	n/a
wrap	1	500	14	3.0	1440	58	3	7	38	n/a	104	6	n/a
Rotisserie-style chicken	6 in	310	6	2.0	760	40	5	6	25	n/a	52	3	n/a
wrap	1	500	15	3.0	1380	54	4	4	38	n/a	104	5	n/a
Spicy Italian	6 in	470	24	9.0	1300	42	3	5	19	n/a	52	3	n/a
wrap	1	820	52	17.0	2430	58	3	4	31	n/a	130	5	n/a
Steak	6 in	360	10	5.0	1040	40	2	5	26	n/a	78	3	n/a
wrap	1	570	20	7.0	1700	55	3	4	43	n/a	130	5	n/a
Sweet onion chicken teriyaki	6 in	350	4	1.0	850	55	5	19	26	n/a	52	4	n/a
wrap	1	590	11	2.0	1540	83	4	31	41	n/a	130	5	n/a
Tuna	6 in	470	25	5.0	690	40	2	5	20	n/a	26	3	n/a
wrap	1	820	54	8.0	1210	53	3	4	33	n/a	104	4	n/a
Veggie Delite	6 in	210	3	0.0	370	39	5	6	10	n/a	26	3	n/a
wrap	1	330	8	1.0	600	57	4	6	10	n/a	130	4	n/a
Subway Series Sandwiches													
Steak													
#1 The Philly	6 in	500	25	9.0	1310	41	2	5	28	n/a	130	3	n/a
#2 The Outlaw	6 in	490	22	9.0	1230	40	2	5	30	n/a	260	3	n/a
#3 The Monster	6 in	580	30	11.0	1270	42	2	6	36	n/a	52	4	n/a
#33 Teriyaki Blitz	6 in	450	14	7.0	1480	53	4	18	30	n/a	130	4	n/a
Italiano													
#4 Supreme Meats	6 in	590	32	12.0	1810	44	3	7	30	n/a	260	4	n/a
#6 The Boss	6 in	650	34	16.0	1690	54	4	8	32	n/a	260	5	n/a
#18 Ultimate B.M.T.	6 in	560	30	11.0	1570	43	3	6	27	n/a	260	3	n/a
#23 Hotshot Italiano	6 in	620	38	14.0	1750	43	3	6	26	n/a	260	4	n/a

RESTAURANT & FAST FOOD CHAINS

Subway

	Amount	Calories	Fat (g)	Saturated Fat (g)	Sodium (mg)	Carbohydrate (g)	Fiber (g)	Sugar (g)	Protein (g)	Vitamin D (mcg)	Calcium (mg)	Iron (mg)	Potassium (mg)
Chicken													
#7 The MexiCali													
w/ smashed avocado	6 in	540	27	9.0	1300	43	5	6	29	n/a	260	3	n/a
w/ sliced avocado	6 in	520	25	9.0	1180	43	5	6	29	n/a	260	3	n/a
#8 The Great Garlic	6 in	570	29	10.0	1260	43	3	6	34	n/a	52	3	n/a
#16 All-Pro Sweet Onion Teriyaki	6 in	430	11	5.0	1260	55	4	20	30	n/a	130	3	n/a
#20 Elite Chicken & Bacon Ranch	6 in	570	29	10.0	1210	43	3	6	34	n/a	52	3	n/a
Club													
#10 All-American Club	6 in	530	28	10.0	1520	43	2	7	27	n/a	130	4	n/a
#11 Subway Club	6 in	500	24	8.0	1550	43	4	8	32	n/a	130	5	n/a
#12 Turkey Cali Club													
w/ smashed avocado	6 in	600	34	10.0	1310	43	6	7	33	n/a	130	5	n/a
w/ sliced avocado	6 in	580	32	10.0	1100	43	6	7	33	n/a	106	5	n/a
#19 Pickleball Club	6 in	500	22	9.0	1700	47	2	10	27	n/a	130	3	n/a
Individual Components													
Bread													
artisan flatbread	6 in	220	4	1.0	360	40	1	2	7	n/a	0	3	n/a
artisan Italian	6 in	200	2	1.0	370	37	1	3	7	n/a	0	2	n/a
mini	1	130	1	0.0	250	24	0	2	5	n/a	0	6	n/a
hearty multigrain	6 in	200	2	0.0	300	36	3	4	9	n/a	26	2	n/a
mini	1	130	2	0.0	240	24	2	3	6	n/a	0	8	n/a
Italian herbs & cheese	6 in	240	5	2.0	560	40	2	3	9	n/a	26	2	n/a
wrap	6 in	300	8	1.0	580	50	2	2	8	n/a	78	3	n/a
Cheese													
American	1 order	40	4	2.0	210	1	0	0	2	n/a	52	0	n/a
BelGioioso fresh mozzarella	1 order	40	3	2.0	55	0	0	0	3	n/a	65	0	n/a
Monterey cheddar	1 order	50	5	3.0	85	1	0	0	3	n/a	78	0	n/a
parmesan	1 order	5	0	0.0	25	0	0	0	1	n/a	26	0	n/a
pepper Jack	1 order	50	4	3.0	140	0	0	0	3	n/a	130	0	n/a
provolone	1 order	50	4	2.0	125	0	0	0	4	n/a	104	0	n/a
Protein													
bacon	1 pcs	80	6	3.0	170	1	0	1	5	n/a	0	0	n/a
Black Forest ham	1 order	70	2	1.0	490	2	0	1	10	n/a	0	0	n/a
capicola	6 pcs	70	4	2.0	480	2	0	2	8	n/a	0	0	n/a
Cold Cut Combo meats	1 order	110	8	3.0	620	1	0	1	9	n/a	52	1	n/a
egg patty	1	180	15	4.0	220	2	0	0	10	n/a	26	1	n/a
white	1	90	4	1.0	290	3	0	1	9	n/a	0	0	n/a
grilled chicken	1 order	80	2	2.0	210	1	0	1	16	n/a	0	0	n/a
Buffalo	1 order	90	2	1.0	900	2	0	0	17	n/a	0	1	n/a
sweet onion teriyaki glazed	1 order	110	2	1.0	350	9	0	8	16	n/a	0	0	n/a
Italian B.M.T. meats	1 order	180	14	5.0	800	3	0	1	11	n/a	26	1	n/a
meatballs	1 order	240	15	6.0	700	13	3	5	13	n/a	52	2	n/a
oven roasted turkey	1 order	60	1	1.0	480	0	0	0	11	n/a	0	2	n/a
pepperoni	3 pcs	80	7	3.0	290	1	0	0	3	n/a	0	0	n/a

RESTAURANT & FAST FOOD CHAINS

Subway	Amount	Calories	Fat (g)	Saturated Fat (g)	Sodium (mg)	Carbohydrate (g)	Fiber (g)	Sugar (g)	Protein (g)	Vitamin D (mcg)	Calcium (mg)	Iron (mg)	Potassium (mg)
roast beef	1 order	90	3	1.0	420	2	0	2	14	n/a	0	0	n/a
rotisserie-style chicken	1 order	90	4	1.0	400	0	0	0	15	n/a	0	0	n/a
spicy Italian meats	1 order	250	22	8.0	920	2	0	0	11	n/a	26	1	n/a
steak	1 order	110	5	2.0	450	2	0	1	17	n/a	0	1	n/a
Subway Club meats	1 order	110	3	1.0	700	3	0	2	18	n/a	0	2	n/a
tuna	1 order	250	23	2.0	310	0	0	0	12	n/a	0	0	n/a
Vegetables													
banana peppers	3 pcs	0	0	0.0	65	0	0	0	0	n/a	0	0	n/a
black olives	3 pcs	0	0	0.0	25	0	0	0	0	n/a	0	0	n/a
cucumbers	3 pcs	0	0	0.0	0	1	0	0	0	n/a	0	0	n/a
green peppers	3 pcs	0	0	0.0	0	0	0	0	0	n/a	0	0	n/a
jalapeños	3 pcs	0	0	0.0	70	0	0	0	0	n/a	0	0	n/a
lettuce	1 order	0	0	0.0	0	0	0	0	0	n/a	0	0	n/a
onions	1 order	0	0	0.0	0	1	0	0	0	n/a	0	0	n/a
pickles	3 pcs	0	0	0.0	160	0	0	0	0	n/a	0	0	n/a
spinach	1 order	0	0	0.0	5	0	0	0	0	n/a	0	0	n/a
tomatoes	3 pcs	5	0	0.0	0	1	0	1	0	n/a	0	0	n/a
Sauces													
Baja chipotle	1 order	70	7	1.0	125	1	0	1	0	n/a	0	0	n/a
Frank's red hot Buffalo sauce	1 order	5	0	0.0	350	1	0	0	0	n/a	0	0	n/a
honey mustard	1 order	60	5	1.0	125	3	0	3	0	n/a	0	0	n/a
mayonnaise	1 order	100	11	2.0	65	0	0	0	0	n/a	0	0	n/a
MVP Parmesan Vinaigrette	1 order	60	6	1.0	150	1	0	1	0	n/a	0	0	n/a
oil	1 order	45	5	0.0	0	0	0	0	0	n/a	0	0	n/a
& vinegar	1 order	45	5	0.0	0	0	0	0	0	n/a	0	0	n/a
peppercorn ranch	1 order	80	8	2.0	100	1	0	1	0	n/a	0	0	n/a
red wine vinegar	1 order	0	0	0.0	0	0	0	0	0	n/a	0	0	n/a
roasted garlic aioli	1 order	80	9	2.0	150	1	0	1	0	n/a	0	0	n/a
sweet onion teriyaki sauce	1 order	30	0	0.0	130	7	0	6	0	n/a	0	0	n/a
yellow mustard	1 order	10	1	0.0	170	1	0	0	0	n/a	0	0	n/a
Protein Bowls													
Black Forest ham	1	170	5	2.0	1050	12	3	6	21	n/a	52	2	n/a
Buffalo chicken	1	380	21	4.0	2080	13	4	7	36	n/a	78	3	n/a
Cold Cut Combo	1	260	16	4.0	1310	9	3	5	20	n/a	130	3	n/a
Grilled chicken	1	200	4	2.0	480	9	3	5	35	n/a	52	2	n/a
Italian B.M.T.	1	410	29	11.0	1670	13	3	5	25	n/a	78	3	n/a
Meatball marinara	1	530	32	13.0	1530	33	8	13	28	n/a	195	5	n/a
Oven roasted turkey	1	150	3	1.0	1020	8	3	5	25	n/a	52	5	n/a
Roast beef	1	230	7	2.0	920	12	3	7	30	n/a	52	5	n/a
Rotisserie-style chicken	1	220	8	3.0	810	8	3	4	31	n/a	52	2	n/a
Spicy Italian	1	550	45	17.0	1910	12	3	4	24	n/a	104	3	n/a
Steak	1	380	19	9.0	1150	12	4	5	42	n/a	260	4	n/a
Sweet onion chicken teriyaki	1	350	5	2.0	1170	46	3	38	34	n/a	78	3	n/a
Tuna	1	550	47	8.0	690	8	3	4	26	n/a	52	2	n/a

RESTAURANT & FAST FOOD CHAINS

Subway

	Amount	Calories	Fat (g)	Saturated Fat (g)	Sodium (mg)	Carbohydrate (g)	Fiber (g)	Sugar (g)	Protein (g)	Vitamin D (mcg)	Calcium (mg)	Iron (mg)	Potassium (mg)
Salads													
Black Forest ham	1	120	3	1.0	570	12	4	6	13	n/a	52	2	n/a
Buffalo chicken	1	300	19	4.0	1180	13	5	7	20	n/a	78	3	n/a
Cold cut combo	1	160	9	2.0	700	10	4	5	12	n/a	104	3	n/a
Grilled chicken	1	130	3	1.0	280	10	4	5	19	n/a	78	2	n/a
Italian B.M.T.	1	240	15	5.0	880	12	4	5	14	n/a	78	3	n/a
Meatball marinara	1	290	16	6.0	780	22	7	9	16	n/a	130	4	n/a
Oven roasted turkey	1	110	2	0.0	550	10	4	5	14	n/a	52	4	n/a
Roast beef	1	150	4	1.0	500	12	4	6	17	n/a	78	4	n/a
Rotisserie-style chicken	1	150	5	2.0	470	10	4	5	18	n/a	78	2	n/a
Spicy Italian	1	310	23	9.0	1000	12	4	5	14	n/a	78	3	n/a
Steak	1	210	9	4.0	740	12	4	6	22	n/a	130	3	n/a
Sweet onion chicken teriyaki	1	250	4	1.0	830	39	4	31	19	n/a	78	3	n/a
Tuna	1	310	24	4.0	390	10	4	5	15	n/a	52	2	n/a
Veggie delite	1	50	1	0.0	75	8	4	5	3	n/a	52	1	n/a
Cookies													
Chocolate chip	1	210	10	5.0	120	30	0	18	2	n/a	0	2	n/a
Double chocolate	1	210	9	5.0	125	29	1	20	2	n/a	26	2	n/a
Oatmeal raisin	1	200	8	4.0	110	30	1	16	3	n/a	26	1	n/a
Raspberry cheesecake	1	210	9	5.0	115	29	0	16	2	n/a	26	1	n/a
White chip macadamia nut	1	210	10	5.0	125	28	0	17	2	n/a	26	1	n/a
Taco Bell													
Breakfast													
Crunchwrap													
bacon	1	670	40	13.0	1300	52	4	3	21	0	350	3	390
California		630	37	12.0	1340	53	5	3	21	19	350	3	500
sausage	1	750	49	16.0	1220	53	4	3	21	0	360	3	400
steak	1	660	38	12.0	1360	53	4	3	24	0	370	4	430
Hash brown	1	160	11	1.0	280	14	1	0	1	0	10	0	190
Quesadilla													
bacon	1	510	27	14.0	1250	41	3	3	25	0	510	3	230
sausage	1	510	29	15.0	1130	40	3	3	23	0	510	3	200
steak	1	510	25	14.0	1310	41	3	4	28	0	520	4	270
Salsa	1 pkt	0	0	0.0	50	0	0	0	0	0	0	0	40
Toasted burrito													
cheesy													
bacon	1	350	16	5.0	880	38	2	3	13	0	150	3	270
fiesta potato	1	340	14	3.5	770	44	3	3	9	0	150	3	350
sausage	1	350	17	6.0	770	38	2	3	10	0	150	3	240

Taco Bell	Amount	Calories	Fat (g)	Saturated Fat (g)	Sodium (mg)	Carbohydrate (g)	Fiber (g)	Sugar (g)	Protein (g)	Vitamin D (mcg)	Calcium (mg)	Iron (mg)	Potassium (mg)
grande													
bacon	1	570	30	11.0	1310	52	4	3	23	0	340	4	470
sausage	1	570	31	12.0	1190	51	4	3	21	0	340	4	450
steak	1	570	28	10.0	1370	52	4	4	27	0	360	4	520
hash brown													
bacon	1	580	32	10.0	1290	52	3	3	20	0	330	3	380
sausage	1	570	33	11.0	1170	52	3	3	18	0	330	3	350
steak	1	570	30	10.0	1350	53	3	3	24	0	350	4	420
Burritos													
Bean	1	350	9	4.0	1040	55	10	3	13	0	210	4	400
Beef	1	430	19	6.0	1000	49	4	3	12	0	150	3	300
Beefy 5-layer	1	490	18	7.0	1260	65	8	5	18	0	270	5	460
Beefy melt	1	620	29	11.0	1190	70	6	4	20	0	360	4	410
Black Bean Crunchwrap Supreme	1	520	18	5.0	1100	77	8	6	13	0	260	5	610
Burrito Supreme													
beef	1	390	14	6.0	1140	51	8	4	16	0	220	4	420
chicken	1	370	11	5.0	1150	49	7	4	19	0	220	4	480
steak	1	380	12	6.0	1160	50	7	5	19	0	230	4	440
Cheesy bean & rice	1	420	16	4.0	920	55	7	3	9	0	160	3	360
Cheesy roll up	1	180	9	6.0	430	17	1	1	8	0	230	1	60
Chicken chipotle melt	1	190	9	3.0	530	16	1	0	12	0	100	1	170
Chipotle ranch grilled chicken	1	510	29	7.0	950	47	4	3	17	0	200	3	350
Fiesta veggie	1	570	28	8.0	1020	65	9	4	14	19	270	4	470
Mexican Pizza													
Regular	1	530	29	9.0	980	49	8	4	19	0	320	3	440
Veggie	1	470	25	7.0	730	46	7	3	14	0	310	3	360
Nachos													
Chips & nacho cheese sauce	1 order	220	13	1.5	280	24	2	1	3	0	60	0	290
Nachos BellGrande													
beef	1 order	730	38	6.0	1130	81	15	4	17	0	200	3	970
chicken	1 order	710	35	5.0	1140	79	14	4	20	0	200	2	1020
steak	1 order	720	36	5.0	1150	80	14	5	20	0	210	3	980
Power Menu Bowls													
Chicken	1	460	21	6.0	1250	41	8	3	26	19	160	2	700
Steak	1	470	23	7.0	1280	42	8	4	25	19	180	3	630
Veggie	1	420	20	5.0	870	47	11	3	12	19	170	3	590

Taco Bell

	Amount	Calories	Fat (g)	Saturated Fat (g)	Sodium (mg)	Carbohydrate (g)	Fiber (g)	Sugar (g)	Protein (g)	Vitamin D (mcg)	Calcium (mg)	Iron (mg)	Potassium (mg)
Quesadillas													
Cheese	1	470	24	13.0	1000	41	3	3	18	0	500	3	160
Chicken	1	520	26	13.0	1260	41	3	3	26	0	500	3	290
Steak	1	520	27	14.0	1270	42	3	4	26	0	510	3	260
Tacos													
Chalupas													
Supreme													
black bean	1	340	18	4.0	460	36	6	4	10	0	140	3	300
beef	1	360	20	6.0	570	31	4	4	12	0	120	2	230
chicken	1	340	17	4.0	580	29	3	4	16	0	120	2	280
steak	1	350	18	4.5	590	30	3	4	15	0	130	2	250
Cheesy gordita crunch	1	490	28	10.0	840	41	5	5	20	0	310	3	250
Crunchy taco	1	170	10	3.5	300	13	3	0	8	0	70	1	140
Supreme	1	190	11	4.5	320	15	3	2	8	0	80	1	200
Nacho Cheese Doritos Locos	1	170	10	4.0	360	12	3	0	8	0	80	1	150
Supreme	1	190	11	5.0	380	14	3	2	8	0	90	1	210
Soft													
beef	1	180	8	4.0	500	18	3	1	9	0	110	2	130
chicken	1	160	5	2.5	510	16	1	1	12	0	110	1	190
spicy potato	1	240	12	3.0	480	28	2	1	5	0	110	1	270
Supreme													
beef	1	210	10	5.0	510	20	3	2	10	0	130	2	200
chicken	1	190	7	3.5	520	18	2	2	13	0	120	1	250
Sides													
Black beans	1 order	50	2	0.0	140	7	4	0	3	0	20	1	150
w/ rice	1 order	100	5	0.0	370	25	5	0	4	0	20	1	190
Cheesy fiesta potatoes	1 order	240	13	2.0	520	28	3	1	3	0	40	0	560
Fries													
Nacho fries	1 order	320	18	1.5	800	35	4	0	5	0	30	1	700
Sauces													
Diablo	1 pkt	0	0	0.0	35	0	0	0	0	0	0	0	10
Fire	1 pkt	0	0	0.0	55	0	0	0	0	0	0	0	20
Hot	1 pkt	0	0	0.0	45	0	0	0	0	0	0	0	10
Mild	1 pkt	0	0	0.0	30	0	0	0	0	0	0	0	10
Desserts													
Cinnabon Delights	2 pcs	170	11	3.5	70	15	0	9	2	0	10	0	30
Cinnamon twists	1 order	170	6	0.5	115	27	0	10	1	0	10	0	20

RESTAURANT & FAST FOOD CHAINS

Taco Bell

	Amount	Calories	Fat (g)	Saturated Fat (g)	Sodium (mg)	Carbohydrate (g)	Fiber (g)	Sugar (g)	Protein (g)	Vitamin D (mcg)	Calcium (mg)	Iron (mg)	Potassium (mg)
Freezes													
Mountain Dew Baja Blast	16 oz	150	0	0.0	45	41	0	41	0	0	0	0	0
Watermelon Berry	16 oz	150	0	0.0	65	40	0	40	0	0	0	0	0
Lemonade	16 oz	170	0	0.0	70	45	0	43	0	0	0	0	0
Wild Cherry	16 oz	150	0	0.0	40	41	0	40	0	0	0	0	0

Tim Hortons

	Amount	Calories	Fat (g)	Saturated Fat (g)	Sodium (mg)	Carbohydrate (g)	Fiber (g)	Sugar (g)	Protein (g)	Vitamin D (mcg)	Calcium (mg)	Iron (mg)	Potassium (mg)
Breakfast													
Hash brown	1	130	7	0.5	280	16	1	0	1	n/a	20	0	n/a
Greek yogurt	1 order	250	5	0.0	110	29	3	21	14	n/a	150	6	n/a
Oatmeal													
maple	1 order	220	3	0.5	220	49	4	20	5	n/a	40	10	n/a
mixed berry	1 order	210	3	0.5	220	44	6	14	6	n/a	40	10	n/a
Bagels													
Four cheese	1	320	5	2.0	580	57	2	3	12	n/a	100	3	n/a
12 grain	1	350	9	1.0	450	55	6	8	11	n/a	80	3	n/a
Blueberry	1	300	3	0.0	450	59	3	8	11	n/a	40	3	n/a
Caramel apple	1	340	4	1.0	520	67	3	16	9	n/a	60	3	n/a
Cinnamon raisin	1	300	2	0.0	390	61	2	10	9	n/a	60	3	n/a
Everything	1	300	3	0.5	450	58	3	6	11	n/a	60	3	n/a
Jalapeño Asiago mozzarella	1	310	4	1.5	730	58	3	2	12	n/a	150	3	n/a
Maple cinnamon French toast	1	350	4	1.5	540	67	2	15	10	n/a	80	3	n/a
Plain	1	300	3	0.0	490	59	3	6	10	n/a	60	3	n/a
Pretzel-style	1	300	3	0.0	850	60	2	4	11	n/a	60	3	n/a
Sundried tomato Asiago parm	1	320	5	2.0	860	59	3	4	12	n/a	150	3	n/a
Toppings													
butter	1 order	100	11	7.0	95	0	0	0	0	n/a	0	0	n/a
Concord grape jelly	1 order	35	0	0.0	0	9	0	8	0	n/a	0	0	n/a
cream cheese													
garden vegetable	1 order	130	12	8.0	270	3	0	2	2	n/a	40	0	n/a
light	1 order	90	7	4.5	240	5	0	4	3	n/a	80	0	n/a
plain	1 order	130	12	8.0	210	3	0	2	2	n/a	40	0	n/a
strawberry	1 order	130	11	7.0	190	7	0	6	2	n/a	40	0	n/a
honey	1 order	45	0	0.0	100	11	0	11	0	n/a	0	0	n/a
margarine	1 order	60	7	2.0	115	0	0	0	0	n/a	0	0	n/a
peanut butter	1 order	120	11	2.0	100	5	2	2	5	n/a	0	0	n/a
strawberry jam	1 order	35	0	0.0	0	9	0	8	0	n/a	0	0	n/a
Baked Goods													
Cinnamon roll													
frosted	1	400	14	6.0	380	60	2	24	7	n/a	40	2	n/a
glazed	1	350	13	5.0	350	51	2	16	7	n/a	40	2	n/a
ultimate cinnamon bun	1	570	21	10.0	670	89	3	50	8	n/a	150	3	n/a

RESTAURANT & FAST FOOD CHAINS

Tim Hortons

	Amount	Calories	Fat (g)	Saturated Fat (g)	Sodium (mg)	Carbohydrate (g)	Fiber (g)	Sugar (g)	Protein (g)	Vitamin D (mcg)	Calcium (mg)	Iron (mg)	Potassium (mg)
Croissant	1	280	15	6.0	280	30	1	3	6	n/a	20	1	n/a
cheese	1	310	17	8.0	330	30	1	3	7	n/a	80	1	n/a
Danish													
cherry cheese	1	370	16	6.0	310	50	1	24	5	n/a	40	1	n/a
maple pecan	1	400	19	6.0	270	53	2	21	7	n/a	20	1	n/a
Nutella pastry pocket	1	150	9	4.0	105	16	1	8	2	n/a	20	0	n/a
Donuts													
Apple fritter	1	290	8	3.5	330	48	2	15	7	n/a	40	2	n/a
caramel	1	300	8	3.5	390	52	2	17	7	n/a	40	2	n/a
Cake													
blueberry	1	370	19	9.0	180	46	1	31	3	n/a	40	1	n/a
chocolate glazed	1	280	14	6.0	320	37	1	19	4	n/a	20	1	n/a
cinnamon sugar	1	220	10	5.0	270	28	1	10	3	n/a	40	1	n/a
double chocolate	1	270	15	6.0	330	32	2	13	4	n/a	20	1	n/a
old fashion	1	210	10	5.0	260	25	1	8	3	n/a	40	1	n/a
dip	1	250	11	5.0	270	33	1	15	4	n/a	40	1	n/a
glazed	1	270	10	5.0	270	41	1	23	3	n/a	40	1	n/a
peanut crunch	1	300	14	5.0	270	39	1	20	5	n/a	40	1	n/a
sour cream	1	270	16	8.0	210	27	1	11	3	n/a	40	1	n/a
cinnamon	1	270	16	8.0	210	29	1	12	3	n/a	40	1	n/a
glazed	1	310	16	8.0	220	46	1	29	3	n/a	40	1	n/a
strawberry double chocolate	1	200	15	6.0	330	33	2	14	4	n/a	20	2	n/a
Filled													
blueberry	1	200	5	2.0	230	34	1	12	4	n/a	20	1	n/a
bloom													
blueberry	1	240	9	4.5	180	37	1	15	3	n/a	20	1	n/a
strawberry	1	350	7	3.5	190	66	1	44	4	n/a	20	1	n/a
Boston cream	1	220	6	2.5	250	35	1	13	5	n/a	20	1	n/a
Canadian maple	1	210	6	2.5	250	35	1	14	5	n/a	20	1	n/a
chocolate caramel	1	280	9	4.0	330	47	1	23	5	n/a	20	1	n/a
Nutella	1	290	14	4.5	180	34	2	14	6	n/a	40	1	n/a
Oreo	1	420	18	7.0	270	60	1	33	5	n/a	20	1	n/a
strawberry	1	200	5	2.0	230	34	1	14	5	n/a	20	1	n/a
cream	1	290	10	4.0	230	45	1	25	4	n/a	20	1	n/a
double	1	230	5	2.5	230	40	1	20	5	n/a	20	2	n/a
Honey cruller	1	310	18	9.0	200	37	0	22	2	n/a	20	0	n/a
Yeast													
dip													
chocolate	1	190	7	2.5	210	29	1	8	5	n/a	20	1	n/a
honey	1	190	6	2.5	210	31	1	11	4	n/a	20	1	n/a
maple	1	190	6	2.5	210	29	1	9	4	n/a	20	1	n/a
strawberry	1	210	6	2.5	210	35	1	14	4	n/a	20	1	n/a
vanilla w/ colored sprinkles	1	270	9	3.5	220	45	1	22	4	n/a	20	1	n/a
sugar loop	1	180	6	2.5	210	28	1	8	4	n/a	20	1	n/a

	Amount	Calories	Fat (g)	Saturated Fat (g)	Sodium (mg)	Carbohydrate (g)	Fiber (g)	Sugar (g)	Protein (g)	Vitamin D (mcg)	Calcium (mg)	Iron (mg)	Potassium (mg)
Timbits													
Apple fritter	1	50	2	1.0	40	9	0	4	1	n/a	0	0	n/a
Cake													
birthday	1	80	3	1.5	60	12	0	8	1	n/a	0	0	n/a
blueberry	1	90	5	2.5	45	11	0	7	1	n/a	0	0	n/a
chocolate glazed	1	70	3	1.5	85	10	0	5	1	n/a	0	0	n/a
cinnamon French toast	1	70	4	1.5	65	8	0	3	1	n/a	20	0	n/a
cinnamon sugar	1	60	3	1.0	75	8	1	3	1	n/a	0	0	n/a
double chocolate	1	70	3	1.5	85	9	0	4	1	n/a	0	0	n/a
old fashion	1	50	3	1.0	75	7	0	2	1	n/a	0	0	n/a
glazed	1	70	3	1.0	75	10	0	5	1	n/a	0	0	n/a
salted caramel	1	70	3	1.5	120	11	0	6	1	n/a	0	0	n/a
sour cream glazed	1	90	5	2.0	55	12	0	7	1	n/a	0	0	n/a
Honey dip	1	45	1	0.5	30	8	0	4	1	n/a	0	0	n/a
Strawberry filled	1	50	1	0.5	35	8	0	4	1	n/a	0	0	n/a
Muffins													
Chocolate caramel	1	410	15	4.0	480	64	2	35	5	n/a	40	2	n/a
Chocolate chip	1	420	16	4.5	330	66	2	35	6	n/a	40	3	n/a
Cran apple walnut bran	1	350	14	2.0	370	54	8	20	5	n/a	40	2	n/a
Cranberry white chocolate	1	370	12	2.5	370	60	2	30	5	n/a	60	1	n/a
Fruit explosion	1	340	10	1.5	470	58	2	25	5	n/a	60	1	n/a
Lemon blueberry Greek yogurt	1	360	12	2.0	400	58	5	24	6	n/a	60	2	n/a
Whole grain													
carrot orange	1	350	11	1.5	360	59	6	26	5	n/a	60	2	n/a
pecan banana bread	1	350	11	1.5	400	60	5	27	6	n/a	40	2	n/a
Wild blueberry	1	340	11	2.0	430	57	2	25	5	n/a	20	1	n/a
Grilled Wraps													
Chicken fajita	1	430	19	8.0	1060	39	3	4	28	n/a	350	2	n/a
Farmer's breakfast	1	680	42	12.0	1150	54	3	3	21	n/a	250	3	n/a
Steak fajita	1	430	20	8.0	1140	40	3	4	26	n/a	350	3	n/a
Sandwiches													
Aged cheddar biscuit	1	540	37	19.0	1220	30	1	4	20	n/a	200	2	n/a
Angus steak & egg	1	400	20	12.0	1200	34	2	5	21	n/a	150	3	n/a
Bacon	1	420	23	13.0	1110	33	2	4	19	n/a	150	3	n/a
Bagel B.E.L.T.	1	560	24	8.0	1140	62	7	11	24	n/a	200	3	n/a
Croissant	1	600	42	18.0	1040	36	2	6	19	n/a	150	2	n/a
Sausage	1	530	34	17.0	1180	33	2	4	19	n/a	150	3	n/a
Steak & four cheese bagel	1	510	17	7.0	1360	62	2	5	27	n/a	250	4	n/a
Turkey sausage	1	350	16	6.0	960	31	1	3	20	n/a	200	2	n/a

RESTAURANT & FAST FOOD CHAINS

	Amount	Calories	Fat (g)	Saturated Fat (g)	Sodium (mg)	Carbohydrate (g)	Fiber (g)	Sugar (g)	Protein (g)	Vitamin D (mcg)	Calcium (mg)	Iron (mg)	Potassium (mg)
Soups & Sides													
Chili	1 order	330	18	7.0	960	18	5	5	23	n/a	100	2	n/a
Homestyle soft bun													
white	1	210	1	0.0	450	42	2	1	7	n/a	0	3	n/a
whole wheat	1	200	1	0.0	430	40	4	1	8	n/a	0	2	n/a
Kettle cooked potato chips	1 order	220	14	1.0	110	22	1	0	2	n/a	20	1	n/a
Mac & cheese	1 order	490	27	10.0	1120	48	1	7	16	n/a	300	1	n/a
Soups													
broccoli cheddar	1 order	180	9	4.0	680	16	2	6	8	n/a	200	0	n/a
chicken noodle	1 order	120	2	0.0	710	21	1	2	5	n/a	20	0	n/a
clam chowder	1 order	190	7	2.0	680	23	1	6	9	n/a	150	1	n/a
hearty vegetable	1 order	80	0	0.0	590	14	2	3	4	n/a	40	0	n/a
potato bacon cheddar	1 order	260	15	8.0	820	22	1	5	7	n/a	150	0	n/a
roasted red pepper & Gouda	1 order	220	14	6.0	680	17	3	11	6	n/a	100	0	n/a
turkey & wild rice	1 order	130	2	0.0	600	25	1	1	3	n/a	20	0	n/a
Drinks													
Apple cider	medium	260	0	0.0	10	66	0	66	0	n/a	0	0	n/a
caramel supreme	medium	350	5	5.0	30	75	0	45	0	n/a	20	0	n/a
Apple juice	10 oz	130	0	0.0	30	33	0	31	0	n/a	0	0	n/a
Brewed iced tea													
sweetened	medium	130	0	0.0	20	34	0	33	0	n/a	0	0	n/a
unsweetened	medium	0	0	0.0	20	0	0	0	0	n/a	0	0	n/a
Café mocha	medium	240	9	8.0	240	38	2	32	2	n/a	20	1	n/a
Cappuccino	medium	100	0	0.0	150	15	0	14	9	n/a	250	0	n/a
Coffee	medium	5	0	0.0	10	0	0	0	0	n/a	0	0	n/a
iced	medium	110	7	4.5	30	11	0	9	1	n/a	40	0	n/a
Espresso shot	1 shot	0	0	0.0	0	1	0	0	0	n/a	0	0	n/a
Frozen													
hot chocolate	medium	570	27	18.0	360	80	2	71	4	n/a	100	1	n/a
lemonade	medium	190	0	0.0	20	46	0	43	0	n/a	0	0	n/a
strawberry	medium	190	0	0.0	20	47	0	43	0	n/a	0	0	n/a
strawberries & cream	medium	530	27	18.0	130	70	0	62	4	n/a	150	0	n/a
sugar cookie & cream	medium	540	28	19.0	135	71	0	63	4	n/a	150	0	n/a
vanilla & cream	medium	530	27	18.0	135	70	0	64	4	n/a	150	0	n/a
Fruit smoothies													
pineapple orange	medium	260	0	0.0	75	56	0	55	8	n/a	80	0	n/a
strawberry banana	medium	230	0	0.0	65	52	1	47	8	n/a	100	0	n/a
Hot chocolate	medium	300	7	6.0	460	57	3	49	2	n/a	20	2	n/a
caramel	medium	400	13	11.0	430	68	3	57	3	n/a	20	3	n/a
Iced Capp	medium	430	22	14.0	55	55	0	50	4	n/a	100	0	n/a
caramel	medium	500	28	19.0	70	60	0	53	4	n/a	100	0	n/a
mocha	medium	550	28	19.0	80	72	1	62	4	n/a	100	1	n/a
Oreo	medium	560	30	19.0	115	69	0	59	4	n/a	150	1	n/a
Orange juice	10 oz	140	0	0.0	30	35	0	33	1	n/a	0	0	n/a

RESTAURANT & FAST FOOD CHAINS

Tim Hortons

	Amount	Calories	Fat (g)	Saturated Fat (g)	Sodium (mg)	Carbohydrate (g)	Fiber (g)	Sugar (g)	Protein (g)	Vitamin D (mcg)	Calcium (mg)	Iron (mg)	Potassium (mg)
Latte	medium	100	0	0.0	160	15	0	15	10	n/a	350	0	n/a
iced	medium	240	7	4.0	170	35	0	34	12	n/a	450	0	n/a
flavored supreme	medium	220	5	5.0	170	34	0	32	10	n/a	350	0	n/a
iced	medium	330	12	9.0	180	43	0	41	12	n/a	450	0	n/a
mocha	medium	230	7	6.0	200	32	0	30	9	n/a	300	0	n/a
flavored	medium	240	6	5.0	220	34	0	31	10	n/a	200	0	n/a
iced	medium	390	9	7.0	330	68	2	56	12	n/a	350	4	n/a
Tea, bagged & steeped	medium	0	0	0.0	10	0	0	0	0	n/a	0	0	n/a

Cookies

Chocolate chunk	1	210	9	5.0	240	32	1	17	2	n/a	20	1	n/a
Double chocolate w/ peanut butter filling	1	360	20	11.0	290	40	2	23	5	n/a	20	2	n/a
Lemon shortbread w/ raspberry filling	1	280	10	7.0	250	44	1	21	3	n/a	0	1	n/a
Nutella filled	1	360	18	7.0	190	44	1	25	4	n/a	40	1	n/a
Oatmeal raisin spice	1	210	8	4.5	190	32	1	19	3	n/a	20	0	n/a
Peanut butter	1	250	15	6.0	240	24	2	14	5	n/a	20	0	n/a
Red velvet w/ cream cheese filling	1	300	13	9.0	250	42	1	23	3	n/a	20	1	n/a
Smile	1	300	12	7.0	370	47	1	27	3	n/a	20	1	n/a
White chocolate macadamia nut	1	220	11	5.0	240	29	1	15	2	n/a	20	0	n/a

Uno Pizzeria & Grill

Appetizers

Bites													
Buffalo boneless	1 order	1450	97	21.0	4460	67	2	4	75	n/a	n/a	n/a	n/a
honey BBQ boneless	1 order	1490	94	19.0	3390	86	2	21	73	n/a	n/a	n/a	n/a
red chili glazed	1 order	1530	95	19.0	3800	98	2	31	73	n/a	n/a	n/a	n/a
Buffalo chicken quesadillas	1 order	860	30	15.0	2610	81	4	11	46	n/a	n/a	n/a	n/a
Cheesy garlic bread	1 order	1180	33	9.0	2330	126	6	10	52	n/a	n/a	n/a	n/a
Giant fried ravioli	1 order	680	37	16.0	1660	63	2	8	26	n/a	n/a	n/a	n/a
Mozzarella sticks	1 order	1090	57	23.0	3340	107	4	9	46	n/a	n/a	n/a	n/a
Muchos nachos	1 order	1700	61	14.0	3930	199	1	13	66	n/a	n/a	n/a	n/a
Pizza skins	1 order	1970	131	43.0	2800	146	7	8	53	n/a	n/a	n/a	n/a
Dips													
shrimp & crab	1 order	1160	84	40.0	2300	66	2	13	32	n/a	n/a	n/a	n/a
spinach artichoke deep	1 order	1710	114	28.0	3250	132	7	7	34	n/a	n/a	n/a	n/a
Wings													
Buffalo	1 order	1130	89	23.0	3890	6	2	4	71	n/a	n/a	n/a	n/a
honey BBQ	1 order	1170	86	21.0	2820	25	2	21	69	n/a	n/a	n/a	n/a

Burgers

Aged cheddar & mushroom burger	1	1120	81	31.0	1250	37	2	3	53	n/a	n/a	n/a	n/a
½ lb	1	1000	72	25.0	1070	35	2	2	46	n/a	n/a	n/a	n/a
cheddar	1	1110	81	30.0	1250	35	2	2	53	n/a	n/a	n/a	n/a
gluten sensitive	1	1140	83	29.0	1340	46	6	7	52	n/a	n/a	n/a	n/a
gluten sensitive	1	1030	74	24.0	1160	46	6	7	45	n/a	n/a	n/a	n/a

RESTAURANT & FAST FOOD CHAINS

Uno Pizzeria & Grill

	Amount	Calories	Fat (g)	Saturated Fat (g)	Sodium (mg)	Carbohydrate (g)	Fiber (g)	Sugar (g)	Protein (g)	Vitamin D (mcg)	Calcium (mg)	Iron (mg)	Potassium (mg)
Bacon cheddar	1	1350	99	36.0	2070	35	2	2	71	n/a	n/a	n/a	n/a
gluten sensitive	1	1380	101	35.0	2160	46	6	7	70	n/a	n/a	n/a	n/a
Classic Beyond	1	560	32	10.0	920	42	4	3	26	n/a	n/a	n/a	n/a
Gluten-free hamburger bun	1	220	6	0.5	360	39	4	5	6	n/a	n/a	n/a	n/a
Pasta													
Chicken Spinoccoli	1 order	1260	62	29.0	2850	105	7	13	77	n/a	n/a	n/a	n/a
Chicken & broccoli Alfredo	1 order	1450	73	26.0	2150	132	7	13	68	n/a	n/a	n/a	n/a
Classic spaghetti & meatball	1 order	1400	79	0.0	2540	111	7	14	51	n/a	n/a	n/a	n/a
Deep dish ravioli lasagna	1 order	1190	65	25.0	3240	3	7	14	60	n/a	n/a	n/a	n/a
Mac & cheese	1 order	1740	103	52.0	2640	140	6	14	70	n/a	n/a	n/a	n/a
Buffalo chicken	1 order	2200	133	58.0	4310	160	6	14	96	n/a	n/a	n/a	n/a
Romano-crusted chicken parm	1 order	1260	39	7.0	2390	125	7	15	82	n/a	n/a	n/a	n/a
Rattlesnake	1 order	1410	70	25.0	2120	126	6	10	67	n/a	n/a	n/a	n/a
Shrimp scampi	1 order	1190	54	18.0	1540	128	6	10	44	n/a	n/a	n/a	n/a
Pizza, Deep Dish*													
Cheese & tomato	1 slice	410	20	3.0	650	27	1	1	13	n/a	n/a	n/a	n/a
Chicago classic	1 slice	540	38	12.0	1070	28	1	2	22	n/a	n/a	n/a	n/a
Chicago meat market	1 slice	570	35	9.0	1240	30	1	3	22	n/a	n/a	n/a	n/a
Farmer's market	1 slice	400	22	4.0	510	31	2	3	10	n/a	n/a	n/a	n/a
Four cheese & pesto	1 slice	476	28	7.0	691	28	0	3	16	n/a	n/a	n/a	n/a
Meatball & ricotta	1 slice	515	33	4.0	818	28	0	3	15	n/a	n/a	n/a	n/a
New York deli	1 slice	454	25	6.0	838	30	0	3	16	n/a	n/a	n/a	n/a
Numero Uno	1 slice	440	28	6.0	820	29	2	3	13	n/a	n/a	n/a	n/a
Prima pepperoni	1 slice	420	23	4.0	690	27	1	1	13	n/a	n/a	n/a	n/a
Pizza, Gluten Sensitive**													
Cheese	1 slice	160	6	3.0	200	23	1	2	6	n/a	n/a	n/a	n/a
Pepperoni	1 slice	200	9	4.0	350	23	1	2	8	n/a	n/a	n/a	n/a
Veggie	1 slice	160	6	3.0	200	24	1	3	7	n/a	n/a	n/a	n/a
Pizza, Thin Crust***													
BBQ chicken	1 slice	130	5	2.0	260	15	0	3	8	n/a	n/a	n/a	n/a
cauliflower crust	1 slice	100	5	2.5	240	8	1	3	7	n/a	n/a	n/a	n/a
Bianco Love	1 slice	149	6	2.0	206	14	0	1	6	n/a	n/a	n/a	n/a
Cheese Please!	1 slice	110	5	2.0	180	13	1	1	6	n/a	n/a	n/a	n/a
cauliflower crust	1 slice	80	5	2.5	170	6	1	1	5	n/a	n/a	n/a	n/a
Margherita	1 slice	103	1	0.0	182	13	0	3	5	n/a	n/a	n/a	n/a
Spicy Hawaiian	1 slice	150	6	2.0	390	19	1	6	7	n/a	n/a	n/a	n/a
cauliflower crust	1 slice	120	6	2.5	380	12	1	6	6	n/a	n/a	n/a	n/a
Super Roni	1 slice	150	8	3.0	310	13	1	1	7	n/a	n/a	n/a	n/a
cauliflower crust	1 slice	120	8	3.5	300	6	1	1	7	n/a	n/a	n/a	n/a

* 8 slices per pie.
** 6 slices per pie.
*** 9 slices per pie.

RESTAURANT & FAST FOOD CHAINS

Uno Pizzeria & Grill

	Amount	Calories	Fat (g)	Saturated Fat (g)	Sodium (mg)	Carbohydrate (g)	Fiber (g)	Sugar (g)	Protein (g)	Vitamin D (mcg)	Calcium (mg)	Iron (mg)	Potassium (mg)
Veggie extravaganza	1 slice	130	5	2.0	200	15	1	2	6	n/a	n/a	n/a	n/a
cauliflower crust	1 slice	100	6	2.5	190	7	1	1	6	n/a	n/a	n/a	n/a
Windy City Works	1 slice	150	7	3.0	270	14	1	1	8	n/a	n/a	n/a	n/a
cauliflower crust	1 slice	120	8	3.5	260	7	1	1	7	n/a	n/a	n/a	n/a
Sandwiches													
BBQ bacon chicken	1	910	43	15.0	2540	52	0	18	74	n/a	n/a	n/a	n/a
Caprese	1	450	18	8.0	770	52	0	3	21	n/a	n/a	n/a	n/a
Chicken parm	1	940	48	12.0	2740	60	0	5	65	n/a	n/a	n/a	n/a
Fish	1	670	35	5.0	1210	68	1	4	21	n/a	n/a	n/a	n/a
Steak, Seafood & Chicken													
Baked haddock	1 order	530	33	6.0	490	12	1	2	48	n/a	n/a	n/a	n/a
Chicken tender platter w/ French fries	1 order	1600	106	18.5	3510	88	7	0	72	n/a	n/a	n/a	n/a
Fish & chips	1 order	1350	93	14.0	2360	106	6	17	32	n/a	n/a	n/a	n/a
Grilled shrimp & sirloin	1 order	690	45	16.0	1400	1	0	0	66	n/a	n/a	n/a	n/a
Lemon basil salmon	1 order	490	38	6.0	700	0	0	0	40	n/a	n/a	n/a	n/a
Mediterranean chicken	1 order	560	21	10.0	1940	43	1	5	49	n/a	n/a	n/a	n/a
Sirloin tips	1 order	470	20	5.0	500	4	1	2	62	n/a	n/a	n/a	n/a
Top sirloin steak	1 order	560	37	15.0	880	0	0	0	52	n/a	n/a	n/a	n/a
Salads													
Antipasto	1	680	48	14.0	3130	29	5	13	32	n/a	n/a	n/a	n/a
Berry & goat cheese	1	340	21	5.0	240	34	3	25	7	n/a	n/a	n/a	n/a
Chicken Caesar	1	560	41	9.0	1280	17	5	5	33	n/a	n/a	n/a	n/a
gluten sensitive	1	440	32	7.0	1140	9	5	5	32	n/a	n/a	n/a	n/a
Chopped honey chicken													
crisp	1	1320	90	24.0	2000	67	5	18	53	n/a	n/a	n/a	n/a
grilled	1	710	45	15.0	1450	36	5	18	42	n/a	n/a	n/a	n/a
House	1	270	13	6.0	510	30	4	6	14	n/a	n/a	n/a	n/a
Side salads													
berry & goat cheese	1	170	10	2.5	130	18	2	13	4	n/a	n/a	n/a	n/a
Caesar	1	220	19	4.5	330	9	3	2	5	n/a	n/a	n/a	n/a
gluten sensitive	1	160	15	3.5	260	5	2	2	4	n/a	n/a	n/a	n/a
house w/o dressing	1	90	5	1.0	95	10	2	3	2	n/a	n/a	n/a	n/a
gluten sensitive	1	25	0	0.0	20	6	2	3	1	n/a	n/a	n/a	n/a
wedge	1	230	19	5.0	550	10	3	5	7	n/a	n/a	n/a	n/a
Dressings													
balsamic vinaigrette	1 order	160	16	2.0	330	3	0	3	0	n/a	n/a	n/a	n/a
bleu cheese	1 order	210	23	4.5	280	1	0	1	1	n/a	n/a	n/a	n/a
Caesar	1 order	200	20	4.5	310	1	0	1	3	n/a	n/a	n/a	n/a
honey mustard	1 order	200	18	3.0	270	9	0	9	0	n/a	n/a	n/a	n/a
low-fat vinaigrette	1 order	60	5	0.0	150	5	0	3	0	n/a	n/a	n/a	n/a
honey	1 order	80	4	0.0	110	13	0	11	0	n/a	n/a	n/a	n/a
ranch	1 order	170	18	3.0	350	3	0	1	0	n/a	n/a	n/a	n/a

RESTAURANT & FAST FOOD CHAINS

Uno Pizzeria & Grill

	Amount	Calories	Fat (g)	Saturated Fat (g)	Sodium (mg)	Carbohydrate (g)	Fiber (g)	Sugar (g)	Protein (g)	Vitamin D (mcg)	Calcium (mg)	Iron (mg)	Potassium (mg)
Soups													
Broccoli & cheddar	1 order	310	21	10.0	1580	18	3	4	11	n/a	n/a	n/a	n/a
French onion	1 order	450	30	14.0	2070	25	2	6	19	n/a	n/a	n/a	n/a
Sides													
French fries	1 order	450	33	4.5	1550	35	7	0	5	n/a	n/a	n/a	n/a
Mashed potatoes													
loaded	1 order	420	26	12.0	860	37	3	4	13	n/a	n/a	n/a	n/a
red bliss	1 order	280	14	4.5	560	36	3	3	5	n/a	n/a	n/a	n/a
Roasted seasonal vegetables	1 order	70	4	0.0	105	8	2	5	2	n/a	n/a	n/a	n/a
Steamed broccoli	1 order	70	6	1.0	420	5	3	0	3	n/a	n/a	n/a	n/a
Sweet potato fries	1 order	430	25	3.5	740	47	7	19	2	n/a	n/a	n/a	n/a
Desserts													
Awesome Chocolate Cake	1 slice	1740	79	32.0	770	241	10	168	20	n/a	n/a	n/a	n/a
Brownies	1 order	520	23	7.0	310	77	3	42	5	n/a	n/a	n/a	n/a
Chocolate brownie sundae	1	1130	53	25.0	480	152	4	113	12	n/a	n/a	n/a	n/a
Chocolate chip cookies	1 order	550	27	13.0	310	78	3	46	7	n/a	n/a	n/a	n/a
Crazy-Good Caramel Cake	1 slice	640	25	6.0	930	96	1	67	8	n/a	n/a	n/a	n/a
Gluten sensitive ice cream sundae	1	890	38	21.0	230	126	0	107	9	n/a	n/a	n/a	n/a
Ooey Gooey Dough Bites	1 order	1370	39	11.0	1080	230	4	107	23	n/a	n/a	n/a	n/a
Shooters													
brownie chocolate	1	230	16	9.0	150	23	1	19	2	n/a	n/a	n/a	n/a
strawberry	1	220	11	7.0	135	30	0	25	2	n/a	n/a	n/a	n/a
Uno deep dish sundae	1	1520	74	39.0	700	206	5	139	19	n/a	n/a	n/a	n/a

Wendy's

	Amount	Calories	Fat (g)	Saturated Fat (g)	Sodium (mg)	Carbohydrate (g)	Fiber (g)	Sugar (g)	Protein (g)	Vitamin D (mcg)	Calcium (mg)	Iron (mg)	Potassium (mg)
Breakfast													
Biscuit													
bacon, egg & cheese	1	420	27	11.0	1240	28	1	3	16	n/a	130	3	188
honey butter	1	310	19	7.0	670	32	1	8	3	n/a	26	2	94
chicken	1	500	29	9.0	1260	44	2	9	14	n/a	52	3	282
sausage	1	450	33	13.0	950	27	1	3	11	n/a	52	2	188
w/ egg & cheese	1	580	43	17.0	1350	28	1	3	19	n/a	130	3	282
w/ sausage gravy	1	400	25	10.0	1230	38	1	3	6	n/a	52	2	188
Breakfast Baconator	1	710	48	19.0	1740	37	1	7	33	n/a	195	4	470
Classic sandwich													
bacon, egg & cheese	1	320	17	6.0	850	25	1	2	18	n/a	130	3	282
sausage, egg & cheese	1	480	33	12.0	960	25	1	3	21	n/a	130	3	376
Croissant													
bacon, egg & Swiss	1	370	19	9.0	700	34	0	6	13	n/a	78	3	188
maple bacon chicken	1	570	31	11.0	1210	52	1	14	22	n/a	26	4	376
sausage, egg & Swiss	1	590	40	16.0	1020	35	0	7	21	n/a	104	4	282
Homestyle French toast sticks	6 pcs	610	25	5.0	570	81	2	25	16	n/a	104	5	188

RESTAURANT & FAST FOOD CHAINS

Wendy's

	Amount	Calories	Fat (g)	Saturated Fat (g)	Sodium (mg)	Carbohydrate (g)	Fiber (g)	Sugar (g)	Protein (g)	Vitamin D (mcg)	Calcium (mg)	Iron (mg)	Potassium (mg)
Burgers													
Baconator	1	960	66	27.0	1540	36	1	7	57	n/a	195	7	705
Son of Baconator	1	630	40	16.0	1210	36	1	7	32	n/a	130	5	470
Big Bacon Classic	1	650	41	16.0	1230	38	2	8	33	n/a	195	5	470
double	1	910	62	25.0	1400	38	2	8	53	n/a	195	7	705
triple	1	1220	86	36.0	1770	38	2	9	75	n/a	260	9	1175
Dave's	1	590	37	15.0	1030	37	2	8	29	n/a	195	5	470
double	1	860	57	23.0	1200	37	2	8	49	n/a	195	7	705
triple	1	1160	81	34.0	1570	38	2	8	70	n/a	260	9	940
Double Stack	1	410	24	10.0	690	26	1	6	23	n/a	104	4	282
bacon	1	440	26	11.0	820	26	1	6	26	n/a	104	4	376
Jr.	1	250	11	4.0	420	25	1	5	13	n/a	52	3	188
cheeseburger	1	290	14	6.0	610	26	1	6	14	n/a	104	3	188
bacon	1	370	23	8.0	650	25	1	5	18	n/a	104	3	282
deluxe	1	340	20	7.0	610	27	1	6	15	n/a	104	3	282
Chicken													
Asiago ranch chicken club	1	600	28	8.0	1710	50	2	5	36	n/a	130	3	470
spicy	1	600	28	8.0	1480	51	3	5	36	n/a	130	5	470
Crispy chicken BLT	1	420	23	6.0	1010	35	1	5	19	n/a	104	2	282
Grilled chicken ranch wrap	1	420	16	5.0	1230	41	2	2	27	n/a	130	3	470
Nuggets													
crispy	6 pcs	270	17	3.5	570	14	1	0	15	n/a	0	0	188
spicy	6 pcs	280	18	4.0	720	13	1	0	15	n/a	0	0	188
Sandwich	1	490	21	3.5	1450	49	2	5	28	n/a	52	3	470
crispy	1	330	16	3.0	680	33	1	4	14	n/a	52	1	188
ghost pepper ranch	1	690	35	8.0	1650	61	3	7	32	n/a	195	5	470
spicy	1	490	20	3.5	1160	50	3	5	28	n/a	52	4	470
Salads													
Apple pecan	1	540	28	11.0	1420	44	5	34	32	n/a	325	2	799
Cobb	1	680	50	12.5	1340	19	3	5	37	n/a	286	3	940
Parmesan Caesar	1	530	38	10.5	1410	15	3	4	34	n/a	377	2	705
Taco	1	690	34	13.0	1870	68	12	16	30	n/a	455	5	1410
Sides													
Apple bites	1 order	35	0	0.0	0	8	1	6	0	n/a	26	0	94
Baked potato	1	270	0	0.0	40	61	7	3	7	n/a	52	3	1645
cheese	1	380	9	5.0	400	63	7	4	12	n/a	195	4	1645
bacon	1	440	13	6.0	600	64	7	4	17	n/a	195	4	1645
chili	1	500	14	7.0	840	74	9	7	20	n/a	195	4	1880
sour cream & chive	1	310	3	1.5	55	63	7	4	8	n/a	78	3	1645

RESTAURANT & FAST FOOD CHAINS

Wendy's	Amount	Calories	Fat (g)	Saturated Fat (g)	Sodium (mg)	Carbohydrate (g)	Fiber (g)	Sugar (g)	Protein (g)	Vitamin D (mcg)	Calcium (mg)	Iron (mg)	Potassium (mg)
Chili	medium	240	11	4.5	910	22	6	6	16	n/a	52	3	470
Fries	medium	350	16	2.5	620	47	4	0	5	n/a	26	1	705
Baconator	1 order	460	26	9.0	1090	43	3	1	14	n/a	130	1	705
cheese	1 order	370	20	7.0	830	38	3	0	9	n/a	130	1	705
chili	1 order	520	27	9.0	1330	53	6	3	17	n/a	195	3	940
ghost pepper	1 order	450	29	5.0	830	42	4	1	5	n/a	26	1	705
Oatmeal bar	1	280	10	4.0	230	45	4	23	3	n/a	26	2	94
Seasoned potatoes	medium	330	14	2.5	900	46	4	1	4	n/a	26	1	705
Desserts													
Cookies													
chocolate chunk	1	330	16	8.0	210	43	2	26	3	n/a	26	3	94
sugar	1	330	16	8.0	300	44	1	24	3	n/a	0	3	0
Frosty, chocolate	medium	390	11	7.0	220	61	1	51	12	n/a	390	1	705

Nutrients

CHOLINE

Choline is necessary for your brain and nervous system to manage functions like mood, memory, and muscle control. Your body can make a small amount of choline in your liver, but most comes from your diet.

Did you know? Most multivitamins, including prenatal supplements, do not contain choline, and most adults do not get enough choline overall. More research is being done to help us better understand how a low choline intake may impact our overall health, especially brain health.

The good news is . . . Choline is found in many foods, and deficiency symptoms are very rare in healthy adults.

Tips

1. Reach for proteins like beef (72 mg in 3 oz lean ground beef), chicken (72 mg in 3 oz chicken breast), turkey (72 mg in 3 oz turkey breast), fish (187 mg in 3 oz salmon), dairy products, and eggs (147 mg in 1 egg).

2. Snack on nuts such as almonds (15 mg in 1 oz).

3. Try veggies like shiitake mushrooms (145 mg in 1 cup), cauliflower (72 mg in 1 cup), brussels sprouts (30 mg in 1 cup), or broccoli (30 mg in 1 cup).

4. Say yes to beans, including soybeans (214 mg in 1 cup), kidney beans (54 mg in 1 cup), and lima beans (75 mg in 1 cup).

5. Choose quinoa (43 mg in 1 cup).

6. Sprinkle wheat germ (153 mg in 3 oz) on yogurt, oatmeal, smoothies, or salads.

Adequate Intake (AI) for Choline

Age	Male	Female	Pregnancy	Lactation
19+	550 mg	425 mg	450 mg	550 mg

Note: Getting too much choline has been linked to higher cardiovascular disease risk. Therefore, there's an upper limit for choline from food and supplements: 3,500 mg for adults over 19.

FIBER

More than 90 percent of Americans do not eat enough fiber. But fiber is important for feeling full after eating, managing weight, lowering cholesterol, keeping blood sugars within a healthy range, and maintaining gut health.

Did you know? Dietary fiber is found in plant foods like fruits, vegetables, beans, lentils, whole grains, nuts, and seeds and includes the parts of plant foods your body can't digest or absorb. Typically, the more a food is refined, the less fiber it has. There are two types of dietary fiber: soluble and insoluble. Both are important for good health.

The good news is . . . You can easily get fiber in your diet by choosing whole unprocessed plant foods. Eating too much fiber too quickly can cause gas, bloating, and discomfort, so increase fiber gradually over a few weeks. Drink plenty of water, too, as fiber works best when it absorbs water.

Tips

1. Reach for foods that are higher in prebiotics (a type of fiber that's beneficial for gut health), like Jerusalem artichokes, asparagus, plantains, onions, garlic, leeks, chicory root, bananas, and chickpeas.
2. Make at least half your grains whole grains.
3. Fill half your plate with fruits and vegetables.
4. Choose fresh veggies and fruits as snacks.
5. Sprinkle nuts and seeds on salads, cereals, and yogurt.
6. Check the food label to find high-fiber foods: 20 percent of the Daily Value in one serving is considered a high source of fiber.

Adequate Intake (AI) The Daily Value for fiber is 14 grams per 1,000 calories a day.

IRON

Your body needs iron to grow, develop, and make hemoglobin—the substance in red blood cells that helps transport oxygen from your lungs throughout your body. Without enough oxygen in your blood, you may experience fatigue, dizziness, lightheadedness, headaches, and/or shortness of breath.

Women of childbearing age are at higher risk for iron-deficiency anemia because of blood loss during their menstrual periods and pregnancy. Health-care providers often recommend a multivitamin or prenatal vitamin with iron to supplement the iron in foods during these stages of life.

Did you know? Iron in food exists in two different forms: heme and nonheme. Heme iron is only found in animal foods like meats, poultry, and seafood. It is more easily absorbed by your body than the nonheme type, which is found in plant foods like nuts, seeds, lentils, beans, fruits, leafy green vegetables, and fortified cereals. If you don't eat animal foods, you need to consume twice as much iron as someone who eats meat.

The good news is . . . Vitamin C can increase how much iron your body absorbs while you're eating iron-rich vegetarian foods.

Tips

1. A cup of iron-fortified hot cereal contains almost 11 mg of iron. Toss in some dried fruit such as raisins (½ cup has 1.5 mg iron) or dried apricots (½ cup has 3.5 mg iron) for an additional boost. Add some blackberries or orange slices for a colorful burst of vitamin C.

2. A cup of iron-fortified cold cereal has about 18 mg of iron. Wash it down with a chilled glass of citrus juice—an excellent source of vitamin C.

3. Leafy greens like spinach, kale, Swiss chard, and collard and beet greens contain 2.5 to 6 mg of iron per cooked cup. Sauté your greens with a vitamin C–rich food like bell peppers or tomatoes.

4. Grab a handful of seeds or nuts for a snack or toss them into a salad or smoothie. Pumpkin seeds contain 2.7 mg of iron in ½ cup, and 30 peanuts have 1.5 mg.

5. Add beans and lentils to soups and skillet dishes. White, lima, red kidney, and navy beans as well as soybeans, chickpeas, and black-eyed peas are all good sources of iron.

6. Satisfy your sweet tooth with an ounce of dark chocolate (2 mg iron in 1 oz).

Recommended Dietary Allowances (RDAs) for Iron

Age	Male	Female	Pregnancy	Lactation
19–50	8 mg	18 mg	27 mg	9 mg
51+	8 mg	8 mg		

Note: Iron toxicity can be caused by taking high doses of iron supplements for prolonged periods of time or taking a single overdose. Check with your health-care provider before taking an iron supplement.

MAGNESIUM

Many people, especially older adults, don't get enough magnesium. This mineral has an essential role in more than three hundred metabolic pathways in the body, including protein synthesis, muscle and nerve function, blood glucose control, and blood pressure regulation.

Fortunately, healthy people are unlikely to experience magnesium deficiency symptoms. However, it's important to speak with your medical provider if you don't regularly eat foods containing magnesium, have chronic health conditions (like high blood pressure, gastrointestinal diseases, type 2 diabetes, or chronic alcoholism), or take certain medications like antacids and laxatives, all of which can put you at higher risk for deficiency due to poor absorption or increased excretion.

Did you know? The Food and Drug Administration (FDA) does not require food labels to list magnesium content unless it has been added to the food in processing.

The good news is . . . You can find magnesium in many healthy foods like whole unrefined grains, beans, peas, nuts, seeds, legumes, and vegetables.

Tips

1. Nuts and seeds are good sources of magnesium. Examples include 1 T of pumpkin seeds (156 mg), chia seeds (111 mg), or almonds (80 mg).
2. Foods rich in magnesium are also good sources of other nutrients like fiber. To get more fiber, try 1 cup of black beans (120 mg), ½ cup of cooked brown rice (42 mg), or 1 slice of whole grain bread (23 mg).

3. Upgrade your greens to dark leafy greens—a magnesium power player—with 1 cup of spinach (156 mg), Swiss chard (121 mg), or kale (58 mg).

4. Dark chocolate (64 mg in 1 square/oz) is nutritious, delicious, and rich in magnesium.

Recommended Dietary Allowances (RDAs) for Magnesium

Age	Male	Female	Pregnancy	Lactation
19–30	400 mg	310 mg	350 mg	310 mg
31–50	420 mg	320 mg	360 mg	320 mg
51+	420 mg	320 mg		

OMEGA-3 FATTY ACIDS

Omega-3 fatty acids are "essential fats," meaning your body cannot make them from other fats. You must get them from the foods you eat, such as fatty fish and other seafood (like salmon, tuna, trout, crab, oysters, and mussels), nuts and seeds (like walnuts, flaxseeds, chia seeds, and hemp seeds), plant oils (like flaxseed, soybean, and canola oil), seaweed, and fortified foods or supplements. Omega-3s keep your cell membranes, heart, lungs, blood vessels, and immune system healthy and reduce inflammation.

Did you know? There are three main omega-3 fatty acids:

1. Alpha-linolenic acid (ALA)
2. Eicosapentaenoic acid (EPA)
3. Docosahexaenoic acid (DHA)

ALA is found mainly in plant oils, while DHA and EPA are found in fish and other seafood. Your body needs all three to function.

The good news is . . . If you do not eat seafood or you follow a vegan diet, you can still get DHA and EPA by eating nuts, seeds, and plant oils because your body can partially convert ALA to EPA and DHA.

Tips

1. Add 1 T of chia or hemp seeds to your favorite smoothie.
2. Toss some chopped walnuts into salads, oatmeal, or yogurt.

3. Use flaxseed (linseed oil) as a salad dressing oil or add it to juices, smoothies, and shakes. (Do not use it for stir-frying or baking, as it does not react well when heated.)

4. Eat a variety of fish containing omega-3 at least twice a week.

Adequate Intakes (AIs) for Omega-3s (as ALA)

Age	Male	Female	Pregnancy	Lactation
19+	1.6g	1.1g	1.4g	1.3g

Note: Recommended daily amounts for omega-3 fatty acids have not been established for EPA and DHA. The FDA recommends no more than 5 g per day of combined EPA and DHA from dietary supplements, as high doses can be harmful and can interact with some medications such as anticoagulants. Check with your health-care provider before taking an omega-3 supplement.

OMEGA-6 FATTY ACIDS

Omega-6 fatty acids are good for heart health and circulation, and they're necessary for your cells to function properly. Our bodies cannot make omega-6 fats—we need to get them from food. They come from vegetable oils (like corn, safflower, soybean, and sunflower oil), sunflower seeds, pumpkin seeds, walnuts, meat, poultry, fish, and eggs. It's recommended that you eat these types of polyunsaturated fats (generally liquid at room temperature) in place of saturated fats (generally hard at room temperature).

Did you know? You won't find omega-6 or omega-3 fats on food labels. Instead, you can read the label for unsaturated fats versus saturated fats and use that as a guide. Subtract grams of saturated fats and trans fat from total fat grams to see how much of the healthy unsaturated variety is present. Most American adults consume about ten times more omega-6 fats than omega-3 fats.

The good news is . . . Experts generally agree that consuming too little omega-3 is a more significant problem than consuming too much omega-6. The goal is to eat more omega-3 fats to bring the two into balance.

Tips

1. Toss walnuts, hemp seeds, or sunflower seeds into a salad.

2. Add 1 T of peanut butter to a smoothie or slice of whole grain bread.

3. Cook with unsaturated fats like avocado oil in place of saturated fats like butter. Avocado oil has a high smoke point, which makes it ideal for roasting, sautéing, and grilling.

Adequate Intake (AI) for Omega-6 Fatty Acids

Age	Male	Female	Pregnancy	Lactation
19–50	17 g	12 g	13 g	13 g
51+	14 g	11 g		

POTASSIUM

Potassium is important for kidney function, heart health, muscle contraction, and nerve transmission.

Did you know? National surveys tracking dietary intake consistently show that people get less potassium than recommended. Why is this important? Getting too little potassium can deplete calcium in bones, increase blood pressure, and increase risk of kidney stones.

The good news is . . . Potassium is found in many foods and is also an ingredient in many salt substitutes.

Tips

1. Try ½ cup of dried fruit like apricots (1,101 mg), prunes (699 mg), or raisins (618 mg) as a snack.

2. Make lentil soup. One cup of cooked lentils has 731 mg potassium, and you can toss in 2 cups of spinach for an extra 334 mg.

3. Have a baked potato (610 mg in 1 medium) or acorn squash (644 mg in 1 cup) as a side dish.

4. Grab a banana (422 mg in 1 medium) when you're on the go.

5. Grill 3 oz of chicken breast (332 mg), salmon (326 mg), or top sirloin (315 mg).

Adequate Intake (AI) for Potassium

Age	Male	Female	Pregnancy	Lactation
19–50	3,400 mg	2,600 mg	2,900 mg	2,800 mg
51+	3,400 mg	2,600 mg		

SODIUM

Your body uses sodium, found in salt, to maintain fluid balance as well as muscle and nerve function. Your body needs some sodium to work properly, but most of us eat too much, which is linked to health problems like high blood pressure, heart disease, and strokes.

Did you know? Most of the sodium we eat comes from processed, packaged, and canned foods, along with condiments, snack foods, and restaurant meals—not just from the salt shaker.

The good news is . . . Because sodium is an acquired taste, once you reduce the amount you eat, your taste buds may actually prefer foods' natural flavors.

Tips

1. Prepare more meals at home, where you can control how much salt is used in cooking and at the table.
2. Remove the salt shaker from your table and replace it with your favorite no salt-added blend of herbs and spices.
3. Buy fresh or frozen vegetables with no added salt instead of canned veggies.
4. Rinse canned beans, tuna, and vegetables to remove some of the sodium.
5. Cut back on portion sizes for condiments and salad dressings or use a low-sodium variety. Oil, flavored vinegars, and citrus juices are low-sodium alternatives to bottled salad dressings.
6. Choose unsalted or low-sodium snacks such as nuts, chips, pretzels, popcorn, and crackers.
7. Read Nutrition Facts labels and select foods with less than 5 percent of the sodium Daily Value per serving, or 140 mg or less per serving.

How much sodium do you need?

The Dietary Guidelines for Americans recommend that adults limit their sodium intake to no more than 2,300 mg per day.

VITAMIN A

Carrots are good for your eyesight because they contain beta-carotene, a red-orange pigment that your body converts into vitamin A. Vitamin A is not only critical for healthy vision; it's also involved in maintaining your immune system, cells, and organs. Vitamin A has antioxidant properties, helping fight cell damage when your body breaks down food or is exposed to pollution, tobacco smoke, or ultraviolet rays.

Did you know? There are two forms of vitamin A: preformed vitamin A found in animal foods like eggs, meat, fish, fish oils, and dairy, and provitamin A carotenoids found in plant foods like orange and yellow vegetables, leafy green vegetables, tomatoes, fruits, and vegetable oils.

The good news is . . . Because your body can convert beta-carotene from plant foods into vitamin A, it is possible to get enough in your diet even if you don't eat animal foods.

Tips

1. Colorize half your plate with red, orange, yellow, green, blue, and purple fruits and veggies.
2. Add one baked sweet potato (1,403 mcg Retinol Activity Equivalent [RAE]) or frozen spinach (573 mcg RAE in ½ cup) to a meal.
3. Cut up cantaloupe (135 mcg RAE in ½ cup), red peppers (117 mcg RAE in ½ cup), or mango (112 mcg in 1 cup) for a snack.

Recommended Dietary Allowances (RDAs) for Vitamin A

Age	Male	Female	Pregnancy	Lactation
19+	900 mcg RAE	700 mcg RAE	770 mcg RAE	1,300 mcg RAE

Note: Because vitamin A is fat soluble, excess amounts are stored in the body and can be toxic. Check with your health-care provider before taking a vitamin A supplement.

VITAMIN B12

Vitamin B12 is naturally found in animal foods like fish, meat, chicken, turkey, eggs, dairy products, and some fortified foods. Plant foods have no vitamin B12 unless it's been added by the manufacturer during processing.

Did you know? After the age of 50, many adults may not have enough hydrochloric acid in their stomach to absorb vitamin B12 from animal foods. If you're older than 50, look for foods fortified with B12 or talk to a medical provider about supplementation.

The good news is . . . Most adults get enough vitamin B12 from their food. However, some may have trouble absorbing it. If you've been diagnosed with pernicious anemia, celiac disease, or Crohn's disease; had stomach or intestinal surgery; or don't consume any animal products, talk to a medical provider about whether you should supplement your current diet with vitamin B12.

Tips

1. Organ meats like liver and kidneys are rich in vitamin B12. 3 oz of beef liver contains 70 mcg.

2. One 3 oz serving of clams has 84 mcg of vitamin B12. Clams are also high in protein, low in fat, and an excellent source of iron.

3. Embrace sardines, a great source of vitamin B12 and calcium. A 100 g serving of canned sardines in oil contains 9 mcg of vitamin B12. Other fish like salmon (4.8 mcg) and trout (3.5 mcg) are good sources, too.

4. Dairy products don't have as much vitamin B12 as meat and fish, but they are still a good source. Try milk (1.2 mcg in 1 cup) or yogurt (1.1 mcg in 1 cup).

5. Nutritional yeast is a great cheese substitute that has 8 mcg vitamin B12 in 2 T. Sprinkle it on pasta dishes or salads.

6. Reach for fortified foods like breakfast cereals, nondairy milk substitutes, meat substitutes, or energy bars. If vitamin B12 has been added to a food, it will be shown on the label.

Recommended Dietary Allowances (RDAs) for Vitamin B12

Age	Male	Female	Pregnancy	Lactation
19+	2.4 mcg	2.4 mcg	2.6 mcg	2.8 mcg

VITAMIN C

Vitamin C is an antioxidant that protects cell health, assists in making collagen, aids in iron absorption, and is important for immune function. Studies have suggested that getting enough vitamin C from fruits and vegetables may reduce your risk of cancer, heart disease, and age-related macular degeneration (a leading cause of vision loss in older adults).

Did you know? Our bodies don't make vitamin C, so you are entirely dependent on food and drinks for this vitamin.

The good news is . . . Most adults get enough vitamin C from their diet. It is rare to see vitamin C deficiencies in developed countries.

Tips

1. Eat five or more servings of fruits and vegetables every day. Citrus fruits (70 mg in 1 medium orange), red and green peppers (95 mg in ½ cup), kiwis (64 mg in 1 medium), broccoli (51 mg in ½ cup), strawberries (49 mg in ½ cup), brussels sprouts (48 mg in ½ cup), tomatoes (17 mg in 1 medium), and cantaloupe (29 mg in ½ cup) are all good sources of vitamin C.

2. Choose raw fruits and vegetables most often. Vitamin C can be destroyed by heat from steaming, boiling, or microwaving food.

3. Select local fruits and vegetables when possible and eat them as soon as you can after purchase. Vitamin C content decreases with prolonged storage.

4. Check food labels—foods and beverages are often fortified with vitamin C.

Recommended Dietary Allowances (RDAs) for Vitamin C

Note: If you smoke, you need 35 mg more vitamin C per day than nonsmokers.

Age	Male	Female	Pregnancy	Lactation
19+	90 g	75 g	85 g	120 g

VITAMIN D

Your body needs Vitamin D to absorb calcium for building and maintaining healthy teeth and bones as well as protecting against weakening bones. Its anti-inflammatory, antioxidant, and neuroprotective properties support your immune system, muscles, nerves, blood vessels, and brain cells.

Did you know? Only a few foods naturally contain vitamin D, including fatty fish (like tuna, salmon, sardines, herring, mackerel, and trout), fish liver oils, beef liver, and egg yolks. Your body can also make vitamin D when your bare skin is exposed to the sun. However, sunscreen, clouds, smog, old age, and having dark skin can limit the amount of vitamin D your body can make.

The good news is . . . Milk and plant-based milk alternatives such as almond, rice, oat, soy, hemp, and coconut milk are generally fortified with about 2.5–3 mcg (100–120 IU) vitamin D. Vitamin D is also added to other foods like breakfast cereals, margarine, some calcium-fortified orange juice, and yogurt.

Tips

1. Start your day with a bowl of vitamin D–fortified cereal and milk (or fortified milk alternative) and two eggs to get almost half of the recommended daily amount of vitamin D.

2. If you are worried about not getting enough vitamin D, you can measure this with a blood test. If your levels are low, your health-care provider can recommend a vitamin D supplement.

Recommended Dietary Allowances (RDAs) for Vitamin D

Age	Male	Female	Pregnancy	Lactation
19–70	15 mcg (600 IU)	15 mcg (600 IU)	15 mcg (600 IU)	15 mcg (600 IU)
71+	20 mcg (800 IU)	20 mcg (800 IU)		

Note: Vitamin D is fat soluble, and excess amounts stored in the body can be harmful and can interact with some medications. Check with your health-care provider before taking a vitamin D supplement.

VITAMIN E

Hailed as one of the big three antioxidant nutrients along with vitamin A (beta-carotene) and vitamin C, vitamin E helps clean up free radicals in your body. Some free radicals are used by immune cells to fight infections; however, too many can increase oxidative stress, which can accelerate aging and a host of diseases. Your immune system also needs vitamin E to fight off infection.

Did you know? Vitamin E is found mainly in fruits and vegetables that contain fat, including nuts, seeds, avocado, vegetable oils, and wheat germ. Some fish (like salmon and tuna) and some leafy green vegetables (such as beets, turnips, and mustard greens) also contain vitamin E.

The good news is . . . As long as you eat a variety of antioxidant-rich foods, you should get enough vitamin E in your diet.

Tips

1. Snack on a handful of almonds or sunflower seeds (over 7 mg per oz) and you'll be more than halfway to meeting your daily goal.
2. Dip into some guacamole or add avocado slices to toast, sandwiches, or dark green salads. One avocado has 4 mg of vitamin E.
3. Enjoy a glass of almond milk with a peanut butter and jelly sandwich for 10 mg of vitamin E.
4. Sprinkle wheat germ on top of your favorite cereal or yogurt (4.5 mg in 2 T).

Recommended Dietary Allowances (RDAs) for Vitamin E

Age	Male	Female	Pregnancy	Lactation
14+	15 mg	15 mg	15 g	19 mg

Note: Because vitamin E is fat soluble, excess amounts are stored in the body and can be harmful. Check with your health-care provider before taking a vitamin E supplement.

WATER

Drinking water every day is critical for overall health. Staying hydrated helps you think clearly, manage mood, avoid overheating, digest food, lubricate joints, keep a normal body temperature, and prevent kidney stones. In fact, every cell, tissue, and organ in your body requires water to work properly. Even mild dehydration can make you feel low on energy.

Did you know? Recommendations for how much water you need vary based on your age, health, eating patterns, body size, activity level, and geographic location. If you're pregnant or breastfeeding, you need even more water every day. Total water recommendations include what you drink as well as the water in foods, which generally makes up about 20 percent of your water intake.

The good news is . . . Your fluid intake is most likely in balance if you don't feel thirsty and your urine is colorless or light yellow.

Tips

1. Make water your beverage of choice.
2. Carry a water bottle and sip it while you're on the go.
3. Keep a glass of water on your nightstand.
4. Stay ahead of your thirst—drink water throughout the day, even if you don't feel thirsty.
5. Substitute water for sugar-sweetened beverages to feel better and reduce your calorie intake.

Adequate Intake (AI) for water

Age	Male	Female	Pregnancy	Lactation
19+	3.7 L (16 cups)	2.7 L (11 cups)	3.0 L (13 cups)	3.8 L (16 cups)

References

Calculator.net, "BMR Calculator," calculator.net/bmr-calculator.html.

Fast food franchise nutrition information, 2023.

Food Processor Nutrition Analysis software, ESHA Research, 2021.

Institute of Medicine, Dietary Reference Intakes for Energy, Carbohydrate, Fiber, Fat, Fatty Acids, Cholesterol, Protein, and Amino Acids (Washington, DC: The National Academies Press, 2005).

Institute of Medicine, *Dietary Reference Intakes for Water, Potassium, Sodium, Chloride, and Sulfate* (Washington, DC: The National Academies Press, 2005).

Johnson, Rachel K., et al., "Dietary sugars intake and cardiovascular health: a scientific statement from the American Heart Association." *Circulation* 120, no. 11 (August 2009): 1011–20.

Parker, Suzi. *1000 Best Bartender's Recipes* (Illinois: Sourcebooks, Inc., 2005).

Soliman, Ghada A. "Dietary Cholesterol and the Lack of Evidence in Cardiovascular Disease." *Nutrients* 10, no. 6 (June 2018): 780.

US Department of Agriculture and US Department of Health and Human Services, "Dietary Guidelines for Americans, 2020-2025," 9th Edition, 2020.

US Department of Health and Human Services, "Body Weight Planner," niddk.nih.gov/bwp.

USDA MyPlate, myplate.gov.

Index

About the Authors

JANE STEPHENSON is a learning and development senior specialist for a globally diversified medical device and health care company headquartered in Chicago, Illinois. She spent the first half of her career as a registered dietitian nutritionist (RDN) and certified diabetes educator (CDE) prior to entering the health care industry. She is the author of several nutrition and fitness educational books and tools targeted to helping people take action to live healthier, happier lives.

REBECCA LINDBERG, MPH, RDN, is a registered dietitian nutritionist, consultant, author, and speaker at Rebecca Lindberg, LLC. With three decades of experience, she's inspired countless individuals to embrace healthier lifestyles through her user-friendly tools and resources. As the co-founder of Rumblings Media®, LLC, Rebecca also empowers midlife women to live well and flourish through transformative online courses, events, travel experiences, and free content. Rebecca is passionate about helping women ditch dieting, simplify eating, achieve goals through a personalized approach, and find joy in food again.

rumblingsmedia.com | ⓘrumblingsmedia
🅧relindberg | 🅕rumblingsmedia